Fire and Life Safety Educator

Second Edition

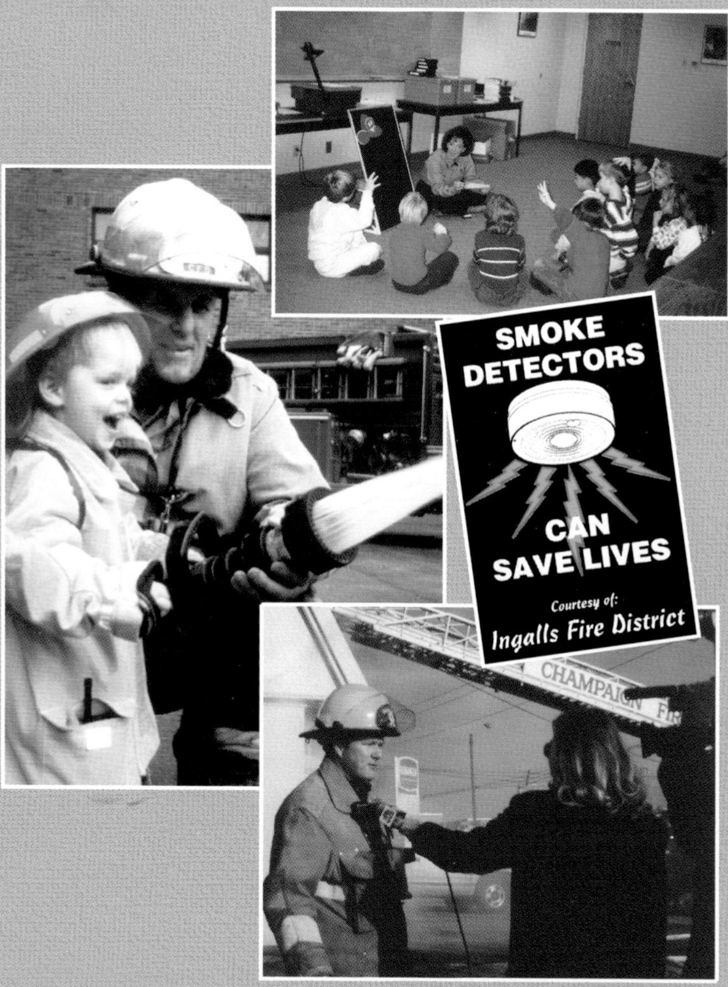

Written by
Pam Powell

Edited by
Marsha Sneed and Richard Hall

Cover photo courtesy of Stillwater Fire Department — A recipient of the 1996 NFPA Learn Not to Burn® Champion Award.

Validated by the International Fire Service Training Association
Published by Fire Protection Publications, Oklahoma State University

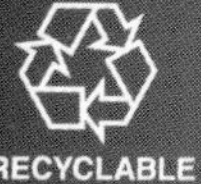

ISBN 0-87939-135-9
Library of Congress 96-61966

Second Edition
First Printing, January 1997
Second Printing, February 2002

Printed in the United States of America

Dedication

This manual is dedicated to the members of that unselfish organization of men and women who hold devotion to duty above personal risk, who count on sincerity of service above personal comfort and convenience, who strive unceasingly to find better ways of protecting the lives, homes and property of their fellow citizens from the ravages of fire and other disasters . . . ***The Firefighters of All Nations.***

Dear Firefighter:

The International Fire Service Training Association (IFSTA) is an organization that exists for the purpose of serving firefighters' training needs. Fire Protection Publications is the publisher of IFSTA materials. Fire Protection Publications staff members participate in the National Fire Protection Association and the International Association of Fire Chiefs.

If you need additional information concerning our organization or assistance with manual orders, contact:

Customer Services
Fire Protection Publications
Oklahoma State University
930 N. Willis
Stillwater, OK 74078-8045
1 (800) 654-4055

For assistance with training materials, recommended material for inclusion in a manual, or questions on manual content, contact:

Technical Services
Fire Protection Publications
Oklahoma State University
930 N. Willis
Stillwater, OK 74078-8045
(405) 744-5723

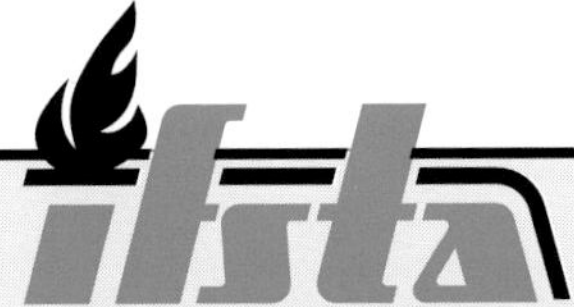

THE INTERNATIONAL FIRE SERVICE TRAINING ASSOCIATION

The International Fire Service Training Association (IFSTA) was established as a "nonprofit educational association of fire fighting personnel who are dedicated to upgrading fire fighting techniques and safety through training." This training association was formed in November 1934, when the Western Actuarial Bureau sponsored a conference in Kansas City, Missouri. The meeting was held to determine how all the agencies interested in publishing fire service training material could coordinate their efforts. Four states were represented at this initial conference. Because the representatives from Oklahoma had done some pioneering in fire training manual development, it was decided that other interested states should join forces with them. This merger made it possible to develop training materials broader in scope than those published by individual agencies. This merger further made possible a reduction in publication costs, because it enabled each state or agency to benefit from the economy of relatively large printing orders. These savings would not be possible if each individual state or department developed and published its own training material.

To carry out the mission of IFSTA, Fire Protection Publications was established as an entity of Oklahoma State University. Fire Protection Publications' primary function is to publish and disseminate training texts as proposed and validated by IFSTA. As a secondary function, Fire Protection Publications researches, acquires, produces, and markets high-quality learning and teaching aids as consistent with IFSTA's mission. The IFSTA Executive Director is officed at Fire Protection Publications.

IFSTA's purpose is to validate training materials for publication, develop training materials for publication, check proposed rough drafts for errors, add new techniques and developments, and delete obsolete and outmoded methods. This work is carried out at the annual Validation Conference.

The IFSTA Validation Conference is held the second full week in July, at Oklahoma State University or in the vicinity. Fire Protection Publications, the IFSTA publisher, establishes the revision schedule for manuals and introduces new manuscripts. Manual committee members are selected for technical input by Fire Protection Publications and the IFSTA Executive Secretary. Committees meet and work at the conference addressing the current standards of the National Fire Protection Association and other standard-making groups as applicable.

Most of the committee members are affiliated with other international fire protection organizations. The Validation Conference brings together individuals from several related and allied fields, such as:

- Key fire department executives and training officers
- Educators from colleges and universities
- Representatives from governmental agencies
- Delegates of firefighter associations and industrial organizations
- Engineers from the fire insurance industry

Committee members are not paid nor are they reimbursed for their expenses by IFSTA or Fire Protection Publications. They come because of commitment to the fire service and its future through training. Being on a committee is prestigious in the fire service community, and committee members are acknowledged leaders in their fields. This unique feature provides a close relationship between the International Fire Service Training Association and other fire protection agencies, which helps to correlate the efforts of all concerned.

IFSTA manuals are now the official teaching texts of most of the states and provinces of North America. Additionally, numerous U.S. and Canadian government agencies as well as other English-speaking countries have officially accepted the IFSTA manuals.

Table of Contents

Tables

Preface

Fire and Life Safety Educator is the second edition of **IFSTA 606, Public Fire Education**. The new title and the updated, greatly expanded text reflect the new broader scope of public education in today's fire service. This manual provides information for those individuals who plan, develop, and deliver fire and life safety education, as addressed in NFPA 1035, *Standard for Professional Qualifications for Public Fire and Life Safety Educator*, 1993 edition.

Acknowledgement and special thanks are extended to the members of the IFSTA validating committee who contributed their time, wisdom, and talents to this manual.

Committee Chairs

Howard Boyd
Consultant
Nashville, TN

Ron Williamson
Edmond Fire Department
Edmond, OK

Committee Secretary

Pam Powell
Custer Powell, Inc.
Wrentham, MA

Committee Members

Cynthia Fuller
North Carolina Fire and Rescue Commission
Raleigh, NC

Ed Kirtley
Colorado Springs Fire Department
Colorado Springs, CO

Bob Moffatt
Consultant
Edmonton, Alberta

Mary Nachbar
Minnesota State Fire Marshal Division
St. Paul, MN

Bruce Piringer
Missouri Fire and Rescue Institute
Columbia, MO

Dena Schumacher
Champaign Fire Department
Champaign, IL

Nancy Trench
Fire Service Training
Stillwater, OK

Special recognition is given to Pam Powell, the primary author of the manual, as well as to Ed Kirtley and Dena Schumacher, who each authored a chapter.

The following individuals and organizations contributed information, photographs, or other assistance that made the completion of this manual possible:

Champaign (IL) Fire Department
City of Bremerton (WA) Fire Department
Colorado Springs (CO) Fire Department
Elk Grove Village (IL) Fire Department
Faye Ann Presnal, Oklahoma State University
Glenn Rousey, Rock Island (IL) Fire Department
Palatine (IL) Fire Department

Peoria, (IL) Fire Department
Plano (TX) Fire Department
Stillwater (OK) Fire Department
Stillwater Central Communications Center
U. S. Forest Service

The divider page photographs were provided by the following individuals:

Brad La Payne, Champaign (IL) Fire Department
Dena Schumacher, Champaign (IL) Fire Department
Todd Haines, Ingalls (OK) Fire Department

Finally, gratitude also is extended to the following members of the Fire Protection Publications staff whose contributions made the final publication of this manual possible:

Cynthia Brakhage, Associate Editor
Susan S. Walker, Instructional Development Coordinator
Pam Griffith, Curriculum Specialist
Don Davis, Coordinator, Publications Production
Ann Moffat, Graphic Designer Analyst
Desa Porter, Senior Graphic Designer
Connie Burris, Senior Graphic Designer
Rick Arrington, Graphic Designer
Ben Brock, Graphics Assistant
Don Burull, Graphics Assistant
Ryan Lewis, Research Technician
Todd Haines, Research Technician

Lynne C. Murnane
Lynne Murnane
Managing Editor

Introduction

Fire and life safety education describes the important role of today's educator. No longer does the fire and life safety educator provide only "fire prevention" education. Today's educator must have basic knowledge and skills in many other life safety and injury-prevention areas, such as burn-injury prevention, electrical safety, baby-sitter training, pedestrian safety, CPR, and water safety. And, no longer is the educator always a member of the fire service. Therefore it is important that today's educator understands certain basic technical background information.

Fire and Life Safety Educator addresses topics such as working cooperatively with other community agencies, working within the legislative process, and finding and using resources (including requesting program funds through grants and in-kind contributions). It also provides the technical background information that the fire and life safety educator needs.

Educators must have a starting point from which to plan their programs. National and local data provide this starting point. National data shows national trends and allows educators to see how their communities compare with other locations nationwide. Local data assists educators in determining trends in their community. This manual addresses data sources and using data for public fire and life safety education planning.

Effective fire and life safety education programs are the result of deciding carefully what to teach and how to teach it. This manual outlines the curriculum development process and gives general guidelines for planning successful presentations. It contains information on what motivates people to learn and how people learn differently. Other topics include educational materials selection and program evaluation.

In some instances, the fire and life safety educator must understand the role of the public information officer as well as that of the public fire and life safety educator. The educator must understand what makes news and how various media fit the needs of the fire service as well as the needs of other injury-prevention agencies. The educator must be able to match the medium with the message and know how to build communication bridges within the department and across the community. This manual introduces the fire and life safety educator to today's media resources and covers techniques for working with the media.

AUDIENCE

This second edition of **Public Fire Education**, now titled **Fire and Life Safety Educator**, is designed to provide the public educator with the knowledge and skills needed to successfully perform as a fire and life safety educator as addressed in NFPA 1035, *Standard for Professional Qualifications for Public Fire and Life Safety Educator*, 1993 edition. The primary audience of the manual is those who practice the multidiscipline profession of fire and life safety educator (including uniformed and nonuniformed fire service personnel and others from outside the fire service).

PURPOSE AND SCOPE

The committee's goal for this manual is for it to be the first document on a public educator's bookshelf, a document that defines the knowledge of the public educator's profession, and a "ready reference" of public education knowledge. The manual is intended to *educate* the educator rather than to *train* the educator. In this way, the educator will be able to apply his or her knowledge and skills to many different areas all under the "umbrella" of injury prevention and control. The manual focuses on fire and burn prevention education as part of the larger discipline of injury prevention and control.

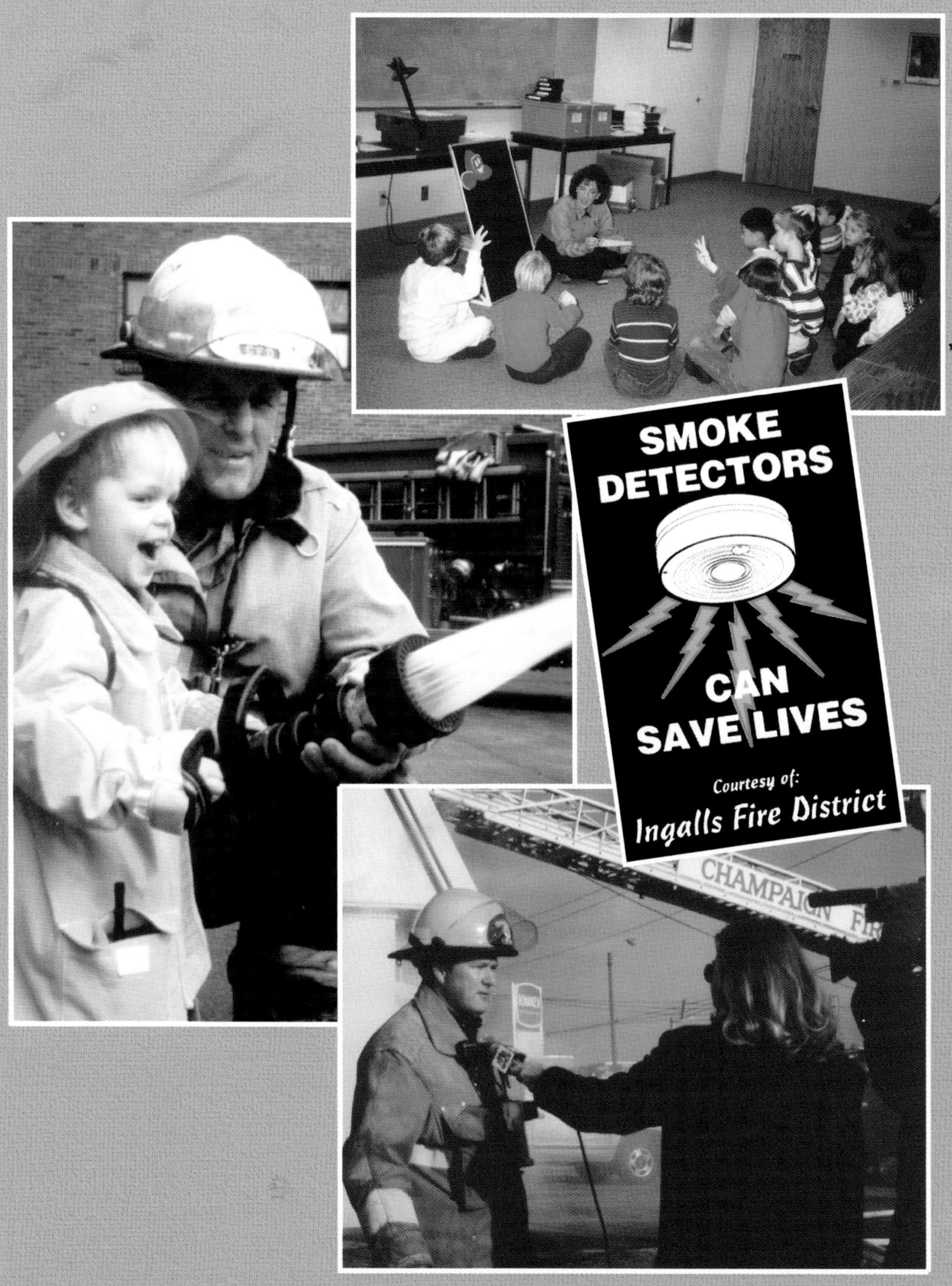
SMOKE
DETECTORS
CAN
SAVE LIVES
Courtesy of:
Ingalls Fire District
CHAMPAIGN

1 Introduction to Fire and Life Safety Education

Chapter 1

Introduction to Fire and Life Safety Education

INTRODUCTION

Fire and life safety education is a growing profession, both inside and outside the fire service. Some educators are uniformed firefighters, and others are civilians working in the fire department. Still other fire and life safety educators work for other state, provincial, and local government agencies, such as state and provincial fire marshal's offices, fire service training organizations, or city health departments (Figure 1.1).

Some fire and life safety educators are full-time educators. Others combine the fire department duties of public education officer and public information officer. Some fire and life safety educators — such as school nurses — are members of allied professions. Whatever their background or position description, fire and life safety educators share a commitment to teaching people how to protect themselves from everyday hazards.

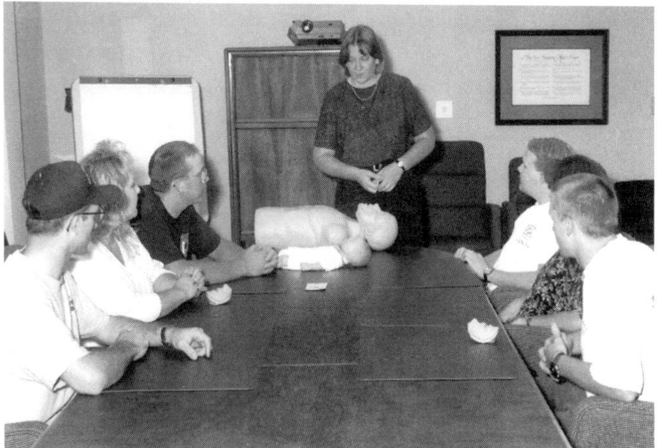

Figure 1.1 Fire and life safety educators come from many different organizations, not just from fire departments.

This chapter briefly reviews the history of "fire safety education" and highlights recent trends in the newer field of "fire and life safety education." The chapter also discusses education's role as an injury-control strategy as well as the role of fire and burns in the larger context of injury prevention.

The growing professionalism of fire and life safety educators is also covered. The chapter concludes with a Canon of Ethics for Fire and Life Safety Educators. (NOTE: A *canon* is a collection of principles or rules.)

Unlike other chapters in this manual, this chapter, "Introduction to Fire and Life Safety Education," concentrates on an overview of the field, rather than on background information and practical skills for the fire and life safety educator.

FIRE AND LIFE SAFETY EDUCATION: THEN AND NOW

A Brief History

Just how old is fire and life safety education? How did today's state of the art evolve?

What is known today as *fire and life safety education* has had several names, including "fire prevention education" and "public fire education." In earlier days, fire was certainly the main subject. More recently, programs have included nonfire topics: how to prevent burn injuries from scalds or fireworks, electrical safety, baby-sitter training, pedestrian safety, CPR, and water safety, to name just a few. In addition, programs have been expanded to include responding to natural hazards (earthquakes, floods, tornadoes, blizzards, etc.) (Figure 1.2). This wider education focus — coupled with the fire service role as the "first responder" to all sorts of emergencies — resulted in fire education becoming "fire and life safety education."

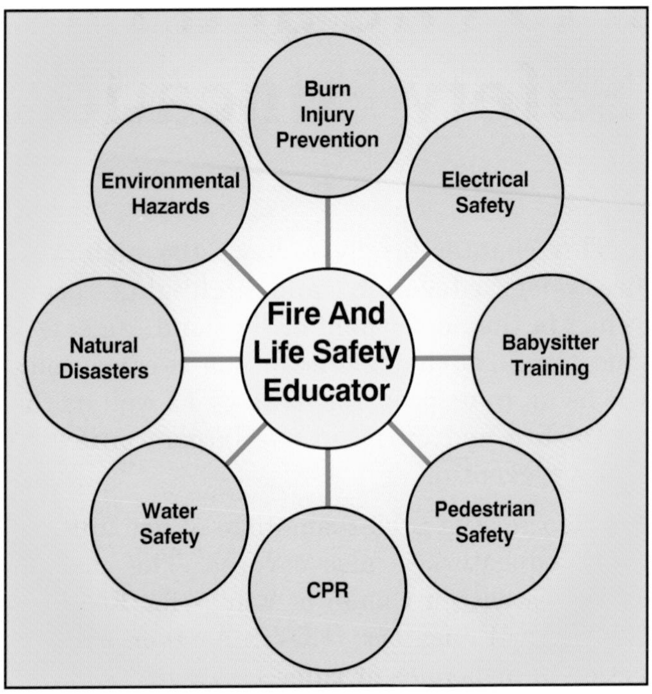

Figure 1.2 Fire and life safety education includes many topics other than fire safety.

Regardless of what it is called, fire and life safety education has a long history. According to one view,[1] "public fire education by the North American fire service goes back to the late 1800s." By 1909, a young member of the National Fire Protection Association (NFPA) staff named Franklin H. Wentworth was recruiting "correspondents" in cities across the continent. From Wentworth, the correspondents received a series of fire prevention bulletins, which they tried to place in local newspapers as news items. The papers were "but mildly responsive" — a reaction that many of today's fire and life safety educators would recognize.

Fire and life safety education marked slow but steady progress throughout the first half of the twentieth century (Figure 1.3).[2] Directly or indirectly, many advances resulted from the work of Percy Bugbee, widely known as "Mr. Fire Protection" and NFPA general manager from 1939 to 1969. School-based programs and a time set aside for fire prevention — whether a day, week, or month — have been core activities for many years. By mid-century, Hartford Insurance Group's Junior Fire Marshal Program and NFPA's Sparky® the Fire Dog had both been born.[3]

Although the 1960s was a fairly quiet decade for fire and life safety education, the 1970s saw an explosion of activity. In 1973, the publication of the report of the National Commission on Fire Prevention and Control, *America Burning,* added its strong voice to those calling for more emphasis on education programs.

Only a year later, NFPA's report *A Study of Motivational Psychology Related to Fire Preventive Behavior in Children and Adults* changed the course of fire and life safety education by focusing on *positive* messages. According to that influential study by Richard Strother, "education programs based on fear of fires, as opposed to danger or consequences of fire, have little educational benefit and can have a negative influence."[4]

The publication of *America Burning* and the *Motivational Psychology* report coincided with another event of great significance to fire and life

America Burning

"Among the many measures that can be taken to reduce fire losses, perhaps none is more important than educating people about fire. Americans must be made aware of the magnitude of fire's toll and its threat to them personally. They must know how to minimize the risk of fire in their daily surroundings. They must know how to cope with fire, quickly and effectively, once it has started. Public education about fire has been cited by many Commission witnesses and others as the single activity with the greatest potential for reducing losses."

America Burning, The Report of the National Commission on Fire Prevention and Control, U.S. Government Printing Office, May 1973, p. 105.

Time Line of Events Affecting Public Fire and Life Safety Education

1909 NFPA's Franklin Wentworth begins sending fire prevention bulletins to correspondents in 70 cities, with the hope that local newspapers will publish the bulletins as news articles.

1911 Fire Marshals Association of North America proposes the October 9 anniversary of the Great Chicago Fire as a day to observe fire prevention.

1912 *Syllabus for Public Instruction in Fire Prevention*—a collection of fire safety topics for teachers to use in the classroom—published by NFPA.

1916 NFPA and the National Safety Council establish a Committee on Fire and Accident Prevention. Communities nationwide organize Fire Prevention Day activities.

1920 President Woodrow Wilson signs first presidential proclamation for Fire Prevention Day.

1922 President Warren G. Harding signs first Fire Prevention Week proclamation.

1923 Twenty-three states have legislation requiring fire safety education in schools.

1927 NFPA begins sponsoring national Fire Prevention Contest.

1942 New York University publishes *Fire Prevention Education.*

1946 U.S. government publishes *Curriculum Guide to Fire Safety.*

1947 Hartford Insurance Group begins the Junior Fire Marshal Program, perhaps the first nationally distributed fire safety program for children.

1948 American Mutual Insurance Alliance publishes first edition of *Tested Activities for Fire Prevention Committees*, based on Fire Prevention Contest entries.

1950 In October, 7,000 newspapers receive the ad, "Don't Gamble with Fire—The Odds are Against You," developed by the Advertising Council and NFPA.

1954 Sparky® the Fire Dog is created.

1965 *Fire Journal* begins a regular column on "Reaching the Public."

1966 "Wingspread Conference" highlights the need for public education.

1967 Three Apollo astronauts die in a fire in their spacecraft, drawing national attention to the need to be prepared for fire emergencies. Later, attacks on firefighters during urban riots attract more public attention.

1970 President Richard Nixon appoints the National Commission on Fire Prevention and Control.

1973 The National Commission on Fire Prevention and Control publishes its report, *America Burning.*

The Fire Department Instructors Conference offers its first presentation on fire and life safety education, delivered by Cathy Lohr of North Carolina.

1974 NFPA and Public Service Council release the first television Learn Not to Burn® public service announcements starring Dick Van Dyke.

Fire Prevention and Control Act establishes the National Fire Prevention and Control Administration.

NFPA report by Richard Strother *A Study of Motivational Psychology Related to Fire Preventive Behavior in Children and Adults* explains the effectiveness of positive educational messages.

1975 The National Fire Prevention and Control Administration holds its first national fire safety education conference.

1977 NFPA 1031, *Standard for Professional Qualifications for Fire Inspector, Fire Investigator, and Fire Prevention Education Officer*, is published.

National Fire Prevention and Control Administration releases *Public Fire Education Planning: A Five Step Process.* National Fire Academy offers its first public education course on the same subject.

National Fire Prevention and Control Administration launches national smoke detector campaign.

1979 J. C. Robertson's *Introduction to Fire Prevention* published by Glencoe Press.

Project Burn Prevention, funded by the Consumer Product Safety Commission, develops educational strategies and materials for reducing burn injuries—a significant milestone in the shift from "fire education" to "all-risk education."

The *Learn Not to Burn® Curriculum* is published by NFPA.

International Fire Service Training Association releases IFSTA 606, *Public Fire Education.*

International Society of Fire Service Instructors establishes its Public Education Section.

1981 NFPA establishes its Education Section.

TriData Corporation releases *Reaching the Hard to Reach.*

1985 The National Education Association recommends the *Learn Not to Burn® Curriculum.*

NFPA publishes *Firesafety Educator's Handbook.*

1986 Learn Not to Burn® Foundation incorporated.

1987 The first edition of NFPA 1035, *Standard for Professional Qualifications for Public Fire Educator*, encourages civilians to become public fire educators in the fire department.

TriData Corporation publishes *Overcoming Barriers to Public Fire Education.*

1990 Oklahoma State University publishes the first issue of the *Public Fire Education Digest.*

TriData Corporation releases *Proving Public Fire Education Works.*

1995 NFPA and National SAFE KIDS® Campaign begin developing all-risk school curriculum called *Safety Sense.*

This time line relies in part on information from Pam Powell's "Firesafety Education: It's Older Than You Think," *Fire Journal*, May1986, pp.13+.

Figure 1.3 This time line shows the variety of events that have affected public fire and life safety education.

safety education. By the mid-1970s, reliable and reasonably priced smoke detectors were available for the home. The combination of *America Burning*'s advocacy, the positive focus from the *Motivational Psychology* report, and smoke detectors as a focus for presentations made the seventies a time of enormous activity in fire and life safety education. Smoke detector education programs resulted in another fundamental change to fire and life safety education: Audiences expanded from school children (often only fifth graders) to include adults (Figure 1.4).

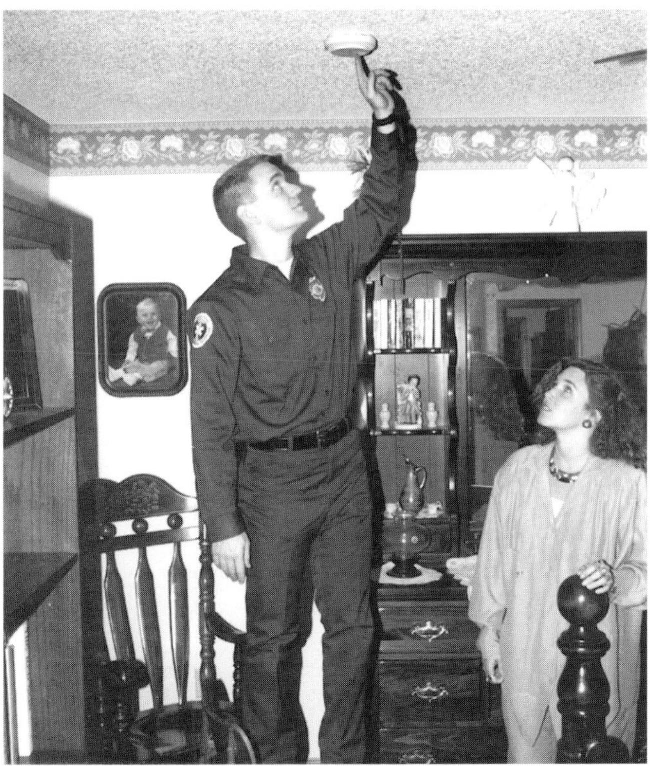

Figure 1.4 Smoke detector education programs include adults as well as children.

By the end of the decade, the National Fire Prevention and Control Administration (later the U.S. Fire Administration) and the National Fire Academy had a number of public education programs in place. Also by this time, the NFPA had begun its Learn Not to Burn® programs[5] and published a professional qualifications standard for fire prevention education officers, and the International Fire Service Training Association published IFSTA 606, **Public Fire Education**.

In the meantime, a number of states conducted their own statewide fire and life safety education conferences. Several of the statewide conferences that began in the 1970s — Massachusetts, North Carolina, and Oklahoma among them — are still held each year in the 1990s. Locally based fire and life safety educators — whether in large urban fire departments or small and isolated volunteer departments — became an integral part of many fire departments and schools.

In the U.S., federal activity in fire and life safety education declined in the 1980s. To a large extent, though, activity shifted to state agencies, not-for-profit organizations, and consulting organizations.

The 1980s also saw a sharpening of the fire and life safety educator's skills. At the same time, educators began demanding higher-quality materials. While in the 1970s fire and life safety educators praised almost any program, the profession seemed to demand more of itself in the eighties. Pilot-testing of materials, market research, more focus on evaluating program results, and efforts aimed at "reaching the hard-to-reach"[6] were hallmarks of education in the eighties.

Throughout the latter half of the 1980s and into the 1990s, fire and life safety education put new energy into finding partners to help with work that seemed somehow harder than in the past. Shrinking budgets for fire departments and other municipal services threatened many fire and life safety programs. In an era of latchkey children, substance abuse, and AIDS, the public demanded classroom instruction in many important subjects — each of which competed with fire and life safety for classroom time. As a result of these challenges, fire and life safety educators turned to "partnerships" and "coalition-building" as a way to extend their resources.

Fire and Life Safety Education Today

The topics of "fire" education have expanded enormously over the past two decades. As fire and life safety education moves toward the twenty-first century, three trends illustrate the increasing growth and sophistication of the field:

- Viewing education as an injury-control strategy

2. Advance the professional competency of other fire and life safety educators through networking and mentoring.
3. Teach only those subjects which the fire and life safety educator is qualified to teach.
4. Prepare for each presentation because a life in the audience depends upon it.
5. Evaluate program results honestly.
6. Continually improve programs and presentations.
7. Use only current and accurate material and information, including statistics.
8. Perform the duties of fire and life safety education with integrity.
9. Respect the work of other educators, through the courtesies of crediting their ideas and materials where appropriate and through compliance with copyright laws.
10. Recognize when your own conduct does not fully meet this canon of ethics, and resolve to improve.

FOR MORE INFORMATION

Several publications have useful information on the costs of various kinds of injuries. These publications include:

Dr. Ted R. Miller, *Medical Care Costs of Injury and Violence, and the Savings Available Through Prevention* (presented before the Senate Finance

What Do Educators Learn From Fires?

Many fire and life safety educators can recite the grim facts of fires that cause large loss of life and major property damage.

Fire	Lessons Learned
Coconut Grove Nightclub (1942) 492 deaths	Overcrowding; the role of interior finish; lack of adequate exits; difficulty in exiting
Our Lady of the Angels School (1958) 95 deaths	Storage of combustible materials; lack of teacher training in emergency response; lack of practiced fire drills; difficulty in exiting
Beverly Hills Supper Club (1977) 165 deaths	Lack of evacuation and planning practice; importance of early detection; difficulty of exiting
MGM Grand Hotel Fire (1980) 85 deaths	Smoke travel in high-rise buildings; evacuation from high-rise buildings; the need to teach people when to evacuate and when to "defend in place" (stay where they are)

These fires and other disastrous fires drew worldwide attention. Published reports told the fire protection community why the fires began and spread, how people died, and how the fire department fought the fires. Newspapers, newsreels, and later television reported on the human interest side of the big fires.

For the fire and life safety educator who is planning programs, however, large loss fires tell only part of the story. Today's fire and life safety educators draw from many other sources of information. Fire and life safety educators can evaluate local, state or provincial, and national data using fire incident reporting systems such as the National Fire Incident Reporting System (NFIRS).* With detailed data, fire and life safety educators are able to more accurately identify high-risk groups and neighborhoods than in the past. Such a localized approach has proven effective in many communities.

*For a description of NFIRS and other data sources, see Chapter 7, "Using Data to Plan Programs."

Committee Hearing on Consequences of Social Behavior on Health Care, October 19, 1993), National Public Services Research Institute, 8201 Corporate Drive, Landover, MD 20785; 301-731-9891.

The Impact of Alcohol-Related Crashes and Health Care, Mothers Against Drunk Driving (National Office), 511 E. John Carpenter Freeway, Irving, TX 75062-8187; 214-744-MADD.

Dr. Ted R. Miller, *Costs of Safety Belt and Motorcycle Helmet Nonuse* (presented before the Subcommittee on Surface Transportation, House Committee on Public Works and Transportation, Hearing on Designating the National Highway System, as required by the Surface Transportation Efficiency Act of 1991, March 3, 1994), National Public Services Research Institute, 8201 Corporate Drive, Landover, MD 20785; 301-731-9891.

Why Employers Should Promote Safety: A Fact Sheet, Children's Safety Network Third Party Payers Injury Prevention Resource Center, c/o the National Public Services Research Institute, 8201 Corporate Drive, Landover, MD 20785; 301-731-9891 or the National Safe Kids® Campaign, 111 Michigan Avenue, NW, Washington, DC 20010-2970; 202-939-4993.

Child Safety Seats: How Large Are the Benefits and Who Should Pay? Children's Safety Network Third Party Payers Injury Prevention Resource Center, c/o the National Public Services Research Institute, 8201 Corporate Drive, Landover, MD 20785; 301-731-9891 or the National Safe Kids® Campaign, 111 Michigan Avenue, NW, Washington, DC 20010-2970; 202-939-4993.

Bicycle Helmets Save Medical Costs for Children, Children's Safety Network Third Party Payers Injury Prevention Resource Center, c/o the National Public Services Research Institute, 8201 Corporate Drive, Landover, MD 20785; 301-731-9891, or the National Safe Kids® Campaign, 111 Michigan Avenue, NW, Washington, DC 20010-2970; 202-939-4993.

The Costs of Poisoning and the Savings from Poison Control Centers: A Benefit-Cost Analysis, Children's Safety Network Third Party Payers Injury Prevention Resource Center, c/o the National Public Services Research Institute, 8201 Corporate Drive, Landover, MD 20785; 301-731-9891, or the National Safe Kids® Campaign, 111 Michigan Avenue, NW, Washington, DC 20010-2970; 202-939-4993.

Injury in America: A Continuing Public Health Problem, Committee on Trauma Research, Commission on Life Sciences, National Research Council, and the Institute of Medicine, National Academy Press, Washington, DC, 1985.

Chapter 1 Notes

1. Mahendra S. Wijayasinghe, "Barriers to Learning Fire Safety in Adults," Fire Prevention Branch, General Safety Services Division, Alberta Labour, Edmonton, Canada (undated).

2. See Pam Powell, "Firesafety Education: It's Older Than You Think," *Fire Journal*, May 1986.

3. *Sparky*® is a registered trademark of the National Fire Protection Association, Quincy, MA 02269.

4. Richard Strother, Foreword to the unpublished report, *A Study of Motivational Psychology Related to Fire Preventive Behavior in Children and Adults*, National Fire Protection Association, 1974.

5. *Learn Not to Burn*® is a registered trademark of the National Fire Protection Association, Inc., Quincy, MA 02269

6. See Ann Kulenkamp, Barbara Lundquist, and Philip Schaenman, *Reaching the Hard-to-Reach: Techniques from Fire Prevention Programs and Other Disciplines*, TriData Corporation, October 1994.

7. *Injury in America: A Continuing Public Health Problem*, Committee on Trauma Research, Commission on Life Sciences, National Research Council, and the Institute of Medicine, National Academy Press, Washington, DC, 1985.

8. Reprinted with permission from *Injury in America*, p. 87. Copyright 1985 by the National Academy of Sciences. Courtesy of the National Academy Press, Washington, DC.

9. These terms are used by the National Fire Academy in its course *Developing Fire and Life Safety Strategies*.

10. See *Child-Resistant Lighters Protect Young Children*, U.S. Consumer Product Safety Commission, Washington, DC, July 1994.

11. *Injury in America*, pp. 37-38.

12. Baker and Waller, *Childhood Injury — State-by-State Mortality Facts*, Johns Hopkins Injury Prevention Center, January 1989.

13. Reprinted with permission from NFPA 1035, *Professional Qualifications for Public Fire and Life Safety Educator*, Copyright ©1993, National Fire Protection Association, Quincy, MA 02269. This reprinted material is not the complete and official position of the National Fire Protection Association, on the referenced subject which is represented only by the standard in its entirety.

Chapter 1 Review

Directions

The following activities are designed to help you comprehend and apply the information in Chapter 1 of **Fire and Life Safety Educator**, second edition. To receive the maximum learning experience from these activities, it is recommended that you use the following procedure:

1. Read the chapter, underlining or highlighting important terms, topics, and subject matter. Read the sidebar material, study the photographs and illustrations, and read the captions with each.
2. Review the list of vocabulary words to ensure that you know the chapter-related meaning of each. If you are unsure of the meaning of a vocabulary word, look up the word in the glossary or a dictionary, and then study its context in the chapter.
3. On a separate sheet of paper, complete all assigned or selected application and review activities before checking your answers.
4. After you have finished, check your answers against those on the pages referenced in parentheses.
5. Correct any incorrect answers, and review material that was answered incorrectly.

Vocabulary

Be sure that you know the chapter-related meanings of the following words and abbreviations:

- all-risk education *(9, 10)*
- canon *(12)*
- IFSAC *(12)*
- NFIRS *(13)*
- NFPA *(6)*

Application of Knowledge

1. Obtain and read one (or more) of the publications listed on pages *13 and 14*. Create a chart similar to the one on page *13,* using several examples from your readings. Be sure to include the headings Fires and Lessons Learned.
2. Create an example for the following statement that shows the most effective use of all three strategies for injury prevention:

   Efforts to control injuries to young children caused by non-fire retardant clothing.

   NOTE: If you need to review an example on how to most effectively use the three strategies for injury prevention, see page *9*.

Review Activities

1. Briefly outline the history of fire and life safety education from the late 1800s through the 1990s. Include important names and organizations that have made significant contributions. *(6-9)*
2. List three trends that illustrate the increasing growth and sophistication of fire and life safety education over the past two decades. *(8, 9)*
3. Name the three phases of injury control. *(9)*
4. Compare terms used to describe the three general injury prevention strategies. *(9)*
5. Explain the most effective use of prevention strategies. *(9)*
6. Explain why education strategy is needed to prevent injuries. *(9)*
7. Discuss how each of the three strategies contributes to an effective comprehensive injury-control program. *(10)*
8. Describe what all-risk education programs should include. *(10)*
9. Outline the evolution of professionalism in fire and life safety education over the past twenty years. *(11, 12)*
10. Define the following terms according to NFPA 1035: *(12)*
    - Public Fire and Life Safety Education
    - Public Fire and Life Safety Educator I
    - Public Fire and Life Safety Educator II
    - Public Fire and Life Safety Educator III

11. List organizations or agencies that are involved with professional certification for fire and life safety education. *(12)*

12. Identify from the list on pages 12 and 13 the professional and ethical conduct commitments to fire and life safety education.

13. Identify from the list on pages 13 and 14 the publications on cost of various kinds of injuries.

14. Explain the educational approach that is taken today by fire and life safety educators on the subject of large-loss fires. *(13)*

15. Review the fire and life safety time line on page *7* from the years 1909 through 1995. *(7)*

Questions and Notes

Information about fuel load and heat release rate can help in distinguishing between more and less hazardous items. If two items have the same fuel load (that is, the total number of Btu is the same) but one of the items releases its heat twice as fast during a fire (in other words, it has a higher heat release rate), then the item with the higher heat release rate is more hazardous. For example, a cotton mattress will tend to smolder slowly, releasing its heat over a long period of time. Once ignited, a foam plastic mattress — containing the same amount of heat energy — burns very quickly and can fill a room with flames in a few minutes (or less).

The fuel load and the heat release rate of the same material can be very different, even though both are measured in Btu. Specifically, the heat release rate can be much higher than one might expect (Table 2.1).

The information in Table 2.1 shows that a polyurethane mattress in a fire will release heat much faster than a cotton mattress the same size. Based on this insight from fire dynamics, the fire and life safety educator might decide to warn the public against attempting to extinguish a mattress fire.

TABLE 2.1
Representative Peak Heat Release Rates*

Sample	Amount Of Fuel	Peak Heat Release Rate
Cotton mattress	26-29 lbs	40-970 kW
Polyurethane mattress	7-31 lbs	810-2630 kW

*Unconfined burning

Portions reprinted with permission from NFPA 921, *Guide for Fire and Explosion Investigations*, Copyright ©1995, National Fire Protection Association, Quincy, MA 02269. This reprinted material is not the complete and official position of the National Fire Protection Association, on the referenced subject which is represented only by the standard in its entirety.

The ignition temperature, surface area, and mass of a material also have a great impact on its ignition behavior.

The lower its ignition temperature, the more likely a material is to ignite. Table 2.2 shows ignition temperatures of materials that are found in most households. Fire and life safety educators can use this kind of information — especially with more technically sophisticated audiences such as homeowner's associations or high school science classes — to generate discussion about issues such as the following:

TABLE 2.2
Ignition Temperatures Of Common Household Materials

Material	Ignition Temperature (°F)	(°C)
Kerosene	410	210
Douglas Fir	500	260
Gasoline (100 octane)	853	456
Cotton	750	400
Propane	842	450
Polystyrene	1063	573
Natural gas	900-1170	482-632
Coal dust	1346	730

Portions reprinted with permission from NFPA 921, *Guide for Fire and Explosion Investigations*, Copyright ©1995, National Fire Protection Association, Quincy, MA 02269. This reprinted material is not the complete and official position of the National Fire Protection Association, on the referenced subject which is represented only by the standard in its entirety.

- How low the ignition temperatures are for some household products (such as kerosene)
- The very small difference in ignition temperatures of gasoline (which most people would consider quite dangerous to have around the house) and polyurethane foam (which many people may not consider dangerous at all)

The fire and life safety educator can illustrate the impact of surface area and mass on a material's ignition potential by describing the differences in lighting equal amounts of newspaper, kindling, and logs for a campfire. Even though the materials are all essentially wood, the newspaper ignites much more readily than the kindling, which ignites much more readily than the logs (Figure 2.2). This example shows that chemically similar materials having a larger surface-area-to-mass ratio ignite more readily than those having a smaller surface-area-to-mass ratio. The ratio of surface area to mass has a direct relationship on the hazards of the storage of combustibles.

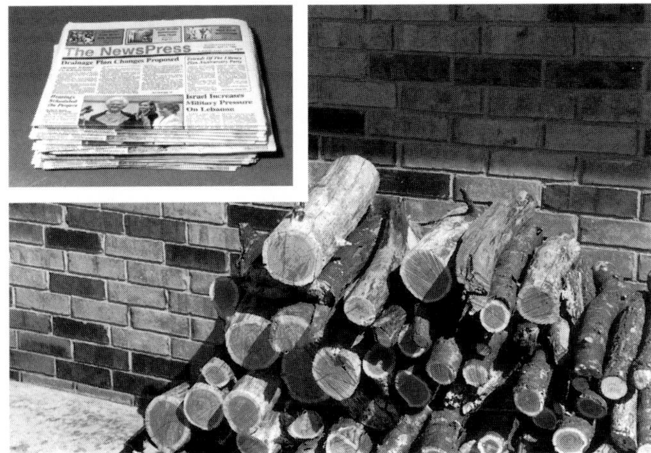

Figure 2.2 Even though it is composed of basically the same material as logs, newspaper ignites much more quickly.

Another area to be considered under ignition is "heat energy applied." *Heat energy applied* is the sum of the temperature of the heat source and the time of exposure. The heat source could be mechanical (from rubbing two sticks together, for example), chemical, nuclear, or solar.

Many common ignition sources are quite hot. With more sophisticated audiences, fire and life safety educators can mention the temperatures of ignition sources, pointing out items of particular interest (such as a cigarette) (Table 2.3).

To explore the idea of "heat energy applied," fire and life safety educators and their audiences can discuss two ways in which a sheet of newspaper can be ignited: by a brief exposure to the high heat of a match or by a longer exposure to the lower heat of a space heater. Like many concepts of fire dynamics, heat applied directly influences fire safety through good housekeeping practices and safety practices such as separating all heat sources from combustible materials (Figure 2.3).

TABLE 2.3
Temperatures Of Common Ignition Sources

Source	Temperature (°F)	Temperature (°C)
Ember from free burning cigarette	930-1300	500-700
Flames from gasoline fire	1798	1026
Flames from wood fire	1800	1027
Mechanical spark from steel tool	2550	1400

Portions reprinted with permission from NFPA 921, *Guide for Fire and Explosion Investigations*, Copyright ©1995, National Fire Protection Association, Quincy, MA 02269. This reprinted material is not the complete and official position of the National Fire Protection Association, on the referenced subject which is represented only by the standard in its entirety.

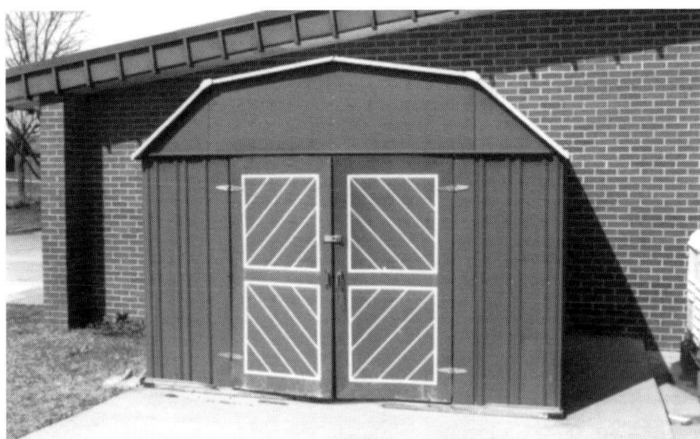

Figure 2.3 A toolshed such as this is a suitable place to store flammable- and combustible-liquid containers outside the home.

Heat Transfer

How is heat transferred from one item or area to another? It is done so by one of three types of heat transfer: radiation, convection, and conduction.

Radiation transfers heat through electromagnetic waves and is especially efficient in heating solid and opaque objects. Radiation from ignition sources is a major factor in accidental ignition.

In convective heat transfer, the energy is transferred by the movement of a medium such as a gas (including air) or liquid. Convective heat transfer is usually not a cause of ignition. However, convection and radiation are major factors in fire growth and spread: Convection moves heated air and smoke upward, which then heat other items from radiation from hot gases and spreads fire.

Conduction transfers heat through direct contact. One example of conduction is the heating of a spoon in a cup of hot soup.

A space heater, a chair, an end table, and curtains hanging above the space heater illustrate the differences between the three types of heat transfer. A chair placed close to the space heater's radiant panel is heated by radiation. An end table that is touching the space heater's casing (but not the radiant panel) is heated by conduction. Air heated by conduction that rises from the space heater to the curtains above is an example of convection (Figure 2.4).

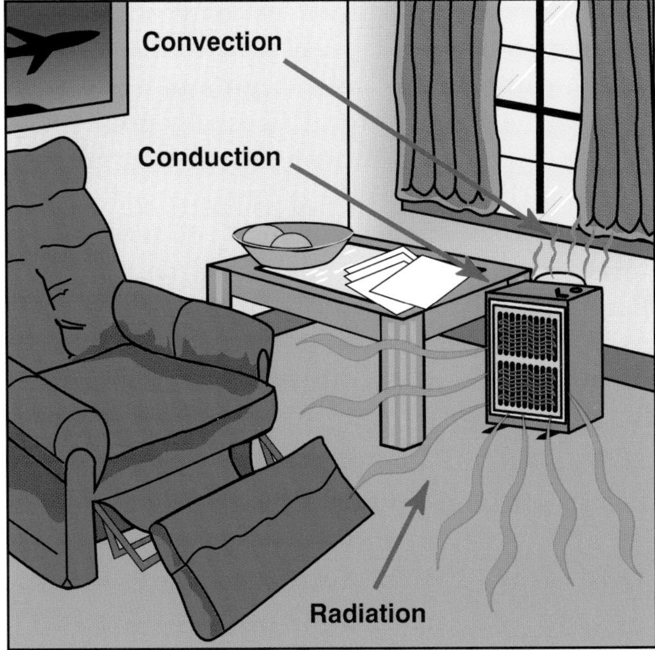

Figure 2.4 A space heater, a chair, an end table, and curtains hanging above the space heater illustrate the differences among the three types of heat transfer.

Fire Growth and Spread

Will the first item keep burning? Early in a fire, the fuel needs the heat from the external heat source to sustain ignition. At some point after ignition, the material will either burn on its own or self-extinguish. When the fuel continues to burn without the external heat source, *established burning* has been achieved. Depending on the material, flame heights may reach 8 to 12 inches before established burning has been reached. Continued fire growth and spread depend on established burning.

Established burning plays a major role in regulating the flammability of clothing and other fabrics. For example, U.S. Consumer Product Safety Commission standards for the flammability of children's sleepwear (sizes 0-6X and 7-14) are based on whether a fabric sample continues burning after a flame is removed.

In the realm of fire dynamics (and the total realm of fire safety!), one of the most critical questions is "Will the fire grow and spread to a second item?" Fire growth is a complex process that is affected by factors as diverse as the following:

- The fuel itself (its ignition temperature, heat release rate, ratio of surface to mass, etc.)
- The orientation of the fuel (Figure 2.5)
- Location of other fuels (that is, those other than the first item ignited) (Figure 2.6)

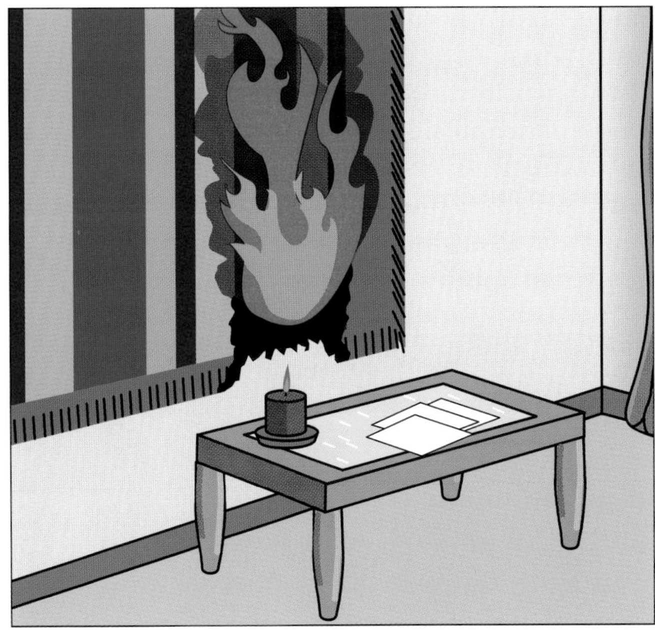

Figure 2.5 Carpet hung vertically, such as for a wall hanging, burns more quickly than does the same carpet on the floor.

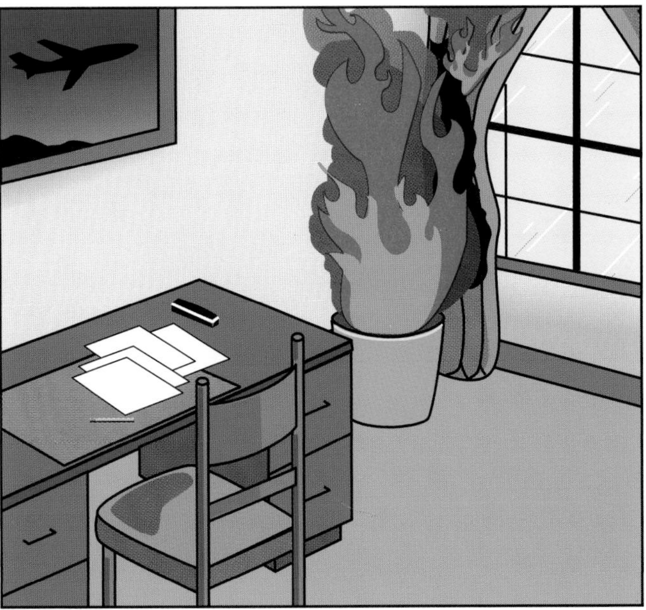

Figure 2.6 Another factor affecting fire growth is the location of other fuels.

- Differences in ventilation (is the door open or closed?)
- Location of the fire in the room
- The geometry of the room

The fire's location and room geometry are two factors that are especially germane to fire educators. For example, a trash can fire in the middle of a room, far away from walls, releases heat at a given rate. That same fire next to a wall has gas temperatures and flame lengths that are twice as large, simply because the wall cuts the airflow in half. When a fire is in a corner — near two walls that block airflow — the effective heat release rate quadruples. As a result, a fire next to a wall or in a corner grows and spreads much faster than a fire in the center of a room. In smaller rooms or in areas with low ceilings, the fire will grow and spread even faster.

Flashover

Regardless of a fire's location or a room's geometry, fires follow a fairly standard pattern during growth and spread. From first ignition and especially after established burning, heat rises toward the ceiling, carrying smoke and gases with it. A hot layer of smoke and gas forms at the ceiling. This layer begins to move down toward the floor (**NOTE:** This is why fire damage is often much greater near the ceiling than near the floor (Figure 2.7). As the smoke darkens and becomes more opaque, its ability to radiate heat increases. Other materials in the room — walls, floor, and furnishings — begin to heat from the radiation. As the materials heat, some of the solid material chemically breaks down and releases combustible gases.

Eventually, all the exposed surfaces in the room reach their ignition temperature at about the

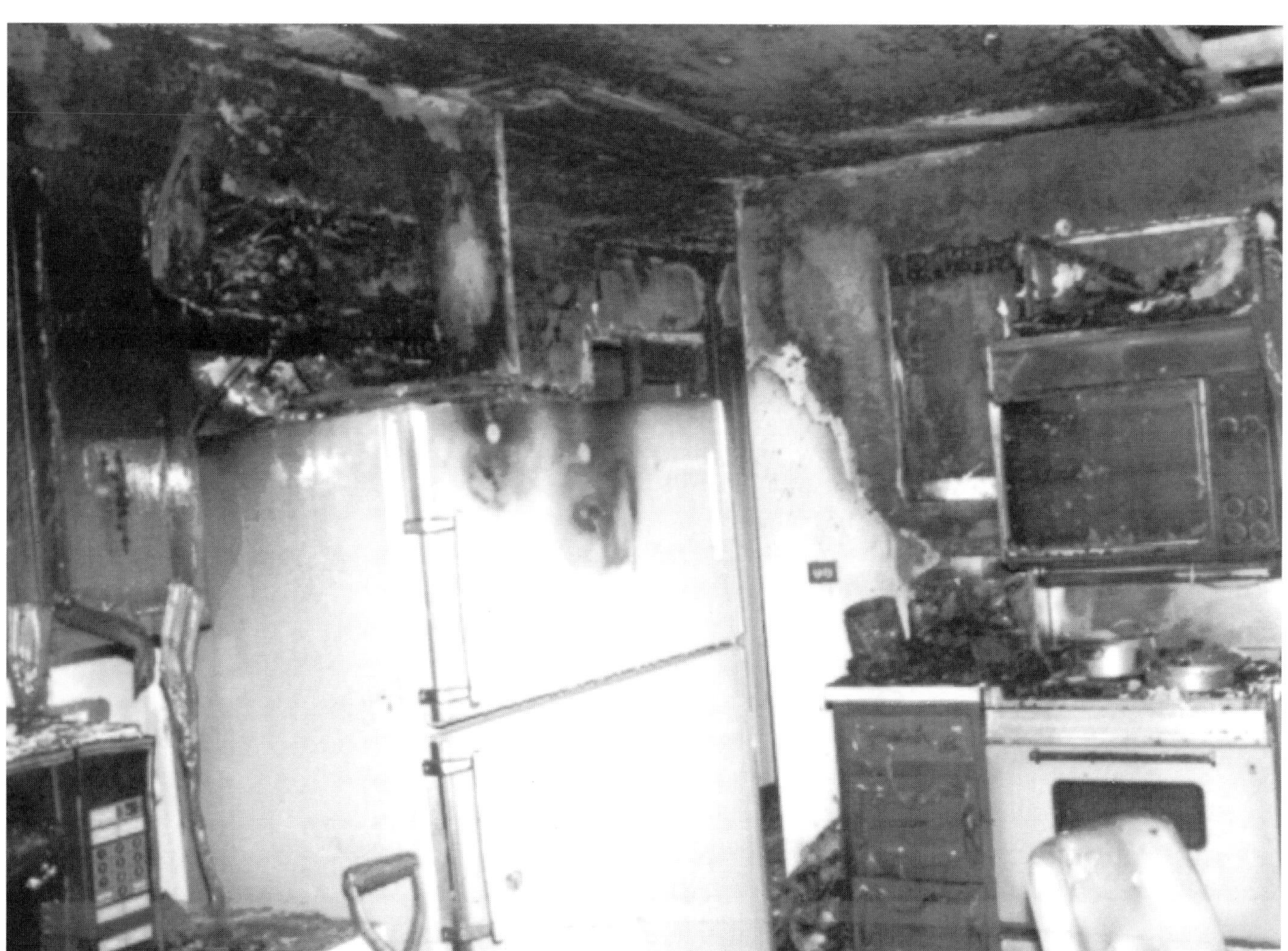

Figure 2.7 The greater amount of fire damage near the ceiling is due to the accumulations of hot smoke and gases. *Courtesy of Elk Grove Village (IL) Fire Department.*

same time. Fire spreads very rapidly, and other items may even appear to burst into flame at this stage of fire spread, which is known as *flashover*. There are several conditions associated with flashover:

- Average temperatures of 930°F to 1,300°F (500°C to 600°C) in the upper part of the room
- Flames flashing over the entire surface of a room or area
- Oxygen levels in the smoke layer dropping to 5 percent or less
- Burning of fire gases outside the room of origin

These conditions are so severe, that people within the room during flashover rarely survive.

Flashover is so dramatic that it is tempting to view it as a single event. More correctly, flashover is one point in fire growth and spread: The point that marks the transition from a fire that is controlled by the first few items ignited to a fully involved room fire.

Flashover can occur in any confined space — in any room, under sinks or desks, in a subway escalator (as it did during the 1987 fire at King's Cross Station in London), or even under the awning of an outdoor stadium (as it did during a soccer match in Bradford, England).

This kind of insight from the science of fire dynamics can enhance and refine fire education's messages. For example, people who place trash cans under the sink, in a corner or a closet, or in the kneehole of a desk need to know that a trash fire can grow and reach flashover with astonishing speed.

TENABILITY

Fire is a very destructive event that can kill people in seconds. The public needs to know how dangerous fire is so that they can take steps to protect themselves.

The term *tenability* refers to whether or not people can remain unhurt in a fire area or escape without serious injury. Although more is being learned all the time, tenability is not a very exact science; neither is tenability ever a simple "yes or no" question. Instead, tenability depends on a number of factors affecting the potential victim, combined with the various hazards produced by the fire.

The Human Factor

Two people could react very differently to the same fire. The same person could have a different physical reaction to a fire today than in a fire a month from now. How well someone can withstand the physical assault of fire's heat, smoke, and gases depends on a combination of the following factors:

- **Age.** In general, very young people and older people will be less physically able to withstand a fire. This is especially true if other factors (such as overall physical condition, respiratory capacity, or the presence of medication, drugs, or alcohol) that diminish physical ability are present.
- **Size.** Larger people can tolerate larger doses of toxic combustion products, just as adults can tolerate larger doses of medication than children can.

  On the other hand, large size may be associated with other factors — a lack of physical conditioning, for example — that reduce the ability to tolerate combustion products (see next paragraph).
- **Pre-existing physical condition.** A person's overall physical condition affects the ability to survive a fire. Heart health, aerobic condition, and mobility (determined by a combination of weight/percentage of body fat, flexibility, or the presence of arthritis, rheumatism, diabetes, or other conditions or injuries that impair mobility) are key factors.
- **Respiratory capacity.** Approximately three out of every four fire deaths are due to smoke inhalation. Because smoke inhalation is such a critical risk, the potential victim's existing respiratory capacity can make an enormous difference in tenability. A number of chronic diseases (such as emphysema, asthma, or asbestosis) can lower respiratory capacity. Acute condi-

tions such as pneumonia, flu, or even a cold can also limit respiratory capacity. Cigarette smoking, which raises the body's level of carbon monoxide, reduces the blood's ability to take up oxygen.

- **Medication, drugs, or alcohol.** Many types of prescribed and over-the-counter medication, drugs, and alcohol can restrict a person's ability to react to a fire or other dangerous condition.

  According to recent estimates, at least 10 percent of those who died in residential fires were impaired by alcohol or other drugs when they died.[3] Those fire victims from 20 to 64 years old were impaired twice as much as the general population. A 1970s study concluded that more than half of fire victims over the age of 20 in Maryland were legally intoxicated. As the population ages, impairment by prescription drugs may become even more significant.

Hazards From the Fire

Fires produce a number of hazardous physical conditions that determine the tenability of a room. These conditions include temperature, heat flux (how fast heat transfers to a surface — such as to the skin), smoke obscuration, oxygen depletion, and exposure to fire gases.

TEMPERATURE

The effects of temperature vary with the length of time of heat exposure, the amount of relative humidity (moisture in the air increases the effects of heat), and the "breathability" of clothing worn. In general, however, temperatures as low as 122°F (50°C) produce severe discomfort in the mouth, nose, and esophagus. As long ago as 1959, a series of school fire tests in Los Angeles known as Operation School Burning concluded that children and teachers could not be expected to enter a corridor in which the temperature was 150°F (65°C). Temperatures above 150°F (65°C) are incapacitating; death from hyperthermia occurs at temperatures above 212°F (100°C). Table 2.4 summarizes other physiological effects of elevated temperatures.

TABLE 2.4
Physiological Effects Of Heat

Physiological Effect	Temperature (°F)	(°C)
Possible heatstroke	140	60
Able to tolerate temperature for 49 minutes	180	82
Very rapid skin burns in humid air	212	100
20-minute tolerance	240	115
Difficulty breathing through nose	260	125
Difficulty breathing through mouth	300	150
Temperature limit for escape	300	150
Rapid, unbearable pain to dry skin	320	160
Ability to tolerate temperature drops to less than 4 minutes	390	200
Respiratory system threshold	390	200

Table courtesy of Southwest Research Institute.

Even ordinary residential fires reach temperatures of 300°F to 400°F (about 150°C to 200°C) very quickly. Temperatures and times recorded in a house fire during the making of the 1986 NFPA film *Fire Power* demonstrate the speed at which untenable temperatures can be reached.[4] The fire began with a simulated cigarette ignition of a wastebasket. For example, temperatures at head level in the room of origin reached 392°F (200°C) only 2 minutes and 30 seconds after flame first appeared in a wastebasket next to the couch. Only three minutes after first flame, the temperature three feet above the floor was 500°F (260°C) — temperatures that no one can survive.

HEAT FLUX AND BURN INJURIES

Heat flux is a scientific measurement of how much heat is available for transfer to a human skin (or any other surface). Generally, the upper limit of heat flux without severe skin pain is 2.5 kW/m^2 for 3 minutes. Holding a hand a few inches from a 100-watt light bulb for 3 minutes would produce a heat flux of about 2.5 kW/m^2.

A simpler way of looking at heat transfer and burn injuries is the "heat energy applied" concept from fire dynamics. In other words, how much heat for how long is required to cause a burn?

The higher the temperature, the more quickly a burn injury will occur. Table 2.5 gives examples of temperatures and exposure times to cause second-degree burns.

TABLE 2.5
Temperature And Time To Second-Degree Burns

Skin Surface Temperature (°F)	(°C)	Time (In Seconds)
160	71	60
180	82	30
212	100	15

Reprinted with permission from *Fire Protection Handbook*, 17th edition, Copyright ©1991, National Fire Protection Association, Quincy, MA 02269.

SMOKE OBSCURATION

Visible smoke has several kinds of negative physical effects during a fire: reduced visibility and the irritation and toxicity caused by inhaling smoke particles. Smoke may also have a marked emotional effect, by causing fear.

Reduced visibility reduces a person's ability to escape. When fire scientists relate smoke obscuration and walking speed, suggested tenability limits for visibility range from 5 feet (for occupants who are in a familiar area) to as much as 40 feet (for occupants in an unfamiliar area). These different limits are based on the assumption that people do not need to see as far in familiar surroundings, but can still find their way out. It is interesting to note that the *Life Safety Code®* (Section 5-10.1.3) allows a distance of 100 feet between an exit sign and an exit access.

OXYGEN DEPLETION

Oxygen normally makes up 21 percent of air on the planet Earth. The human respiratory and nervous systems are designed to function with that concentration of oxygen — not more and not less. When the percent of oxygen drops even a few points, physiological effects are felt. Table 2.6 summarizes how reduced oxygen harms people.

TABLE 2.6
Physiological Effects Of Reduced Oxygen (Hypoxia)

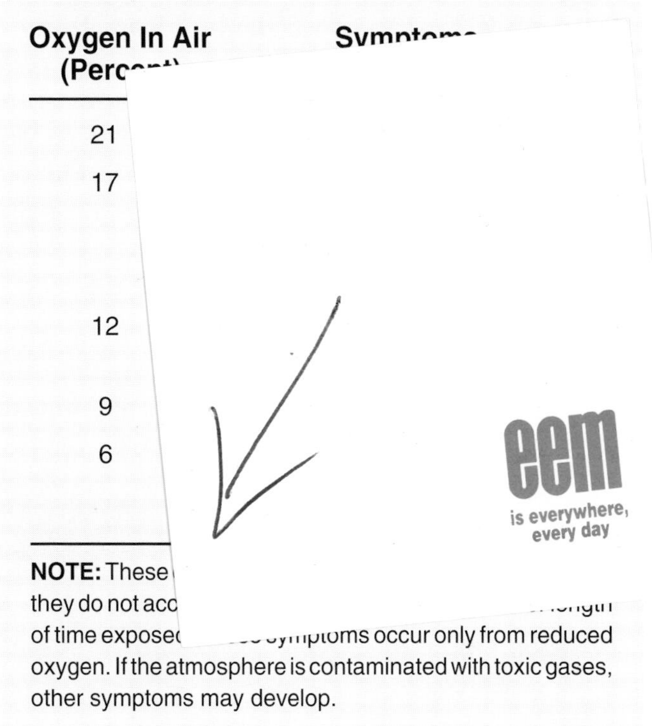

Oxygen In Air (Perc	Symptom
21	
17	
12	
9	
6	

NOTE: These they do not acc ngth of time expose symptoms occur only from reduced oxygen. If the atmosphere is contaminated with toxic gases, other symptoms may develop.

EXPOSURE TO FIRE GASES

Carbon monoxide is the primary culprit in fire deaths. Carbon monoxide poisoning alone accounts for about half of all fire deaths, and carbon monoxide combined with other factors is responsible for another 30 percent of all fire fatalities. Carbon monoxide easily attaches itself to hemoglobin (red blood cells), decreasing the blood's ability to carry oxygen. In other words, carbon monoxide prevents oxygen from going to red blood cells.

Carbon monoxide is so dangerous that even relatively small amounts may be incapacitating or even lethal. One measure of toxicity is the exposure concentration (abbreviated C) in parts per million (ppm) times the time of exposure (in minutes [T]) and is expressed as the CT product or ppm per minute.

Any concentration above 35,000 parts per million (ppm) per minute is hazardous. *However, higher concentrations for even very short times can be incapacitating or lethal.* Table 2.7 outlines some of the effects of carbon monoxide poisoning.

Members of the fire service may be more familiar with another way of viewing carbon monoxide — by the percentage of carboxyhemoglobin (COHb) saturation in the blood. In general, carboxyhemoglobin levels below 30 percent will not harm a person's ability to escape a fire. By 40 percent saturation, however, escape becomes much more difficult. At saturation levels of 50 to 60 percent, severe symptoms and even death occur, as Table 2.8 illustrates.

It is important to note that carboxyhemoglobin levels, while a valuable tool in measuring toxicity, do not consider the length of exposure. The CT measurement, on the other hand, does account for how long a victim is exposed to a hazard.

HUMAN BEHAVIOR DURING FIRES

Human behavior is the raw material of fire and life safety education. Changing human behavior is what the fire and life safety educator does, by developing and sharing safety skills and information. At the same time, human behavior is what the educator has to work with — because education builds on pre-existing positive and helpful behaviors.

Despite its importance, human behavior during fires was unstudied until about a generation ago. New findings about how people act during fires challenge many old myths.

The Myth of Panic

As reported in newspapers and on television news and as shown in movies, fire and panic are very closely linked. A lay person, when asked what happened at fires at the Coconut Grove nightclub, the MGM Grand Hotel, or the Happyland Social Club, will likely respond, "People panicked."

TABLE 2.7
Toxic Effects Of Carbon Monoxide

Carbon Monoxide (CO) (ppm*)	Carbon Monoxide (CO) In Air (Percent)	Symptoms
100	0.01	No symptoms — no damage
200	0.02	Mild headache; few other symptoms
400	0.04	Headache after 1 to 2 hours
800	0.08	Headache after 45 minutes; nausea, collapse, and unconsciousness after 2 hours
1,000	0.10	Dangerous — unconsciousness after 1 hour
1,600	0.16	Headache, dizziness, nausea after 20 minutes
3,200	0.32	Headache, dizziness, nausea after 5 to 10 minutes; unconsciousness after 30 minutes
6,400	0.64	Headache, dizziness, nausea after 1 to 2 minutes; unconsciousness after 10 to 15 minutes
12,800	1.26	Immediate unconsciousness, danger of death in 1 to 3 minutes

*parts per million

TABLE 2.8
Consequences Of Carboxyhemoglobin (COHb) Saturation

COHb Saturation (Percent)	Symptoms In Humans
0-10	None
10-20	Tension in forehead, dilation of skin vessels
20-30	Headache and pulsating temples
30-40	Severe headache, weariness, dizziness, weakened sight, nausea, vomiting, prostration
40-50	Same as above, plus increased breathing and pulse rates, asphyxiation, and prostration
50-60	Same as above, plus coma, convulsions, Cheyne-Stokes respiration
60-70	Coma, convulsions, weak respiration and pulse; death possible
70-80	Slowing and stopping of breathing, death within hours
80-90	Death in less than 1 hour
90-100	Death within a few minutes

From *Advances in Combustion Toxicology*, Volume One, Gordon E. Hartzell (ed.), Technomic Publishing Company, Inc., 1989, p. 23. Used with permission.

Just what is panic? How real is it during fires? What can fire and life safety educators do to prevent it?

As long ago as 1958, Dr. John L. Bryan of the University of Maryland described panic as "a sudden and excessive feeling of alarm or fear, usually affecting a body of persons, originating in some real or supposed danger, vaguely apprehended, and leading to extravagant and injudicious efforts to secure safety."[5] By the 1970s, however, Dr. Bryan and other behavioral experts had begun to conclude that panic was rare — not widespread — during fires. In 1982, Dr. John Keating, a psychology professor at the University of Washington, crystallized his colleagues' ideas in the influential *Fire Journal* article, "The Myth of Panic."[6]

In that article, four elements were identified as essential to panic behavior:

- A hope for escape, even with closing escape routes
- Contagious behavior, especially if keynoted by leaders of the group affected by the fire
- "Aggressive concern" by the individual for his or her own safety, as opposed to concern for others in the same fire
- Irrational, illogical response to the fire situation

Dr. Keating argued that one or more of those elements were missing in most fire evacuations:

- For example, there is usually no evidence of panic when there is no hope of escape (from a submarine fire, for example).
- Contagious behavior is very common in emergencies or ambiguous situations simply because people tend to "follow the leader" in times of stress or when they need reassurance about the right thing to do. Panic occurs when a rare individual does not follow the actions (and rely on the collective information) of the group.
- In many types of emergencies, people often help others — even at great personal risk. People are even more likely to help others when they feel somehow linked. Dining room staff at the Beverly Hills Supper Club, for example, led the patrons from "their" tables to safety.
- Escape strategies that are unsuccessful, such as using the stairs at the MGM Grand Hotel, are not necessarily irrational or illogical. On the contrary, using the stairs instead of the elevator was exactly what placards instructed people to do.

What may appear as panic behavior from the comfortable perspective of an outsider after the fire probably seemed very logical and rational at the time — especially given the incomplete and confusing information available during the fire emergency.

Just how often does true panic happen in fires? As few as one-third of the victims of the Coconut Grove fire actually panicked, and there was no panic behavior among the 164 people who died at the Beverly Hills Supper Club fire. Interviews of 100 survivors of single-family dwelling fires revealed no panic behavior whatsoever.

What Happens During a Fire?

Human behavior during a fire is just as complex as the fire itself. A first step in understanding this behavior is cataloging what people do first. Table 2.9 outlines the first, second, and third actions (expressed as percentages) that people take during a fire. The table is based on interviews with more than 500 fire survivors in the United States.

As Table 2.9 reveals, there are patterns in the order in which people take specific actions during a fire. For example, "notifying others" ranked high as a first action (15 percent) but dropped off to less than 6 percent as a third action. By contrast, actions such as "called fire department," "left building," and "fought fire" are more common as a third action than as a first act.

Men and women do act differently during a fire. Table 2.9 shows that men are much more likely to engage in fire fighting activities (such as "searched for fire" and "got extinguishers") than women. On the other hand, women are more likely to take the lead in warning and evacuation activities ("got family" and "called fire department"). It is also interesting that more women than men left the building as their first action.

Interviews with survivors of residential fires in the United Kingdom show similar patterns.[7] For example, people notice fire cues very early in a fire but find them ambiguous (misinterpreting or ignoring strange noises, or perhaps discussing them with others). If the cues persist, people will investigate and will even enter a room with smoke or fire in it. Both men and women misinterpreted ambiguous cues before investigating fires in the United Kingdom study, but men were more likely to delay investigation.

The U.K. interviews showed that gender differences affected fire behavior. Women are more likely to warn others or to wait for instructions than men (especially if husband and wife are both present). Women will close the door, leave the home, and seek help from neighbors more often than men. Men are more likely to fight the fire. Male neighbors tend to search for and try to rescue victims.

Making Sense of Human Behavior During Fires

The complex patterns of human behavior during fire can be grouped together. These groupings often describe the decision processes of the individual or sociopsychological concepts of human response. Through these groupings, fire and life safety educators can better understand why people do what they do during a fire.

People use six basic techniques to decide what to do in a fire.[8] They are recognition, validation, definition, evaluation, commitment, and reassessment.

- **Threat recognition.** For lay people, the first cues of a fire can be very ambiguous and unclear. In fact, people may worry that "something isn't right" and — at the same time — optimistically hope that the threat is false. For many people, fire's threat is unrecognized until large quantities of smoke, heat, or flame appear. Children who have received fire and life safety instruction may recognize fire's threat much earlier than adults.

  A main job of the fire and life safety educator is countering the delayed recognition of a fire's immediate threat. Messages such as "Always leave the building when the fire alarm sounds" help audiences overcome their "built-in" tendency to not recognize threats.

- **Validation.** When people are unsure about how serious a threat is, they want reassurance that the threat is mild. When threats seem more serious, people ask others for information. Seeking more information proves or validates that there is, indeed, a

TABLE 2.9
Occupant Actions During A Fire

Action	1st Action	2nd Action	3rd Action	Male 1st Action	Female 1st Action
		(Percent Of Participant Population)			
Notified others	15.0	9.6	5.8	16.3	13.8
Searched for fire	10.1	2.4	0.8	14.9	6.3
Called fire department	9.0	14.6	12.7	6.1	11.4
Got dressed	8.1	1.8	0.3	5.8	10.1
Left building	7.6	20.9	35.9	4.2	10.4
Got family	7.6	5.9	1.4	3.4	11.0
Fought fire	4.6	5.7	11.5	5.8	3.8
Got extinguisher	4.6	5.3	1.6	6.9	2.8
Left area	4.3	2.8	1.1	4.6	4.1
Woke up	3.1	0.0	0.0	3.8	2.5
Nothing	2.7	0.0	0.0	2.7	2.8
Had others call fire department	2.2	4.0	4.1	3.4	1.3
Got personal property	2.1	3.8	0.8	1.5	2.5
Went to fire area	2.1	1.0	0.0	1.9	2.2
Removed fuel	1.7	1.0	1.1	1.1	2.2
Entered building	1.6	0.8	1.1	2.3	0.09
Tried to exit	1.6	2.4	0.5	1.5	1.6
Went to fire alarm	1.6	1.8	1.1	1.1	0.19
Telephoned others	1.2	0.6	1.1	0.8	1.6
Tried to extinguish	1.2	1.8	1.9	1.9	0.6
Closed door to fire area	1.0	0.2	0.3	0.8	1.3
Pulled fire alarm	0.9	0.6	0.5	1.1	0.6
Turned off appliances	0.9	0.6	0.3	0.8	0.9
Checked on pets	0.9	1.4	0.5	0.8	0.9
Awaited fire department arrival	0.0	1.0	3.6	Not reported	Not reported
Went to balcony	0.2	0.8	2.7	Not reported	Not reported
Removed by fire department	0.0	0.0	1.6	Not reported	Not reported
Opened doors and windows	0.2	0.4	1.1	Not reported	Not reported
Other	3.9	8.0	6.6	6.5	2.5

serious problem. Questions such as "Do you think we really need to evacuate the building?" or "Do you smell smoke?" are examples of validation questions.

Validation is a natural, human process. However, fire and life safety educators need to explain how questioning takes valuable time that may be needed for escape.

- **Definition.** Through definition, people structure or even quantify what they know about a threat. Defining how much smoke people smell, how much heat they feel, or how many flames they see helps people relate a threat to their own situation.

- **Evaluation.** During evaluation, people decide whether to use fight or flight to reduce their danger. The decision often happens very quickly — within seconds — and under great stress and threat. The actions of other people greatly influence the evaluation process.
- **Commitment.** Through the commitment process, people begin to act on the decision made during evaluation.
- **Reassessment.** If an action does not appear to be working, the person in the fire becomes more threatened and more frustrated. Decisions become less rational. The likelihood of injury increases with reassessment.

Another way to understand how people act in fires is to view actions in the light of four sociopsychological concepts.[9] These concepts are avoidance, commitment, affiliation, and role.

- **Avoidance.** People feel that they can protect themselves — psychologically — by denying unpleasant situations. This kind of denial is very common during the first moments of a fire, when people search for other, safer explanations for the cues they see, smell, and hear.

  Avoidance explains why people delay their response to a fire. Messages such as "Treat alarms as real fires — not as false alarms or drills" are designed to overcome avoidance.
- **Commitment.** People are often very committed to what they are doing — standing in line at the supermarket, watching television, or working at a desk — when they pick up their first cues that something is wrong. Because of commitment, people continue what they are doing, despite warnings of danger. Many people, for example, may notice flashing fire warning lights on their way into a hotel or office building but continue into the building.
- **Affiliation.** People are social animals. They tend to act as a group, even with people they do not know very well. Affiliation explains why it takes so long for evacuation to start. No one leaves until everyone can leave together. Once a group has started to evacuate, the slowest member determines the speed of movement for the whole group.

  Affiliation is a strong concept. No matter how strong the threat, parents will not leave without their children; children are reluctant to go without their siblings. People will wait for their co-workers and even for strangers.
- **Role.** The role or status someone has in a building determines that person's response to a fire or other emergency.

  For example, visitors are more passive during an emergency than residents or employees. Simply because they are unfamiliar with a building under normal conditions, visitors are likely to spend more time on threat recognition and validation. People turn to supervisors and others in authority for instruction. People also turn to those "in the know" about the building, such as maintenance personnel or long-time employees. For example, employees followed their supervisors during the 1991 multiple-fatality fire at the Imperial Foods Processing Plant in Hamlet, North Carolina.

  The concept of role makes it critical that a building's natural leaders receive fire and life safety training.

What Do People Really Do When the Alarm Sounds?

In an ideal world, all occupants of a building would begin to evacuate as soon as a fire alarm sounds. In the real world, though, the action can be very different.

Researchers at the National Fire Laboratory at the National Research Council Canada study human behavior during actual emergencies (including the bombing at the World Trade Center in New York City) and evacuation drills. Canadian research on evacuation drills in four apartment buildings resulted in the following findings[10,11]:

- Many occupants in two buildings (as many as 17 percent in one building) failed to hear the alarm. They only began to evacuate when firefighters knocked on apartment doors.
- The mean (average) time to start evacuation (the time between the first alarm sound and people leaving the apartment unit) in the buildings where the alarm was not heard was 9:02 minutes after the alarm. The time to start evacuation in these two buildings ranged from 1 (one) minute to more than 21 minutes in one building and from less than a minute to more than 24 minutes in another building.
- In the two buildings where the alarm was heard, the mean time to start evacuation was 2:49 minutes. The time to start in these two buildings ranged from about 34 seconds to more than 14 minutes in one building and from less than a minute to more than 12 minutes in another building. It is interesting to note that the first person to start to exit (at 34 seconds after the alarm) was visually impaired.
- Before starting their evacuation, people dressed, gathered valuables, and got their children or pets.
- Most occupants evacuated in groups, and the speed of the slowest person determined the speed of the entire group.
- Gender, age, and limited mobility had little impact on the timing and movement of the evacuations. Older people, for example, tended to move more slowly but started their evacuation sooner.
- People used familiar stairwells or a staircase that led to a familiar area (such as the main entrance).
- It took 25 minutes to evacuate the buildings in which the alarm was not heard, compared to 13 minutes to evacuate the buildings in which the alarm was heard.

This Canadian evacuation research has some very significant messages for fire and life safety educators. For example, not hearing the alarm was clearly a problem that slowed down evacuation. (**NOTE:** The alarms were audible in the hallways but not in the individual living units.) Fire and life safety educators may need to include checks on alarm audibility in living units in future programs.

Even if they hear the alarm, people do not just "drop everything" and start to evacuate. (**NOTE:** This finding reflects the "commitment" concept discussed earlier.) As a result, fire and life safety educators must reinforce the speed of fire growth and spread and the need for immediate action after an alarm.

BUILT-IN FIRE PROTECTION SYSTEMS

Built-in fire protection systems, as used in this chapter, include detection and alarm (or signaling) systems, automatic suppression systems, compartmentation systems, evacuation systems, and smoke-control systems.

As a rule of thumb, complex buildings (manufacturing, health care, or multi-use buildings, for example) have more of these systems — and the systems are more complicated — than do homes. Because the public spends time away from home, fire and life safety educators need to be able to explain how built-in fire protection systems work. Stated another way, educators must tell their audiences how to take advantage of the protection that built-in systems offer.

This portion of the chapter focuses on detection and alarm systems and on evacuation systems because those topics are especially relevant to the fire and life safety educator's job.

Detection and Alarm Systems

Once ignition has occurred, detection and alarm systems provide the first chance for the effects of fire to be mitigated. There are seven kinds of detection and alarm systems[12]:

- Fire department emergency communications systems
- Protective signaling systems
- Waterflow alarms and sprinkler system supervision

- Household warning systems
- Automatic fire detectors
- Gas- and vapor-testing systems
- Guard services/fire protection surveillance

FIRE DEPARTMENT EMERGENCY COMMUNICATIONS SYSTEMS

Fire department emergency communications systems transfer information from whomever reports a fire to fire service personnel. The fire report may come from an individual (using a regular telephone or a coded system such as wired telegraph-type box or telephone-type voice system), from a municipal fire alarm system, from a commercial automatic alarm company, or via two-way radio. Many fire reports are automatically recorded, along with all radio and voice messages from the fire department (Figure 2.8).

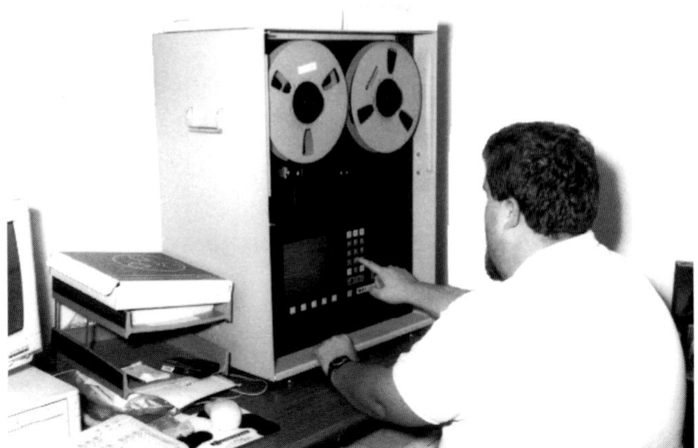

Figure 2.8 A technician reviews recorded reports.

The time it takes for the fire department to receive an alarm and have firefighters arrive on the scene is surprising to many people. Fire and life safety educators could describe the steps (and time needed for each step!) to receive and process an alarm, to dispatch firefighters, to travel to the fire scene, and to set up to begin fire fighting operations. The steps and time vary from department to department. Educators can use this kind of information to explain why prompt, accurate fire reporting is so essential.

Sample Time Line

The relative effectiveness of fire suppression crews is directly related to response time. This does not imply that faster fire engines are the answer. Response times are normally based on factors occurring after notification.

The following sample time line does not include one of the most critical times involved in fire damage and injury — the time between fire inception and discovery/notification. This time period is impossible to calculate and is often the longest span fire crews must overcome. Early detection systems greatly reduce the discovery/notification time.

Function	Approximate Time (In Minutes)
Receiving caller information	0.5 to 1
Alerting suppression crews	0.5 to 1
Suppression crews leaving stations	0.5 to 1
Travel time for suppression crews	2 to 5
Set-up time for fire fighting	1 to 2
Total	4.5 to 10

Of course there is a myriad of variables involved in each of these functions. The times reflected are estimates based on annual averages.

PROTECTIVE SIGNALING SYSTEMS

The term *protective signaling systems* describes systems that transfer information from a specific place in a fire-involved building to some remote monitoring station. The information may be in either voice or data format. Protective signaling systems send out supervisory signals and trouble signals, in addition to fire alarm signals. There are several subsets of protective signaling systems, including:

- Central station systems, which receive signals from protected buildings at a location that is constantly attended. Central station systems are available on a subscription basis through commercial companies.
- Local systems, whose function is to sound a local alarm. Local systems do not communicate with a commercial alarm company or the fire department.
- Auxiliary systems, which have circuits that connect the building's fire alarms to a public fire reporting system. This is often done through a phone line that goes directly to the fire department communications center switchboard.
- Remote station systems, which have alarms that are received at a remote location (usually a public fire service commu-

nications center, police station, or answering service). The remote station must be acceptable to the authority having jurisdiction and be staffed round-the-clock with trained personnel.

- Proprietary systems, which are central station systems with the central station on-site, rather than remote.
- Emergency voice/alarm communications systems, which send voice messages giving specific instructions about leaving the building, going to another area of the building, or staying in place.

From time to time, fire and life safety educators may be involved in training employees in facilities with protective signaling systems. One message for such programs is "Trust what the system tells you." Misinterpreting trouble signals delayed fire reporting for more than an hour — contributing substantially to the losses — at the Illinois Bell Telephone central office facility in Hinsdale, Illinois, in 1988. That fire ultimately cost at least $60 million in losses, injured 45 firefighters, and interrupted telephone service to 35,000 local customers and 118,000 trunk lines.

WATERFLOW ALARMS AND SPRINKLER SYSTEM SUPERVISION SYSTEMS

Waterflow alarms and sprinkler system supervision systems detect sprinkler activation or water supply interruptions. These systems would rarely appear in fire and life safety education programs for the general public. However, the topic might be included in workplace fire safety education programs.

HOUSEHOLD FIRE WARNING SYSTEMS

Household fire warning systems include simple single- and multiple-station smoke detectors as well as the more complicated "household fire warning systems" (which may have a control panel, be integrated with security alarms, and automatically call the fire department).

The way in which smoke detectors operate has changed relatively little. (**NOTE:** The units have become smaller and less expensive, however.) The public needs to know certain basic facts about smoke detectors:

- Smoke detectors can be wired together electrically so that all units sound the alarm when one unit in the home senses smoke. Some jurisdictions require that smoke detectors be interconnected.
- Batteries or household current can power smoke detectors. Electrically powered units with battery backup are available.
- Smoke detectors are required to have a sound level output of at least 85 decibels (dB) at 10 feet. Many factors can interfere with a person's ability to hear the alarm, however. These factors include background noise, sleeping heavily, closed bedroom doors, and even slight hearing loss.

  Emphasizing the importance of actually hearing the alarm is a primary job of the fire and life safety educator. Having interconnected detectors and having detectors on every level of the home are steps the public can take to increase their chances of hearing their smoke detector. People can also install smoke detectors in their bedrooms (especially if there is any question about hearing the alarm).
- Homes need one smoke detector on each level of the residence, outside each sleeping area. If people sleep in a bedroom and nap in a living room at the opposite end of the home, for example, two smoke detectors are needed.
- An estimated 92 percent of households in the U.S. have smoke detectors. Unfortunately, about 20 percent of those households have nonoperational smoke detectors. Dead, missing, or disconnected batteries account for almost all of the nonoperational detectors.[13]

  Without maintenance and testing, smoke detectors may not operate in a fire. Detectors must be maintained and tested regularly, according to the manufacturer's directions. Smoke detector testing and maintenance is always a top fire and life safety education message.
- The types of smoke detectors are ionization, photoelectric, or a combination of

Five Questions and Answers About Smoke Detectors

Q. Why does my family need smoke detectors?

A. Smoke is produced very early in a fire's development, usually before significant heat or flames. Smoke detectors sense the presence of smoke very quickly, often before people see or smell smoke. These lifesaving devices are especially helpful at night, when most fatal fires happen and when people sleep.

Q. How do I choose a smoke detector?

A. Always select a smoke detector that has a UL label. Check the box to make sure that the device is a smoke detector rather than a heat or gas detector.

After knowing that a smoke detector is UL listed, there are two other choices to consider: the kind of detector and the power source.

There are two basic kinds of smoke detectors. Photoelectric detectors alarm when smoke particles scatter light inside the detector; ionization detectors alarm when smoke particles reduce how much electricity is conducted inside the detector. Either kind of detector works well. Some detectors even combine the two methods of operation.

Smoke detectors can be either battery-operated or wired into the electrical system. Some hard-wired detectors have a backup battery.

Q. How many detectors do I need? Where do I put them?

A. Every level of a home needs at least one smoke detector. Protecting sleeping areas — including places where people nap — is especially important. Some homes may need more than one detector per level. For example, a ranch-style home with family bedrooms and an in-law suite at opposite ends should have at least two detectors: one in the hall outside the family bedroom area and another in the in-law suite.

Because smoke rises, detectors are usually placed on the ceiling. Follow the manufacturer's specific instructions.

Q. Why do smoke detectors have false alarms? What can be done?

A. Smoke detectors are really particle detectors. As a result, smoke detectors sense all kinds of particles — smoke from cooking or cigarettes, steam, or even small insects in the unit — besides smoke from a fire.

Locating detectors as far away as possible from the kitchen or bathroom will help reduce these nuisance alarms. Some household smoke detectors have a built-in delay to reduce nuisance alarms.

Q. Why do smoke detectors need maintenance? How do I take care of my smoke detectors?

A. Like any appliance, smoke detectors do need some maintenance. Because smoke detectors are life safety devices, though, maintenance cannot be put off. Detectors always need to be in working condition. Working smoke detectors in a home reduce the risk of dying in a fire by about 40 percent.

Taking care of smoke detectors is fairly simple. Detectors need to be vacuumed from time to time in order to remove insects that may interfere with the detector's operation or cause nuisance alarms. Detectors need to be tested, which usually involves pressing a test button. Most important, battery-operated detectors need fresh batteries twice a year.

Smoke detectors come with maintenance information from the manufacturer.

ionization and photoelectric. Combination units are slightly more expensive than detectors that just use one way to sense smoke.

Ionization smoke detectors. During combustion, minute particles and aerosols too small to be seen by the naked eye are produced. These invisible products of combustion can be detected by devices that use a tiny amount of radioactive material (usually americum) to ionize air molecules as they enter a chamber within the detector. These ionized particles allow an electrical current to flow between negative and positive plates within the chamber. When the particulate products of combustion (smoke) enter the chamber, they attach themselves to the electrically charged molecules of air (ions), making the air within the chamber less conductive. The decrease in current flowing between the plates initiates an alarm signal (Figure 2.9).

An ionization detector responds to most fires; however, this detector generally responds faster to flaming fires than to smoldering ones. It automatically resets when the atmosphere has cleared.

What Does 85 dB Sound Like?

Source of Noise	*Typical Noise Level (dBA)*
Siren	105
Passing truck	100
Subway, machine shop	90
Home smoke detector, 10 feet away	85
Noisy restaurant	80
Inside car with closed windows	70
Office	60
Average home	50

NOTE: These noise levels are expressed in decibels on the A weighted scale (dBA), where 0 dBA is the weakest sound that can be heard in an extremely quiet location and where 140 dBA is a person's threshold of pain.

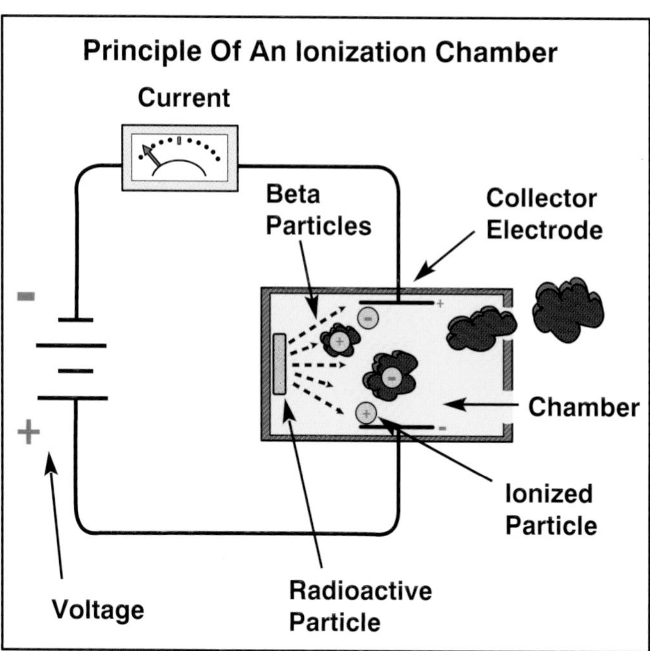

Figure 2.9 Principle of an ionization smoke detector.

Photoelectric smoke detectors. A photoelectric detector, sometimes called a *visible products-of-combustion detector*, uses a photoelectric cell coupled with a specific light source. The photoelectric cell functions in two ways to detect smoke: beam application and refractory application.

The beam application uses a beam of light focused across the area being monitored onto a photoelectric cell. The cell constantly converts the beam into current, which keeps a switch open. When smoke obscures the path of the light beam, the required amount of current is no longer produced, the switch closes, and an alarm signal is initiated (Figure 2.10 a).

The refractory photocell uses a light beam that passes through a small chamber at a point away from the light source. Normally, the light does not strike the photocell, and no current is produced. This allows the switch to remain open. When smoke enters the chamber, it causes the light beam to be refracted (scattered) in all directions. A portion of the scattered light strikes the photocell, causing current to flow. This current causes the switch to close and initiate the alarm signal (Figure 2.10 b).

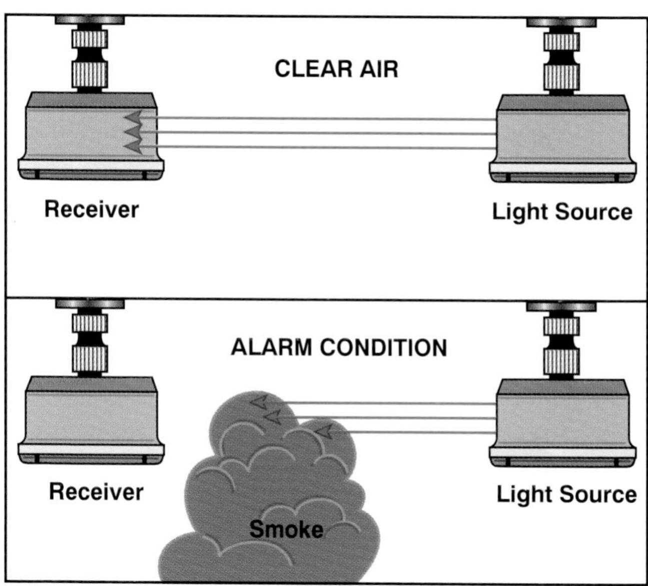

Figure 2.10 a Principle of a beam-application photoelectric smoke detector.

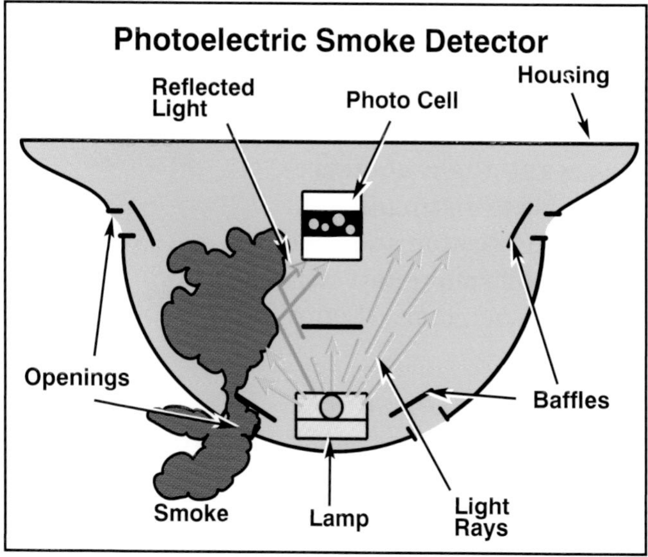

Figure 2.10 b Principle of a refractory photoelectric smoke detector.

A photoelectric detector works satisfactorily on all types of fires and automatically resets when the atmosphere is clear. Photoelectric detectors are generally more sensitive to smoldering fires than are ionization detectors. *Although there are differences in how fast the different types detect smoke, the important thing is that there be enough properly located and operating UL-listed detectors.*

AUTOMATIC FIRE DETECTION SYSTEMS

Automatic fire detection systems are for use in nonresidential buildings. The basic types of automatic fire detectors (apart from smoke detectors) are heat detectors, gas-sensing detectors, and flame detectors.

Heat detectors. *Heat detectors* are fixed-temperature (which alarm at a specific point, usually 135°F [about 60°C] or higher), rate-compensated (which alarm at a low preset temperature, even though the temperature rises slowly), rate-of-rise (which alarm when the temperature changes at a preset value, such as 12°-15°F per minute), sealed pneumatic line-type (which depend on the presence of normal pressure at normal temperatures), or thermoelectric-effect detectors (rate-of-rise or fixed-temperature detectors which measure changes in electrical resistance that go along with temperature changes).

Heat detectors are usually inexpensive and have a low false-alarm rate. However, they respond late in a fire's growth. The public should not rely on heat detectors for life safety protection at home. Fire and life safety educators want their audiences to be able to distinguish the level of protection and overall value of smoke detectors and heat detectors (Figure 2.11).

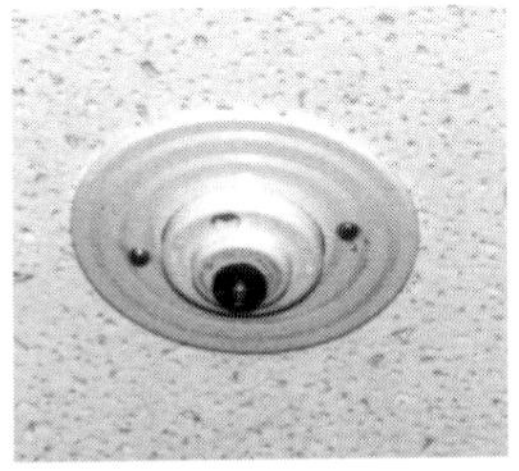

Figure 2.11 An alarm activated by a heat detector such as this usually sounds later in a fire's growth than does an alarm activated by a smoke detector.

Gas-sensing detectors. *Gas-sensing detectors* use either a semiconductor principle or a catalytic-element principle to detect fire gases. Changes in electrical conductivity or in temperature, respectively, operate these detectors. Carbon monoxide (CO) detectors operate on the semiconductor principle. CO detectors have somewhat limited use in fire safety simply because carbon monoxide develops fairly late in a fire. However, carbon monoxide detectors are useful in other life safety areas, such as sensing dangerously high levels of carbon monoxide caused by faulty furnaces or space heaters.

In the home, heating and cooking equipment are possible sources of carbon monoxide (an invisible, odorless, colorless gas caused by incomplete combustion of fossil fuels). Vehicles running in an attached garage could also produce dangerous levels of carbon monoxide.

When CO replaces oxygen in the bloodstream, a condition known as *carboxyhemoglobin (COHb)* develops. This leads to carbon monoxide poisoning. Mild CO poisoning feels like the flu, but more serious poisoning leads to difficulty in breathing and even death.

The number of estimated deaths from accidental carbon monoxide poisoning varies a great deal — about 290 per year, according to the Consumer Product Safety Commission, or 400 in 1993, according to the National Safety Council — but the deaths are fairly rare, whichever estimate is used. About 60 percent of these deaths involved vehicles, and another 20 percent involved heating or cooking equipment.

Household carbon monoxide detectors measure how much CO has accumulated. Currently, CO detectors sound an alarm when the concentration of CO in the air corresponds to a 10 percent carboxyhemoglobin level in the blood (for a healthy adult). Because a 10 percent COHb level is at the very low end of CO poisoning (see Table 2.8), the alarm may sound before people feel particularly sick.

In fact, pollution, atmospheric conditions in some areas, or even operating gas ranges can cause low levels of CO. It is not unusual for these nonhazardous conditions to increase the COHb level to over 10 percent, causing CO detectors to alarm. As a result, many fire departments receive calls from anxious people whose CO detector has just given off a nuisance alarm.

Many fire departments are developing standard operating procedures for responding to CO detector alarms. These procedures often involve responding differently for households where people have symptoms of CO poisoning or establishing a separate phone line to report CO alarms.

The fire and life safety educator should be prepared to explain the differences between smoke detectors and carbon monoxide detectors — and why both are needed. The public must know the different sounds that the two detectors make and how to respond.

Flame detectors. *Flame detectors* sense either infrared (IR) or ultraviolet (UV) light. Their use is generally restricted to high-hazard areas, such as transformer vaults or petrochemical plants.

GAS- AND VAPOR-TESTING SYSTEMS

Gas- and vapor-testing systems use either semiconductors (sensors) or catalytic elements (heated platinum wire) to sense gas and trigger an alarm. These types of systems are used mainly in industry and manufacturing, where there is a potential for large collections of combustible or flammable gases.

Automatic Suppression Systems

Automatic suppression systems include automatic sprinkler systems, standpipe systems, and fire pumps.[14] In addition, automatic suppression systems include carbon dioxide systems, halogenated systems, dry chemical agents and their systems, foam extinguishers, combustible metal agents, and other special systems.[15] The fire and life safety educator generally does not discuss standpipes, fire pumps, carbon dioxide systems, halogenated systems, dry chemical agents, foam extinguishers, combustible metal agents, and other special extinguishing systems for the simple reason that the general public is not exposed to them.

However, automatic sprinkler systems are a topic for fire and life safety education. The public should know the following important facts:

- Sprinklers are essentially heat-activated devices with water pipes and sprinkler heads (spray devices) connected to them. As a result, a sprinkler head only sprays when it senses heat. As a result, a sprinkler head only operates when it reaches certain temperatures. *The myth "If one sprinkler head operates, then they all do" is simply wrong.*
- For sprinklers to work properly, the pipes and sprinkler heads must be free of paint or hanging decorations. Stored materials should not block sprinkler heads.

Residential sprinkler systems are the latest technology for residential fire safety. Of course, standard or conventional sprinklers have been used for more than 100 years to provide reliable property protection.

In the 1980s, however, fast response sprinklers were developed that were far more sensitive than conventional sprinklers. (**NOTE:** Fast response sprinklers include residential sprinklers, quick response sprinklers, early suppression fast response sprinklers, quick response/high challenge large-drop sprinklers, and quick response/early suppression sprinklers.[16]) Sensitivity is measured by the Response Time Index (RTI), with lower RTIs indicating faster sprinkler response. For example, the RTI of residential sprinklers is 50-90 $\text{sec}^{1/2}\text{ft}^{1/2}$, compared to an RTI of 225-700 $\text{sec}^{1/2}\text{ft}^{1/2}$ for standard response sprinklers.

In developing residential sprinklers, two goals were paramount. Residential sprinklers needed to do the following:

- Control fires quickly, before lethal conditions could develop in homes (which are generally smaller than large spaces where conventional sprinklers are used).
- Control fires with as little water as possible, to account for the 20 to 30 gpm water supply in most residences.

With these goals in mind, Factory Mutual Research Corporation (with funding from the U.S. Fire Administration) conducted full-scale fire tests that resulted in prototype residential sprinkler systems that could control or suppress residential fires with only two sprinkler heads and operate while conditions in the room of origin were still survivable. Survivable conditions were maximum gas temperature at eye level of 200°F (93°C), maximum ceiling surface temperature of 500°F (260°C), and maximum CO concentration of 1,500 ppm. In other words, the residential sprinklers were linked to tenability in the room of origin.

The development of sprinkler standards paralleled the improvements in technology. The first edition of NFPA 13D, *Installation of Sprinkler Systems in One- and Two-Family Dwellings and Mobile Homes,* was issued in 1975, and by 1980 this standard required "listed residential sprinklers." By 1990, Underwriters Laboratories listed 35 models of residential sprinklers.

Residential sprinklers have proven their value in actual fires many times. Operation Life Safety maintains a list of residential sprinkler "activations" and provides information on residential sprinklers to fire departments and others. (**NOTE:** Operation Life Safety is operated by the International Association of Fire Chiefs and may be reached at IAFC, 4025 Fair Ridge Road, Fairfax, VA 22033.)

While the value of residential sprinklers in traditional housing construction — "stick-built" homes — is increasingly accepted by the fire service and others, the role of residential sprinklers in manufactured homes is more of an open question. Information on the status of requirements for residential sprinklers in manufactured homes is available from the National Fire Sprinkler Association (P.O. Box 1000, Patterson, NY 12563; 914-878-4200) or from Operation Life Safety.

Compartmentation Systems

A *compartmentation system* is a series of barriers designed to keep flames, smoke, and heat from spreading from one room or floor to another. The barriers may be extra walls or partitions, fire-stopping materials inside walls or other concealed spaces, or floors.

Doors are a vitally important form of compartmentation — if they are closed. Closed fire doors, for example, protect exit routes such as stairwells and corridors. *Fire and life safety educators should always emphasize the need to keep fire doors closed.*

Evacuation Systems

Evacuation systems are intended to allow people to escape to safety during a fire. They include egress systems (exit access, exit, and exit discharge) as well as doors, panic hardware, horizontal exits, stairs, smokeproof towers, fire-escape stairs, escalators, moving sidewalks, elevators, windows, and exit lighting and signs (Figure 2.12). For the fire and life safety educator, egress systems and exit lighting and signs are of particular interest.

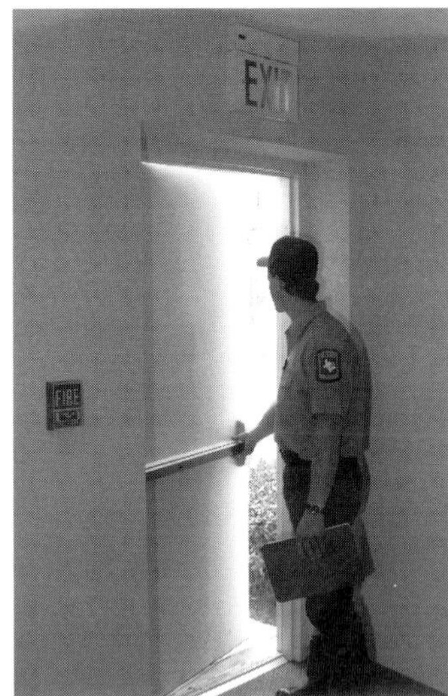

Figure 2.12 A properly identified exit is an important part of an evacuation system.

The NFPA *Life Safety Code®*, building codes, and fire codes pay careful attention to the egress system. These codes specify how wide doors and corridors must be, how long a dead-end corridor may be, how wide and steep stairs may be, etc. Detailed calculations that predict factors such as how fast people walk or how long it takes to evacuate a building are the basis for the specifications.

Two facts about these predictions are important for the fire and life safety educator:

- The predictions assume *unobstructed* egress systems.
- The predictions for evacuation times are longer than actual, observed evacuation times. Said another way, people actually take longer than predicted.

In other words, the design of egress systems is more optimistic than real-world conditions.

For the fire and life safety educator, there are two implications of this optimism:

- People must insist on clear egress systems.

  Exits and the paths to them (access and discharge) are not storage places. Extra merchandise in stores, extra files in offices, or spare furniture and baby carriages or bicycles in homes cannot block the way

- Never use butter or similar products to treat a burn. Butter and other products like petroleum jelly trap heat on the skin, which continues to burn. Never administer analgesics, alcohol, or narcotics for pain relief. Cool water or cool, wet dressings and treatments prescribed by a doctor will be much more soothing.
- Do not touch an electrical burn victim who is still in contact with the electricity; you may endanger yourself. Call 9-1-1 (or the emergency number in your area).
- Whenever there are questions about burns, ask a doctor or nurse.

IDENTIFYING THE FIRE HAZARDS OF MATERIALS

The public may ask fire and life safety educators to "translate" hazard warning signs on buildings. NFPA 704 is the basis for markings on buildings; this standard does not apply to markings on vehicles that transport hazardous materials.

NFPA 704M identifies three kinds of hazards: health, flammability, and reactivity. The severity of a hazard is given by a number, with 0 indicating "no hazard" and 4 indicating "severe hazard" (Table 2.12).

The rating numbers are arranged on a diamond-shaped marker or sign (Figure 2.29). The health rating is located on a blue background at the nine o'clock position. The flammability hazard rating is positioned on a red background at the twelve o'clock position. The reactivity hazard rating appears on a yellow background and is positioned at three o'clock. As an alternative, the backgrounds for each of these rating positions may be any contrasting color, and the numbers (0 to 4) may be represented by the appropriate color (blue, red, and yellow) (Figure 2.30). Special hazards are located in the six o'clock position and have no specified background color; however, white is most commonly used.

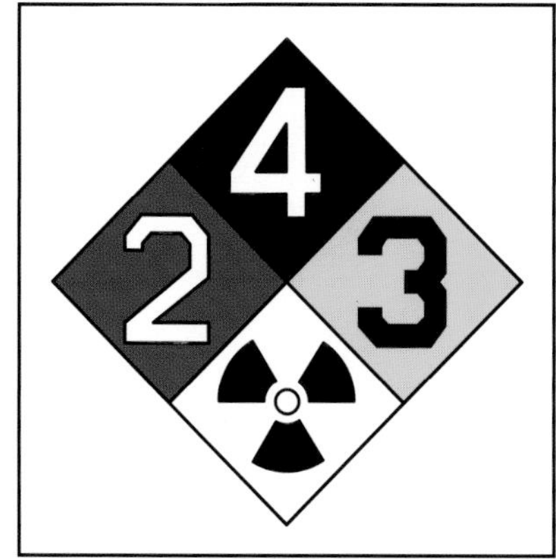

Figure 2.29 Most 704 symbols have colored blocks and black or white numerals.

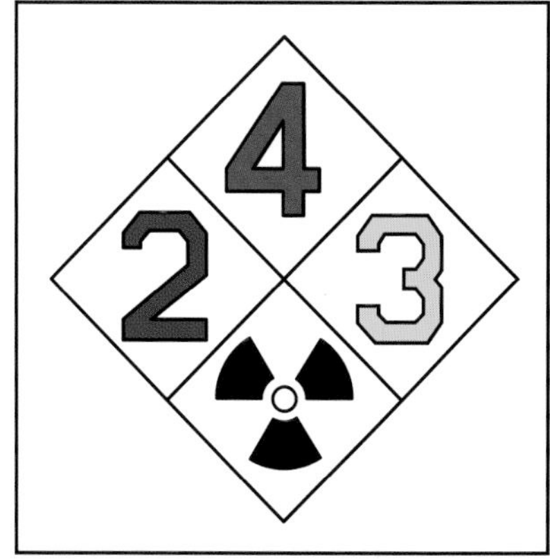

Figure 2.30 Some 704 symbols have white blocks and appropriately colored numerals.

CONCLUSION

The technical knowledge that fire and life safety educators need is indeed quite broad and often complex. Nonetheless, fire and life safety educators are ethically bound to grasp the technical intricacies of their profession. Consider what could happen if the following situations occurred:

- A fire and life safety educator failed to understand how quickly flashover happens and how deadly it is.
- A fire and life safety educator told an audience "Don't panic" but did not give concrete steps to take.
- A fire and life safety educator was confused about the differences between smoke detectors, heat detectors, and carbon monoxide detectors.
- A fire and life safety educator encourages people to gather their belongings before starting an evacuation.
- A fire and life safety educator gives wrong information.

At best, these shortcomings could be embarrassing for the educator. At worst, the wrong messages could be dangerous or even deadly for the audience.

Learning the technical foundation for fire and life safety education is worth the effort — it makes the educator better prepared and more confident. In other words, doing the homework ultimately makes the fire and life safety educator's job easier.

TABLE 2.12
NFPA 704 Rating System

Identification Of Health Hazard		Identification Of Flammability		Identification Of Reactivity	
Type Of Possible Injury		Susceptibility Of Materials To Burning		Susceptibility To Release Of Energy	
Signal		Signal		Signal	
4	Materials that on very short exposure could cause death or major residual injury.	4	Materials that will rapidly or completely vaporize at atmospheric pressure and normal ambient temperature, or that are readily dispersed in air and that will burn readily.	4	Materials that in themselves are readily capable of detonation or of explosive decomposition or reaction at normal temperatures and pressures.
3	Materials that on short exposure could cause serious temporary or residual injury.	3	Liquids and solids that can be ignited under almost all ambient temperature conditions.	3	Materials that in themselves are capable of detonation or explosive decomposition or reaction but require a strong initiating source or which must be heated under confinement before initiation or which react explosively with water.
2	Materials that on intense or continued but not chronic exposure could cause temporary incapacitation or possible residual injury.	2	Materials that must be moderately heated or exposed to relatively high ambient temperatures before ignition can occur.	2	Materials that readily undergo violent chemical change at elevated temperatures and pressures or which react violently with water or which may form explosive mixtures with water.
1	Materials that on exposure would cause irritation but only minor residual injury.	1	Materials that must be preheated before ignition can occur.	1	Materials that in themselves are normally stable, but which can become unstable at elevated temperatures and pressures.
0	Materials that on exposure under fire conditions would offer no hazard beyond that of ordinary combustible material.	0	Materials that will not burn.	0	Materials that in themselves are normally stable, even under fire exposure conditions, and which are not reactive with water.

FOR MORE INFORMATION

Gordon E. Hartzell, "Combustion Products and Their Effects on Life Safety," *Fire Protection Handbook*, 17th ed., National Fire Protection Association, Quincy, MA, 1991.

For a very technical discussion of tenability, see "Tenability Limits," *HAZARD I Technical Reference Guide* (Version 1.1), NIST Handbook 146, National Institute of Standards and Technology, Gaithersburg, MD, 1991.

For a theoretical introduction to panic, see "The Concept of Panic," by Jonathan D. Sime in David Canter (ed.), *Fires and Human Behavior*, 2nd ed., David Fulton Publishers, Ltd., London, 1990.

Chapter 3, "Basic Fire Science" in NFPA 921, *Fire and Explosion Investigations*, National Fire Protection Association, Quincy, MA, explains the fundamentals of fire dynamics.

Dr. Robert W. Fitzgerald, "Fundamentals of Firesafe Building Design," *Fire Protection Handbook*, 17th ed., National Fire Protection Association, Quincy, MA, 1991.

IFSTA **Essentials Of Fire Fighting**, 3rd ed., 1992.

IFSTA **Private Fire Protection and Detection**, 2nd ed., 1994.

"The Healing Touch," *Newsweek*, March 23, 1992, pp. 68-71. This is a photo essay on burn treatment.

"CO," *The Building Official and Code Administrator*, January/February 1995.

Chapter 2 Notes

1. This section is based on presentations by Richard L.P. Custer, Custer Powell, Inc., at the Massachusetts Association of Fire Instructors, Massachusetts and Arizona Chapters of the IAAI, Oklahoma Public Fire Education Conference, Missouri Winter Fire School, and the New York State Fire Academy. His contributions are gratefully acknowledged.

2. This definition of *fire* is from NFPA 921, *Guide for Fire and Explosion Investigations*, 1995 ed.

3. Christopher J. Conley and Rita F. Fahey, "Who Dies in Fires in the United States?" *NFPA Journal*®, May/June 1994, p. 103. (**NOTE:** *NFPA Journal*® is a registered trademark of the National Fire Protection Association, Inc., Quincy, MA 02269.)

4. See the *Fire Power Instructor's Guide*, NFPA FL-76, National Fire Protection Association, Quincy, MA, 1986.

5. Dr. John L. Bryan, "Psychology of Panic," Thirtieth Annual Fire Department Instructors Conference, Memphis, Tennessee, February 1958.

6. Dr. John P. Keating, "The Myth of Panic." Reprinted with permission from *Fire Journal* (May 1982, Vol. 76, No. 3), Copyright ©1982, National Fire Protection Association, Quincy, MA 02269.

7. See David Canter (ed.), "Human Behaviour in Fire," *Fires and Human Behaviour*, 2nd ed., Fulton Publishers, Ltd., London, 1990.

8. This summary is based on John L. Bryan, "Human Behavior and Fire," *Fire Protection Handbook*. Reprinted with permission from *Fire Protection Handbook*, 17th edition, Copyright ©1991, National Fire Protection Association, Quincy, MA 02269.

9. See Dr. Guylene Proulx, "Human Response to Fires," *Fire Research News*, National Research Council Canada, Winter 1994.

10. Guylene Proulx, John Latour, and John MacLaurin, *Housing Evacuation of Mixed Abilities Occupants*, National Research Council Internal Report No. 661, July 1994.

11. Guylene Proulx, "The Time Delay to Start Evacuating Upon Hearing a Fire Alarm," *Proceedings of the Human Factors and Ergonomics Society 38th Annual Meeting (1994)*, Human Factors and Ergonomics Society, Santa Monica, CA.

12. A chapter on each of these seven kinds of systems is included in Section 4, "Detection and Alarm," *Fire Protection Handbook*, 17th ed., National Fire Protection Association, Quincy, MA, 1991.

13. John R. Hall, Jr., "The U.S. Experience with Smoke Detectors," *NFPA Journal*®, September/October 1994, p. 39.

14. For a full description of these systems, see IFSTA **Private Fire Protection and Detection**, 2nd ed., 1994.

15. For a full description of these systems, see Section 5, "Suppression," *Fire Protection Handbook*, 17th ed., National Fire Protection Association, Quincy, MA, 1991.

16. For a discussion of this technology, see Arthur E. Cote and Russell P. Fleming, "Fast Response Sprinkler Technology," *Fire Protection Handbook*, 17th ed., National Fire Protection Association, Quincy, MA, 1991.

17. For a detailed discussion of extinguishers, see David P. Demers, "Selection, Operation, Distribution, Inspection, and Maintenance of Fire Extinguishers," *Fire Protection Handbook*, 17th ed., National Fire Protection Association, Quincy, MA, 1991.

18. Dr. Alexander J. Patton, P.E., and Dr. John C. Russell, *Fire Litigation Sourcebook*, Garland Publishing Inc., 1989, p. 8-2.

19. Wendy Daly, Shriners Burns Institute, Boston, private conversation.

Chapter 2 Review

Directions

The following activities are designed to help you comprehend and apply the information in Chapter 2 of **Fire and Life Safety Educator**, second edition. To receive the maximum learning experience from these activities, it is recommended that you use the following procedure:

1. Read the chapter, underlining or highlighting important terms, topics, and subject matter. Read the sidebar material, study the photographs and illustrations, and read the captions with each.
2. Review the list of vocabulary words to ensure that you know the chapter-related meaning of each. If you are unsure of the meaning of a vocabulary word, look up the word in the glossary or a dictionary, and then study its context in the chapter.
3. On a separate sheet of paper, complete all assigned or selected application and review activities before checking your answers.
4. After you have finished, check your answers against those on the pages referenced in parentheses.
5. Correct any incorrect answers, and review material that was answered incorrectly.

Vocabulary

Be sure that you know the chapter-related meanings of the following words and abbreviations:

- chemistry of fire *(21)*
- compartmentation system *(35)*
- egress system *(42)*
- exothermic *(22)*
- fire *(21)*
- fire dynamics *(21)*
- fire load *(22)*
- hazard *(22)*
- heat energy applied *(24)*
- heat flux *(28)*
- heat release rate *(22)*
- kW *(22)*
- MW *(22)*
- oxidation *(21)*
- panic *(30)*
- tenability *(21)*
- UL *(44)*
- ULC *(44)*

Application of Knowledge

Outline information to include pertinent facts and statistics that you would present to an adult audience during a presentation on the following topics:

- smoke detectors
- CO_2 detectors
- automatic sprinkler systems
- firefighter personal protective equipment
- emergency burn treatment

Review Activities

1. List the raw materials needed for an exothermic reaction. *(22)*
2. Explain how the fire triangle and fire tetrahedron can be used for introducing basic fire safety messages. Illustrate your explanation with examples. *(22)*
3. Name the key factors that determine fire ignition. *(22)*
4. Discuss how ignition temperature, surface area, and the mass of a material impact its ignition behavior. *(22, 23)*
5. List and describe the ways heat is transferred. Provide examples to illustrate each. *(24)*
6. Explain what is meant by established burning and its role in fabric flammability. *(25)*
7. State factors that affect fire growth and spread. *(25, 26)*

8. Describe the conditions associated with flashover. *(26, 27)*
9. Explain the following factors in regard to withstanding the physical assault of fire's heat, smoke, and gases:
   - age *(27)*
   - size *(27)*
   - pre-existing physical condition *(27)*
   - respiratory capacity *(27, 28)*
   - medication, drugs, or alcohol *(28)*
10. List hazardous physical conditions produced by fire. *(28)*
11. State the temperatures for each of the following situations: *(28)*
    - discomfort to mouth, nose, and esophagus
    - incapacitation
    - death from hypothermia
    - residential fires
12. Explain the "heat energy applied" concept using Table 2.5. *(29)*
13. Discuss smoke obstruction and the allowed *Life Safety Code®* distance between exit sign and exit access. *(29)*
14. Using Table 2.6 identify the physiological effects of oxygen at normal to reduced levels in the earth's air. *(29)*
15. Interpret the following abbreviations associated with toxicity measurements:
    - C *(29)*
    - T *(29)*
    - ppm *(29)*
    - COHb *(30)*
16. Describe the effect that carbon monoxide has on the bloodstream. Include what constitutes a dangerous to lethal dosage. *(30, 31 Table 2.8)*
17. List four elements essential to panic behavior. *(31)*
18. Explain the myth of panic behavior. *(30-32)*
19. Describe human behavior in a fire incident. Include the reaction differences between men and women. *(32)*
20. Explain the following techniques used by people to decide what to do in a fire:
    - threat recognition *(32)*
    - validation *(32)*
    - definition *(33, 34)*
    - evaluation *(34)*
    - commitment *(34)*
    - reassessment *(34)*
21. Discuss the following sociopsychological concepts in regard to understanding how people act in fires: *(34)*
    - avoidance
    - commitment
    - affiliation
    - role
22. Summarize the research from the National Fire Laboratory at the National Research Council Canada pertaining to human behavior in an evacuation drill. *(35)*
23. List and briefly describe the seven kinds of detection and alarm systems. *(35, 36)*
24. State the approximate response times for the following functions: *(36)*
    - receiving caller information
    - alerting suppression crews
    - suppression crews leaving stations
    - travel time for suppression crews
    - set-up time for fire fighting
25. Define protective signaling systems. *(36)*
26. Describe the following protective signaling systems and their subsets:
    - central station systems *(36)*
    - local systems *(36)*
    - auxiliary systems *(36)*
    - remote station systems *(36, 37)*
    - proprietary systems *(37)*
    - emergency voice/alarm communications systems *(37)*
27. List basic facts the public should know about smoke detectors. *(37, 38)*
28. Distinguish among the following automatic fire detectors:
    - heat detectors *(40)*
    - gas-sensing detectors *(40)*
    - flame detectors *(41)*
29. Explain the differences between smoke detectors and CO detectors and why each is needed. *(40, 41)*
30. Explain the importance of barriers and doors in a compartmentation system. *(42)*
31. Explain the differences between automatic fire detection and automatic suppression systems. Where are each used? *(42)*

32. Discuss the implications for the fire and life safety educator of the NFPA *Life Safety Code®* specifications on an egress system. *(42)*
33. Distinguish among the following exit lighting and signs: *(43)*
    - exit lighting
    - emergency lighting
    - exit signs
34. Using Table 2.10 identify the different classes of fires and the types of extinguishers used on each. *(43)*
35. List and explain the three levels of hazard occupancy. *(43, 44)*
36. List the two key points to emphasize when choosing a portable fire extinguisher. *(44)*
37. Define the following catagories of fire: *(44)*
    - Class A
    - Class B
    - Class C
    - Class D
38. Interpret the following portable fire extinguisher rating: 4-A 20-B:C. *(45)*
39. Explain why Class C and D portable fire extinguishers are not given numerical ratings. *(45)*
40. Explain the rating system for Class A, B, C, and D extinguishers. *(45, 46)*
41. Describe the two marking systems used to label portable fire extinguishers. *(45, 46)*
42. Discuss factors to consider prior to purchase and after the purchase of a portable fire extinguisher. *(45, 46)*
43. Distinguish among the following types of burns: *(48)*
    - thermal
    - chemical
    - electrical
44. Discuss the differences among first-, second-, and third-degree burns. *(48, 49)*
45. Interpret the types and significance of hazards indicated by NFPA 704 hazard warning signs. *(51)*

Questions and Notes

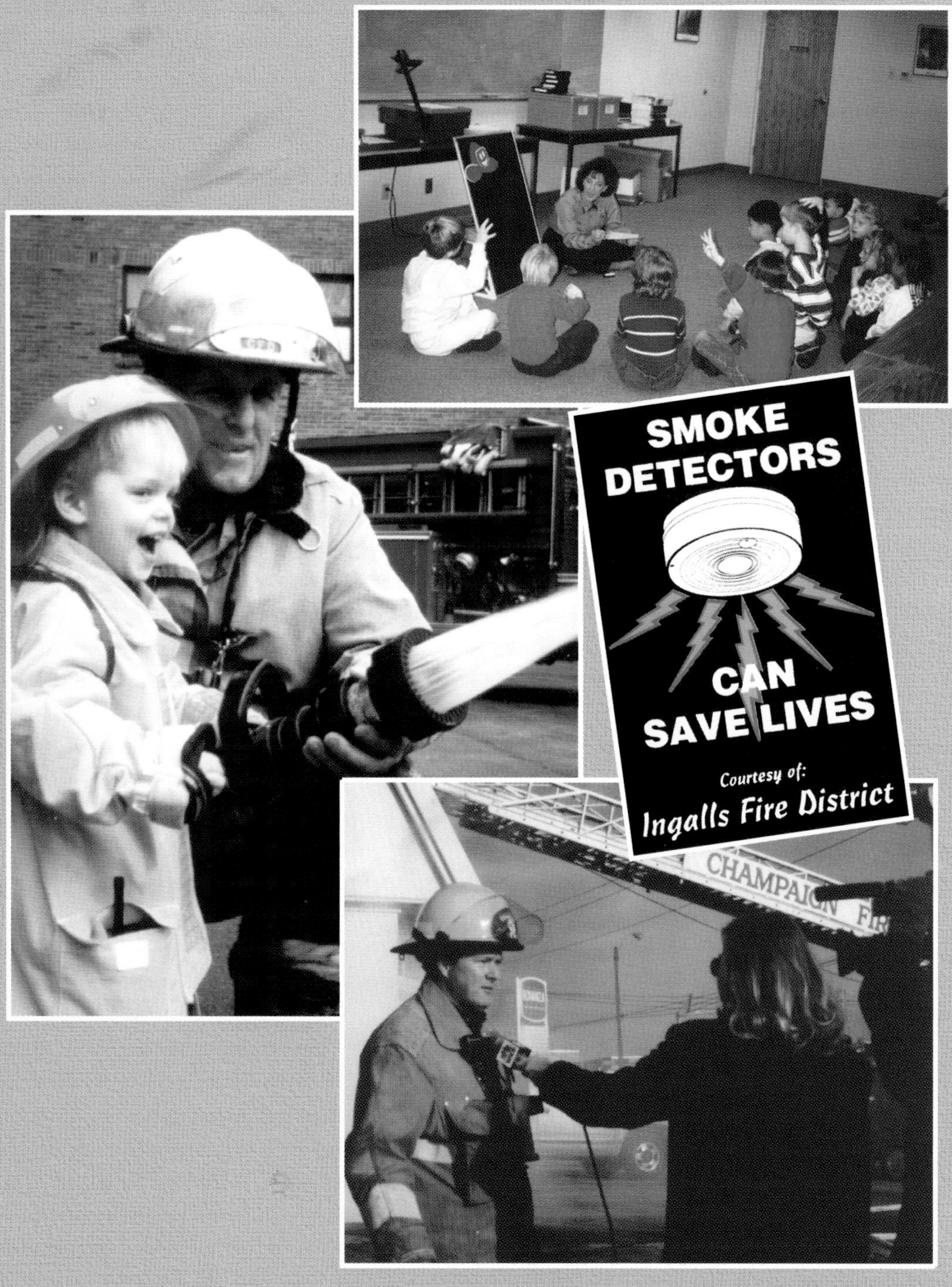
SMOKE
DETECTORS
CAN
SAVE LIVES
Courtesy of:
Ingalls Fire District
CHAMPAIGN

3 Managing Fire and Life Safety Resources

LEARNING OBJECTIVES

This chapter provides information that addresses the following objectives of NFPA 1035, *Standard for Professional Qualifications for Public Fire and Life Safety Educator* (1993 edition):

Public Fire and Life Safety Educator I

3-2.2 Prepare written reports, given appropriate forms or formats, so that all elements of the format are addressed in the report.

3-2.3 Maintain a work schedule, given a list of events, program requests, preprogram requirements, and time allotments, so that all activities are scheduled and completed without conflict.

3-2.3.1 *Prerequisite Skills:* Time management, scheduling, organizing, and planning.

Public Fire and Life Safety Educator II

4-2.1 Prepare a budget request, given budget guidelines, program development, and delivery expense projections, so that all guidelines are followed.

4-2.1.1 *Prerequisite Knowledge:* Budgetary process.

4-2.2 Project program budget expenditures, given program needs, past expenditures, current materials, personnel cost, and guidelines, so that the projections are within accepted guidelines.

4-3.4 Prepare a plan for the use of human or material resources, given policies on soliciting, previous solicitation efforts, and specific program needs, so that resources are identified and program needs are addressed.

Public Fire and Life Safety Educator III

5-2.1 Create public fire and life safety education goals and objectives, given an organization's mission statement, available resources, and local loss statistics, so that the goals are consistent with the organization's mission and reflect the public's need for education.

5-2.1.1 *Prerequisite Skills:* Organizational planning, resource management, and data analysis.

5-2.2 Create a program budget, given organizational goals, community needs, and budget guidelines, so that overall program needs are met within budget guidelines.

5-2.2.1 *Prerequisite Knowledge:* Budgeting methods, cost allocation breakdown, local budget guidelines and requirements, and budget administration issues.

Chapter 3
Managing Fire and Life Safety Resources

INTRODUCTION

Management is sometimes called "the art of accomplishing organizational objectives through and with people." Planning, organizing, implementing (directing and controlling), and evaluating the work of other people — Those are the traditional activities of managers.[1] Some fire and life safety educators are managers in this very traditional sense. Yet many more fire and life safety educators are responsible for using scarce resources — people, time, money, and materials — as effectively as possible; these educators are also accountable for how well the resources are used (Figure 3.1). Any fire and life safety educator who decides how scarce resources are used are "managers," regardless of their title or rank.

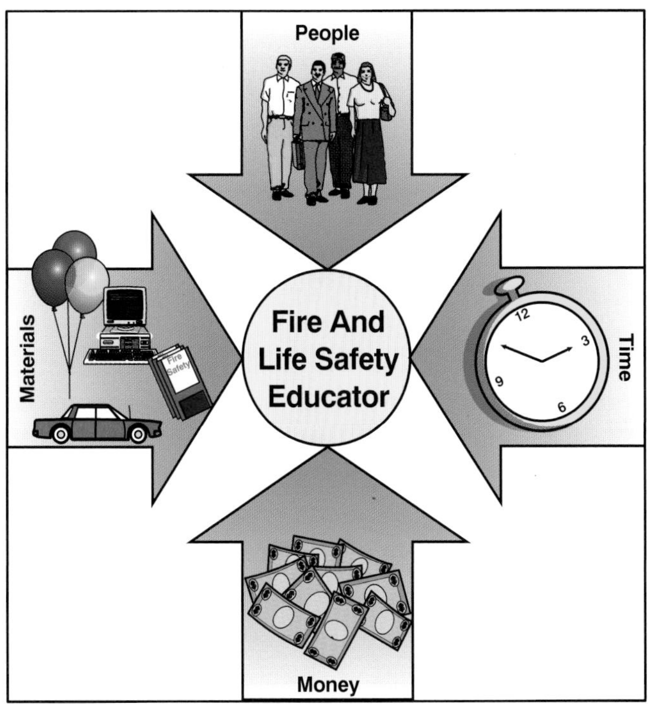

Figure 3.1 Fire and life safety educators not only manage people but also manage limited resources.

This chapter introduces ideas for educators to use in managing the people, time, money, and materials for which they are responsible. This chapter also introduces the ways in which computers can help the manager. Because people management is so important, Chapter 4, "Managing Fire and Life Safety Personnel," covers that subject in more detail.

> **Committing Resources**
>
> Fire and life safety educators are often optimistic people! In fact, they are sometimes so optimistic that they overcommit their people, time, money, and materials.
>
> Effectively managing the resources of people, time, money, and materials helps prevent overcommitment.

MANAGERS

The word *manager* brings many images to mind: the people higher up in the organization who must approve the public educator's plans, the people caught between the needs of those above and below them in the chain of command, or even the compassionate bosses who are mentors to their staffs. Whatever their rank, all managers are accountable to someone for how they use resources. In much the same way, fire and life safety educators are accountable to someone higher in the organization. Stated another way, everyone is responsible for managing the department's resources effectively. Management is not a chore for a few high-ranking people, but rather it is a central part of the fire and life safety educator's job.

"Management is official, sanctioned leadership. Management is decision-making about a variety of resources — whether those resources are budgets, buildings, apparatus, equipment, or people. Personnel management is decision-making about specific human resources."

Reprinted with permission from *Managing People: Fire Service Personnel Strategies*, copyright © 1984, National Fire Protection Association, Quincy, MA 02269 p. 7.

MANAGING PEOPLE

A few fortunate fire and life safety educators have a staff that reports directly to them. More rely on the cooperation of others in the department (such as firefighters, the public information officer, or the staff from the training division and the fire prevention bureau) to help get the public education job done. Many educators rely on people outside the department (classroom teachers, school nurses, human service staff, or members of civic organizations for example). These valuable human resources may be paid staff (on the educator's payroll or paid by another department) or may be community volunteers.

Because the fire and life safety educator has to use these different resources effectively, all must be "managed." *Note that "managed" does not necessarily mean "supervised"*; some human resources are outside the educator's span of direct control.

Effective managers know that achieving the most from the "people power" available involves much more than simply telling people what to do. Getting the best performance depends on the fire and life safety educator's ability to lead. *Leadership* is "the knack of getting other people to follow you and to do willingly the things that you want them to do."[2]

Leadership Styles

There are three broad styles of leadership: autocratic, laissez-faire, and democratic or participative (Figure 3.2).

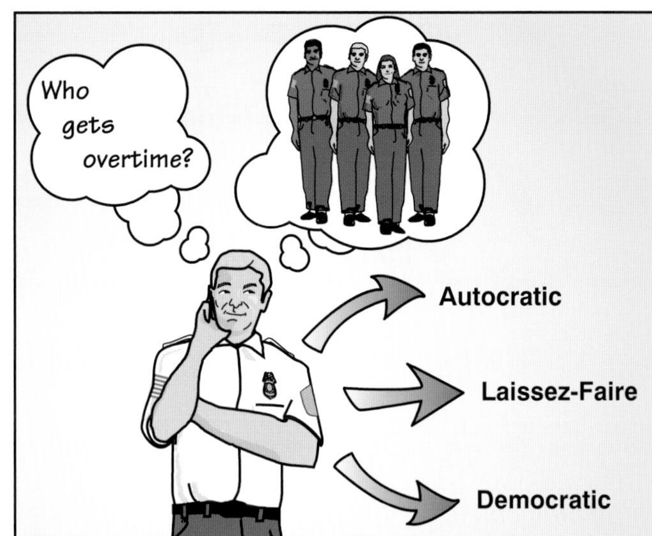

Figure 3.2 Depending on the situation, three broad styles of leadership may be used.

Under the autocratic style, the leader relies very little (if at all) on suggestions from others. Autocratic leaders usually make decisions independently, informing people after the decision is made. Autocratic leadership is often speedy, but it shuts out the viewpoint and experience of other people.

The laissez-faire leader shares responsibility with the group. This type of leader often relies on other people for suggestions and delegates some (usually a fairly limited amount) of the decision making. The laissez-faire leader may set an objective but leave the method for meeting the objective up to the others.

The democratic leader is team-oriented and gives authority to the group. The group — whether a planning team or paid staff — gives suggestions. The group, rather than the leader, makes decisions.

The "right" style varies with the situation and the group. Laissez-faire or democratic leadership styles are not well-suited for emergencies. Decision making probably takes longer under the laissez-faire and democratic styles than under the autocratic style. Delicate or unpleasant decisions (Who gets overtime? Who gets re-assigned? Who gets the new vehicle or slide projector?) call for an autocratic approach. Untrained or inexperienced staff may force a leader to be autocratic, at least temporarily.

On the other hand, laissez-faire and democratic leadership are very appropriate when it is important to have people agree with a decision. These leadership styles are also effective when many people are involved in implementing a decision. Deciding how to organize a major new fire and life safety education program or how to organize major events (such as Fire Prevention Week) are examples of when to use laissez-faire or democratic leadership.

Another View of Leadership

So much has been written about leadership in the fire service and in other fields that it is not surprising that there are other views of leadership. For example, a leader's style could be described as bureaucratic, single-issue, middle-of-the-road, or dual-issue. These four leadership styles describe how a leader balances concern for workers (whether paid or volunteer) and a concern for production (Figure 3.3). (**NOTE:** For a more complete discussion of these styles, see IFSTA **Fire Department Company Officer**, 2nd ed.)

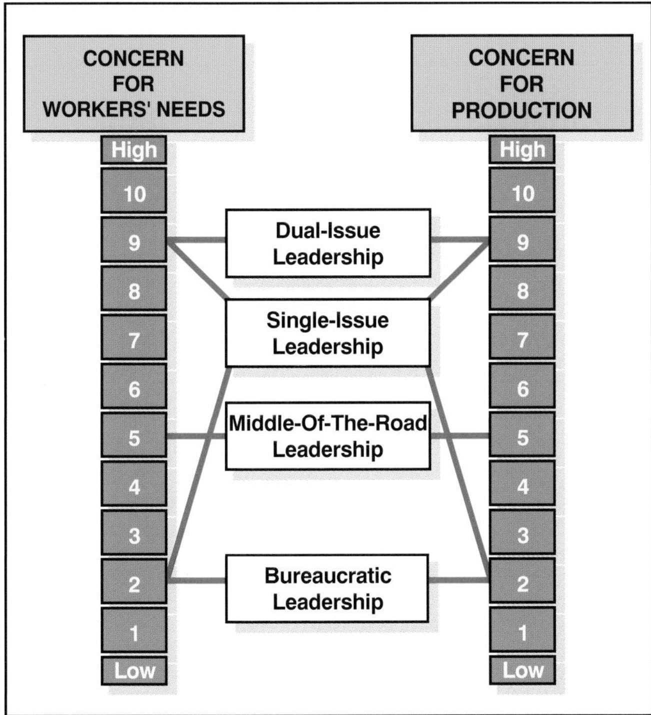

Figure 3.3 Some leadership styles are based on the amount of concern that leaders place on production and on their workers needs.

BUREAUCRATIC

Bureaucratic leaders have a low degree of concern for workers and a low degree of concern for production. Bureaucratic leadership is likely to be found in large organizations — or in smaller ones with an extensive merit system or labor contracts. Under this style of leadership, production is limited to the minimum needed to get by. A bureaucratic fire and life safety education leader might say: "Under the contract, we don't have to work on Saturday, so my people will not work at any Fire Safety Fair on a Saturday." Bureaucratic leaders do not reward — and they even discourage — extra effort.

SINGLE-ISSUE

Single-issue leaders, on the other hand, are very concerned about *either* production needs or worker needs. This style of leadership results in a very production-oriented or a very worker-oriented working atmosphere. For example, "We've got to get into every classroom in this town, so the education staff will just have to work harder" reflects the point of view of a production-oriented, single-issue leader. A worker-oriented, single-issue leader might say, "My people are too valuable and talented to be pushed around by a quota system for classroom visits." Whether production-oriented or worker-oriented, the single-issue leader tends to create workers who are unsatisfied in their work.

MIDDLE-OF-THE-ROAD

A moderate concern for production and a moderate concern for workers characterize middle-of-the-road leaders. At first glance, this style seems like a reasonable approach to leadership. However, the *results* of middle-of-the-road leadership are also middle-of-the-road, not exceptional.

DUAL-ISSUE

In dual-issue leadership, the leader has a high degree of concern for workers as well as a high degree of concern for production (Figure 3.4). This kind of leader encourages workers to "be all they can be." The dual-issue leader knows that job satisfaction is also personally satisfying. "Putting this new preschool program together is really important, and it's going to take some real skill to get it done. You'll have to work hard, but you're perfect for this assignment." This type of expression is typical of a dual-issue leader.

Today's managers try to avoid three "leadership land mines"[3]:

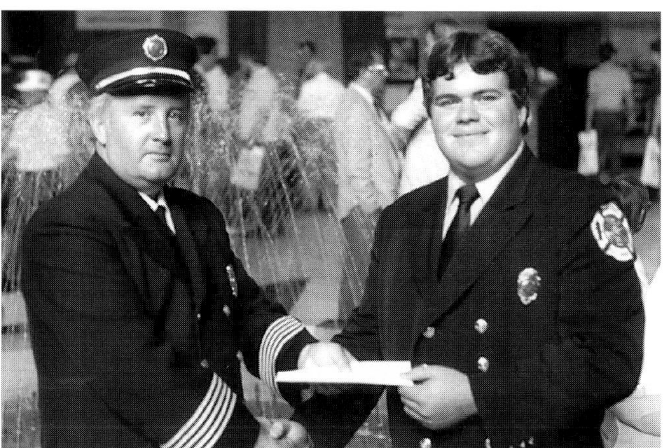

Figure 3.4 A dual-issue leader gives recognition for quality work.

- The belief that one leadership style fits every person
- A tendency to be overly autocratic or dictatorial
- A tendency to adopt the same approach to leadership used by impressive former managers

In other words, leadership is not an exact science, but an art. Like other fire and life safety education skills, leadership calls for judgment and practice.

Using Controls

With whatever style of leadership the manager uses, the manager needs a system of controls. Typical controls in fire and life safety education include time sheets, written reports, copies of important letters, public education requests (Figure 3.5), logs of presentations delivered, assignment forms, formal or informal meetings to check status (Figure 3.6), observations of presentations, and standard operating procedures. Controls help managers monitor progress by providing information.

Controls need to be used with *everyone* involved in the fire and life safety education program — not be reserved for a few people. Managers must monitor the progress of everyone who can deter-

PUBLIC EDUCATION REQUESTS

NUMBER________ ENGINE/SHIFT______ / ______

SCHEDULED DATE________ SCHEDULED TIME________

NAME ________

ADDRESS ________

POINT OF CONTACT________

PHONE________ TYPE OF PRESENTATION ________ AGE ____

NUMBER OF PARTICIPANTS ______ / ______ EDUCATOR ________

OTHER PERSONNEL ______ / ______ / ______ / ______

COMMENTS ________

____

PLEASE CALL POINT OF CONTACT LISTED ABOVE IF ANY SCHEDULING CONFLICTS OCCUR!

REQUESTED______ CONFIRMED______ FILED______ RETURNED______

Figure 3.5 A typical control in a fire and life safety education program is a public education request. *Courtesy of Colorado Springs (CO) Fire Department.*

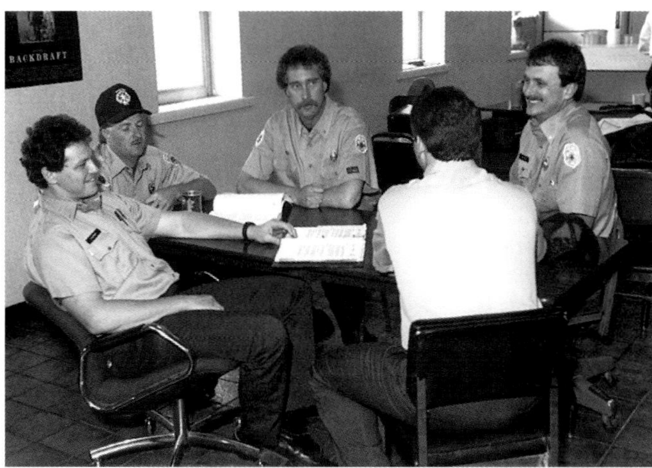

Figure 3.6 Educators meet to check the status of fire and life safety education program projects.

mine a program's success or failure, even when there is no direct supervisory relationship. Obviously, the fire and life safety educator needs to be diplomatic in monitoring people who are not in the educator's chain of command.

The best controls have the following characteristics[4]:

- Identify and report problems without delay
- Are objective
- Are easy to understand
- Are cost-effective

MANAGING TIME

Managers are accountable for using two kinds of time: their own and the time of other people who work in fire and life safety education. The other people can include supervised fire and life safety educators, cooperating people from other agencies, and community volunteers.

Managing time is closely related to managing money. Time has value. For example, managers who try to do something in-house — such as create a brochure — to save money may ultimately spend so much time that it would have been less expensive to buy the brochures.

Managing the Manager's Time

A manager's time is a very scarce resource. Practicing time management is an all-important favor that managers can do for themselves.

Most libraries and bookstores have books on time management. These books describe several well-known techniques on time management:

- Set priorities for answering mail — and stick to them.
- As much as possible, handle each piece of paper only once.
- Go through the "in" box every day to make sure that time-sensitive material does not get "buried" (Figure 3.7).

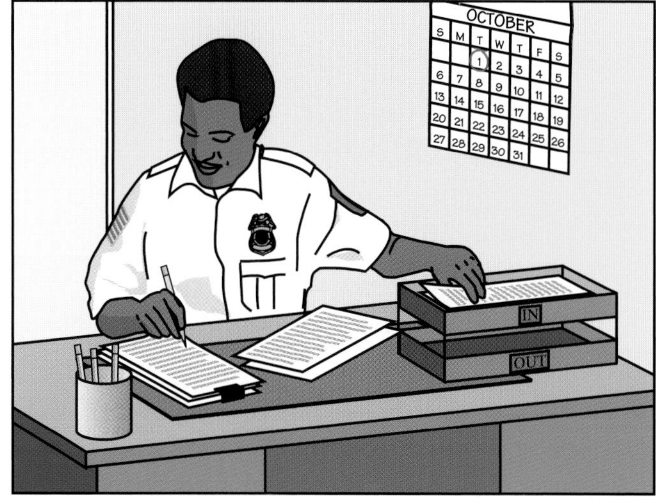

Figure 3.7 A time-wise manager checks incoming information daily.

- Pick one standard time (first thing in the morning or just after lunch, for example) to go through the "in" box.
- Skim material to see if it even needs to be read. Discard junk mail right away.
- Adopt boilerplate responses to routine correspondence; put these responses into your word processor.
- As much as possible, answer mail the day it arrives.
- Use charts and graphs to track progress on major, important, or complicated projects.
- Establish categories for files. Avoid the "miscellaneous" file, which can quickly grow too large to be useful.
- Use fragmented time well. While waiting for a meeting to start, for example, draft a "to do" list for the next day.

- Schedule a time for returning calls.
- Know your most productive time (first thing in the morning, after a coffee break, etc.). Schedule especially important work for your most productive time.

Fire and life safety educators have their own specialized techniques for managing time. Here are some of their time-management guidelines (Figure 3.8):

- Reserve the first half hour of each workday for making — and prioritizing — an agenda for the day.
- Begin and complete the most important task first thing after arriving at work.
- Hold staff meetings with everyone standing up; this helps to keep meeting times to a minimum.
- List tasks, make sure that each task is in line with the overall goals, and identify who will do each task.
- Know your time limitations, and be willing to say "no," accepting only tasks that can be accomplished with the time available. Do a few tasks well rather than many tasks poorly.

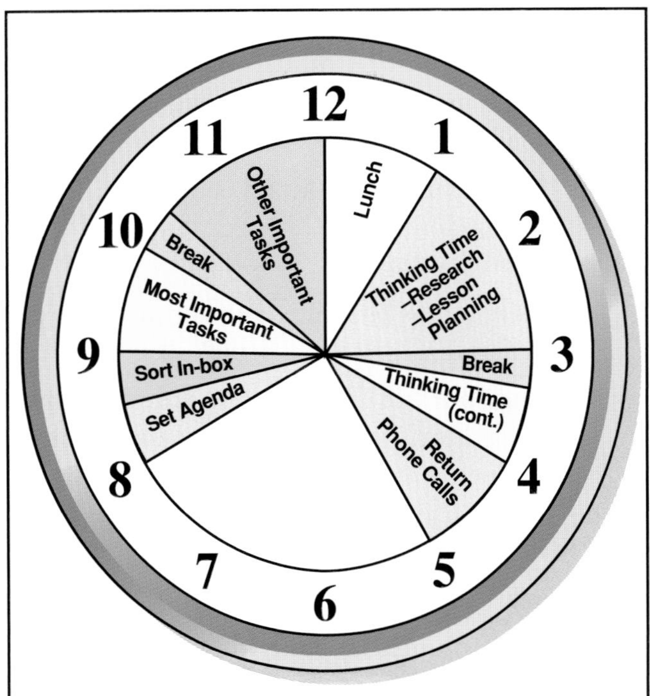

Figure 3.8 One time-management technique is to follow a daily agenda.

- List the tasks for each week, and number them in order of importance. Focus on the most important tasks, beginning and completing task 1 before beginning task 2. Carry uncompleted tasks forward to the next week.
- Delegate tasks (including returning phone calls) to others, as much as possible.
- Collect reading materials, and catch up on professional reading during downtime.
- Use a Franklin Day Planner®, or similar daily calendar (Figure 3.9).

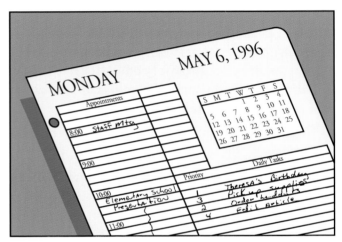

Figure 3.9 A daily calendar can be used by the fire and life safety educator to help plan activities and manage time.

- Schedule "thinking time" in fairly large blocks (two to three hours). Use that time for research, overall program planning, writing lesson plans, and other activities that call for concentration.
- Use electronic mail (E-mail) for routine questions and answers, especially if you are frequently away from the office setting.
- Use the computer to manage schedules and contact lists as well as for repetitive correspondence (Figure 3.10).

Managing Other People's Time

As long as the fire and life safety education manager relies on other people for successful programs, the manager needs to know how their time is spent.

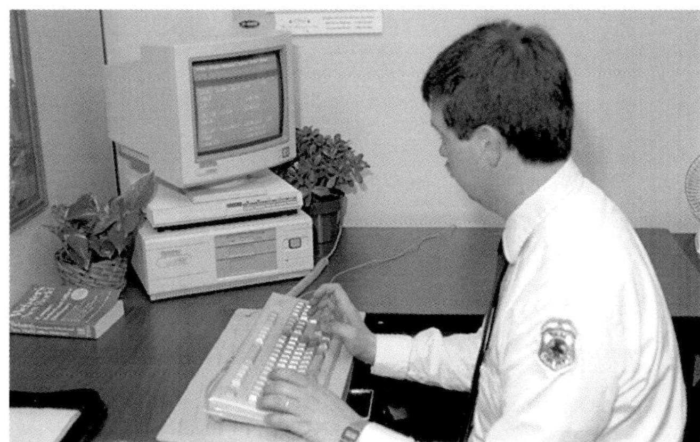

Figure 3.10 An educator uses the computer to manage schedules.

Time management is fairly straightforward to supervised fire and life safety education staff. Time sheets, logs, the manager's own observations, and other control techniques reveal whether or not the staff is using time wisely. The manager can then act. Possible actions range from counseling or training in time management techniques, to setting more specific (perhaps short-term) work assignments, and to making time management a measurable job performance objective. For example, work assignments may start as very short term (maybe a day completed in a day's time and requiring daily monitoring by manager) and change to longer term (perhaps completed within a week and requiring weekly monitoring); this technique, however, does require more of the manager's time.

Managing the time of people not on the fire and life safety education staff (those not supervised by the fire and life safety education manager) is a more delicate matter. Using some control techniques, such as requiring time sheets or written reports from other fire department personnel who are involved in education programs, is difficult. In other cases, techniques such as oral reports at meetings and observation can be used quite effectively. Actions to correct time management problems include counseling/training and setting specific, short-term work assignments. Realistically, the manager can rarely make time management a job performance issue for unsupervised workers, whether paid or volunteer.

MANAGING MONEY

Two distinct skills are involved in managing money for fire and life safety education. They are budgeting and monitoring expenditures (Figure 3.11).

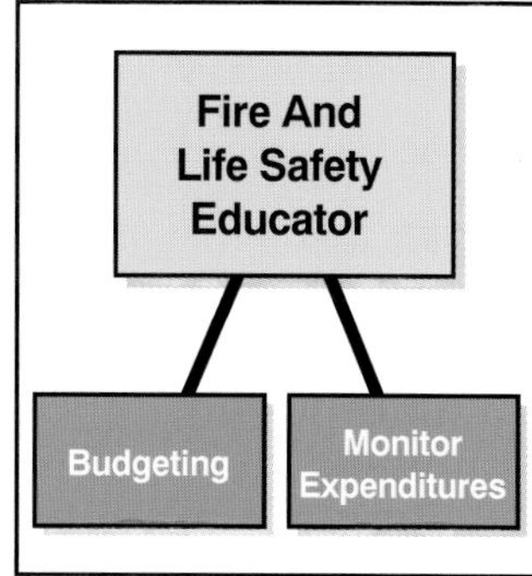

Figure 3.11 The fire and life safety educator must be skilled in budgeting and monitoring expenditures.

Fire departments and other organizations may have special requirements for accounting for donated funds, as compared to funds from tax revenues. Anyone who deals with donated dollars should check with the department attorney and the funder to make sure that these special requirements are met.

Budgeting

Most fire departments and other organizations have specific requirements for the format used for budget requests. These SOPs may require that specific forms be filled out or that projected expenses above a certain dollar amount or percent of increase must be justified in writing. They may also require that the budget manager make oral or written presentations to the fire chief, city council, state/province fire marshal, legislative staff, or governor's staff (Figure 3.12). Fire and life safety education managers are responsible for knowing and following their organization's procedures.

A budget, though, is more than creating numbers that add up and fall within limits set by

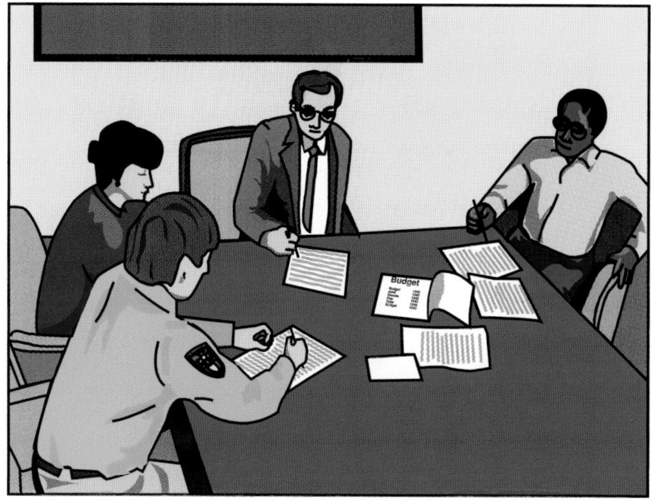

Figure 3.12 The fire and life safety educator must be prepared to make oral or written presentations about the budget request.

upper management. A *budget* is a plan for action, with associated costs, for the coming year. In other words, *a budget results from setting program goals and objectives and then deciding which goals and objectives can be met with the financial resources available* (Figure 3.13). For a budget to be meaningful, program plans must come first.

Developing this budget plan is much like other planning activities. Some fire and life safety educators use a structured planning process, such as that described in Chapter 6, "Planning Fire and Life Safety Education." Others may use another planning process or create their own. The important point is to start the budget by planning the program (Figure 3.14). This sort of planning process changes budgeting from "Here's what I want to spend" to "Here's what the spending will accomplish."

In developing the dollar costs for the budget, fire and life safety educators can use guidelines set down by their organization, suggestions from Chapter 9, "Funding Programs Through Outside Sources," or some combination of the two.

In planning for next year's budget, the educator should follow these guidelines:

- **Do a self-critique of last year's budget**. Is the budget clearly linked to a program plan? Did written or verbal presentations link dollars to programs?

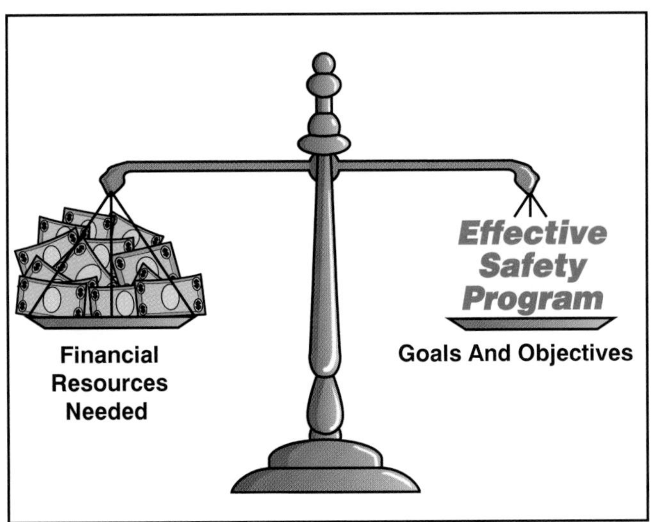

Figure 3.13 The financial resources needed to meet the goals and objectives for the year are reflected in the educator's budget.

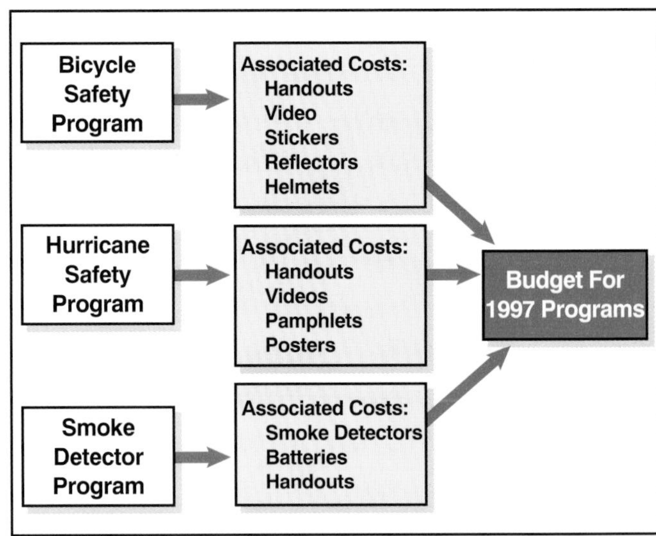

Figure 3.14 Planning the upcoming fire and life safety programs is the first step in budgeting.

- **Start a file of cost information**. Include catalogs of fire and life safety materials, ads for computers, cameras, and other equipment, and announcements of fire and life safety conferences. Use this cost information, rather than guess about costs.
- **Keep accurate records about this year's costs**. Which costs were higher than planned? Which were lower? What percentage of total costs were a complete surprise?
- **Learn to use a computer spreadsheet before the next budget cycle**. Make the learning simpler by investing in a community college course or practicing at home.

Try to review the written budget justification or attend the budget presentation of very successful departments (within the city or in other jurisdictions). Adopt their techniques.

- **Use graphs and visuals in written or oral budget justifications**. Keep presentations simple, clear, and linked to program plans.
- **Document the successes of education**. Use the results of evaluation efforts (see Chapter 11, "Evaluating Presentations and Programs"). Keep an annual file of clippings, letters from grateful citizens, etc. In presentations, link those successes to specific program objectives.

- **Review your materials before submitting them**. "Here's what the spending will accomplish" is a better message than "Here's what I want to spend."

Monitoring Expenditures

Managers are accountable for spending money wisely. Their first step is knowing exactly how the money was spent.

In the past, accounting was usually centralized, in part because computer power was concentrated in the accounting area. Now, personal computers and a general trend of decentralization are moving bookkeeping to the education program level.

Whether or not computers are available, fire and life safety education managers need to know how they are spending their money. Is spending ahead of schedule or behind schedule? Will the money last throughout the year? What adjustments will need to be made? Does higher management know that public education spending is higher or lower than planned?

Answering these questions demands doing some paperwork. A log of invoices, purchase orders, mileage reimbursements, or other expenses should be kept. The log can be manual or computer-driven and can take almost any form (Figure 3.15). The educator should include enough information so that the log will make sense a year later. Copies of invoices and other documentation should also be kept.

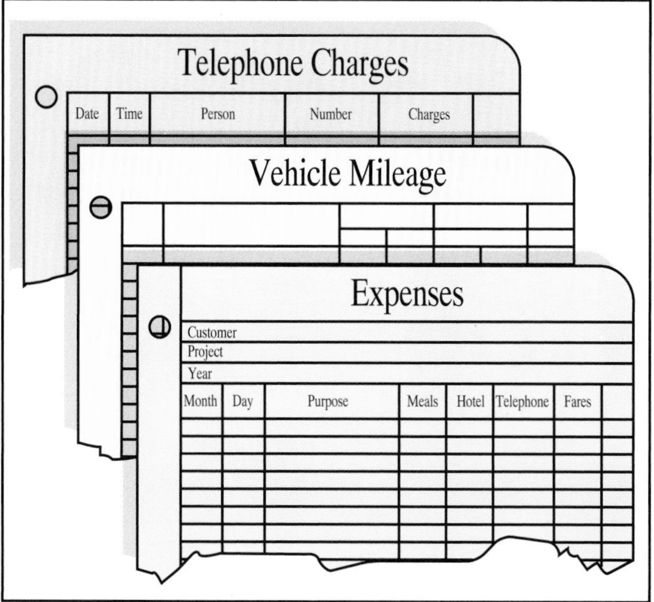

Figure 3.15 Expenses entered into logs such as these are more easily accounted for.

Follow these guidelines to keep the expense log useful:

- Keep the log as simple as possible. Record only information that will be used.
- Make the log clear. Entries that no one can understand are not helpful — and may even cause needless confusion.
- Enter expenses regularly. Falling behind on an expense log is like falling behind in balancing a checkbook: the longer you wait, the harder it gets. Pick a time, such as the first of each month, to enter expenses (Figure 3.16).
- Log expenses by project: school programs, Fire Prevention Week, etc. This helps in planning future efforts.

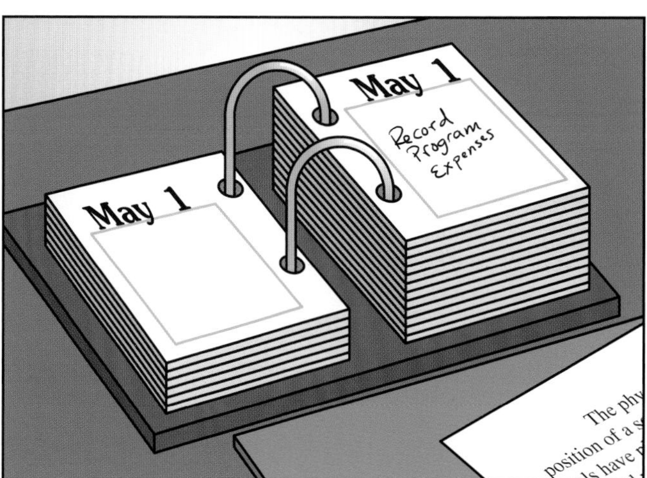

Figure 3.16 Educators may pick a specific time each month so that they remember to enter expenses regularly.

MANAGING MATERIALS

The fire and life safety educator is entrusted with a great deal of expensive equipment and consumable materials. Equipment for fire and life safety education includes vehicles (cars and vans), cameras, a wide range of audiovisual equipment, computer hardware and software, and demonstration equipment (such as firefighter personal protective equipment, puppets, "safety houses" or other scale models, and even remotely controlled talking fire hydrants). Consumable materials include handouts, toy helmets, films, videotapes, and slides (Figure 3.17). (**NOTE**: These last three are consumable in that after a certain amount of usage they must be replaced.)

About an Inventory

An accurate and current inventory of equipment and consumables is essential to managing materials. The inventory should be written and as detailed as possible. For example, the brand name, model, serial number, cost, and purchase date for each piece of equipment should be on the equipment. The inventory for consumable materials includes the number of each type of item on hand. Including information on when and how to reorder is especially helpful.

To make sure that the inventory is current, the fire and life safety education manager must decide who will update the inventory. Will one person be responsible for updating the inventory? Will each educator note when consumables are used?

The purpose of the inventory is simple: The inventory helps prevent the loss of valuable equipment or the sudden discovery that there are no handouts left in the cabinet (Figure 3.18). The fire and life safety education manager may have an inventory system that must be followed. When such a system is not in place, one should be instituted.

Personal Use of Equipment

Many fire departments and other organizations have a written policy on the personal use of equipment. Policies are especially important for vehicles, cameras, and personal computers. Fire and life safety educators who are responsible for equipment should know and follow the department's policy on personal use. If a policy

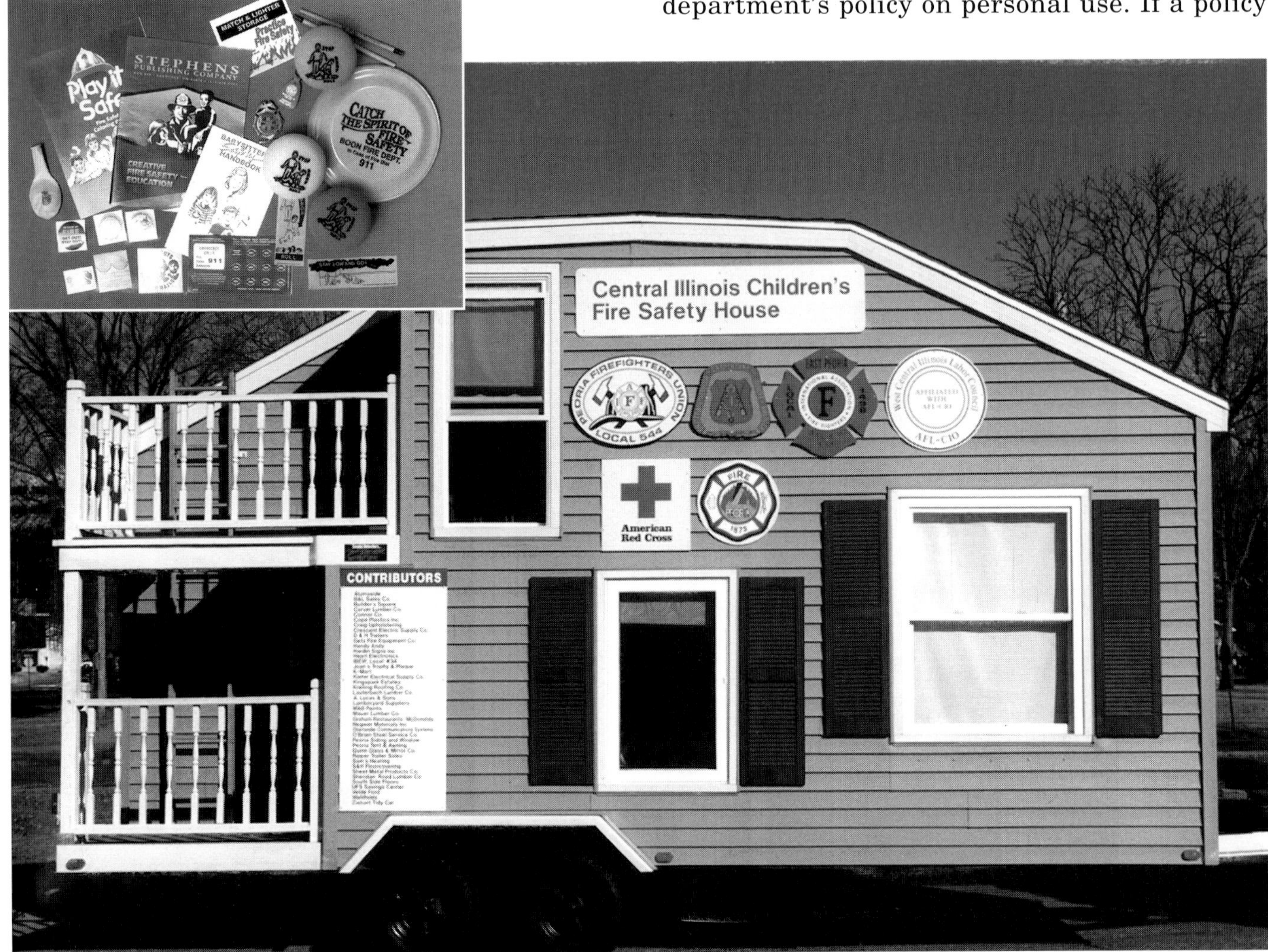

Figure 3.17 Educators may be responsible for items ranging from large training aids to small consumables. *Courtesy of Peoria (IL) Fire Department.*

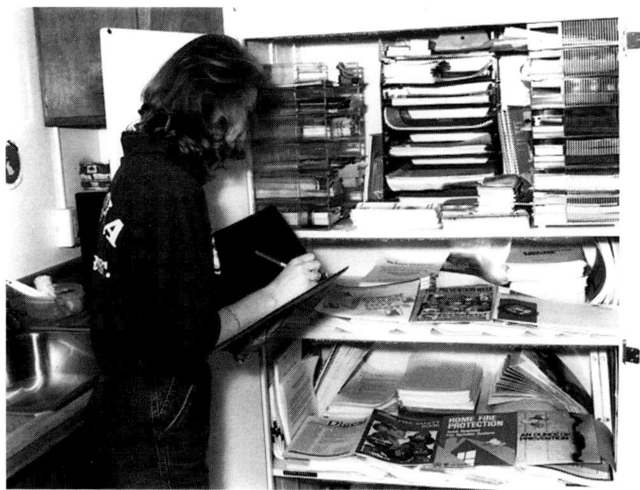

Figure 3.18 An educator checks the availability of supplies and equipment.

does not exist, the educator should establish one. The educator should post the policy where camera and computer equipment are stored. Where personal use is permitted, a sign-out sheet may be needed for cameras and computers.

Use of Personal Equipment

On the other hand, personal equipment is sometimes used at work. It is a good idea for educators to find out whether the organization will, for example, pay for film used in personal cameras for work purposes.

COMPUTERS AS MANAGEMENT TOOLS

Over the last ten years or so, personal computers have revolutionized the way people work. For fire and life safety education managers, personal computers are valuable tools for managing people, time, money, and materials.

Selecting computer hardware and software is an enjoyable — but sometimes intimidating — job. Be sure to consider the following guidelines when selecting hardware and software:

- Ask “computer-literate” people you know for advice. Ask for a demonstration. Sit at the computer, trying hardware and software, before making a selection.
- Decide what work you will perform on computer, and select hardware and software based on those needs.
- Read computer magazines. They have articles for the novice and expert users, as well as pages of ads for hardware, software, and accessories (Figure 3.19).
- Know about and follow organization standards (using only MS-DOS® or only Macintosh®, for example).

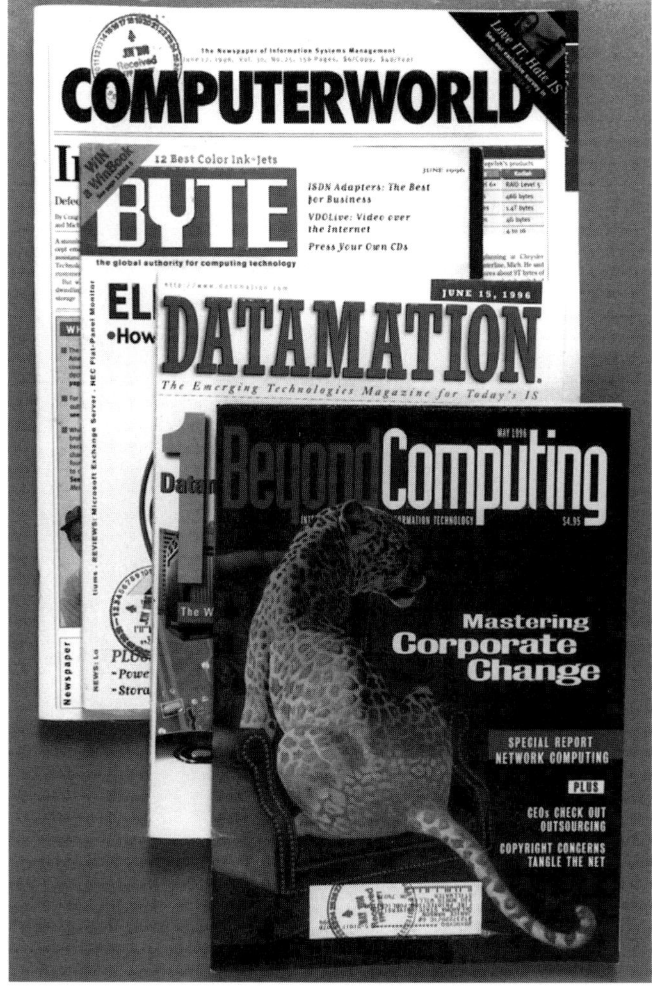

Figure 3.19 Computer magazines are excellent sources of information on hardware and software.

The fire and life safety educator could consider taking a computer course at a local community college. By doing so, the educator can become familiar with a program before making a purchasing decision. Typically, many courses covering the basic kinds of software (word processors, spreadsheets, databases, and graphics programs) are available.

Computer Hardware

Computer hardware includes computers themselves, monitors, printers, and modems (or fax-modems). Scanners and CD-ROM technology are also available. When budgeting for computer hardware, include computers, monitors, printers, modems, scanners, and CD-ROMs (Figure 3.20).

Computers are available in two basic formats: MS-DOS® (Microsoft Disk Operating System) and Macintosh®. As computer hardware becomes more sophisticated, the differences between the two formats are less and less important.

Storage capacity and speed are the two main decision points in buying a computer. Storage capacity or memory is measured in megabytes (MB); one megabyte equals one million characters. Two kinds of storage capacity are important: hard drive and random-access memory (RAM). A typical hard drive can store one gigabyte (one billion characters). RAM automatically saves data for instant accessibility and retrieval. Computers with 4, 8, or even 16 megabytes of RAM are available for under $2,500 — compared to only 1 MB RAM for about the same price a decade or so ago. With more memory, the computer can accommodate more software programs. Many software programs — especially graphics packages and the Windows™ application for MS-DOS® machines — need a certain amount of memory in order to function (Figure 3.21). *The cost of storage, RAM, and accessories are dropping dramatically. The fire and life safety education manager should see that the organization buys the most it can afford.*

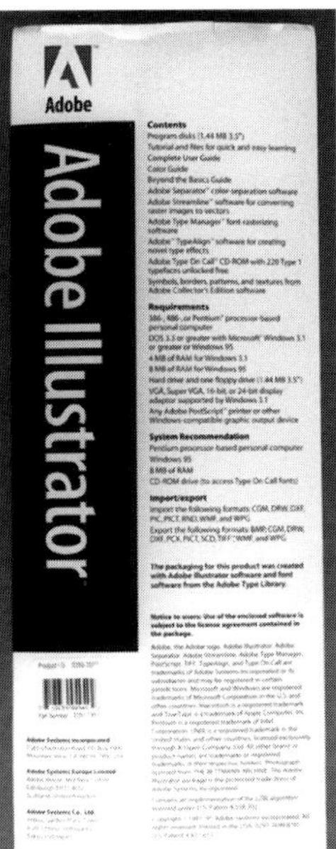

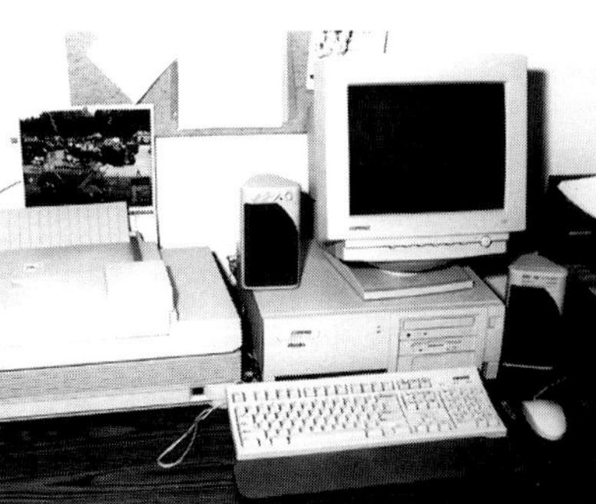

Figure 3.20 A budget for computer hardware should include everything necessary to do the job.

Figure 3.21 This package lists the requirements for using this software. *Adobe® and Adobe Illustrator® are trademarks of Adobe Systems Incorporated.*

Computer speed is determined by a combination of available (that is, unused) memory and processing time (which is sometimes called *clock speed*). Processing time determines how quickly a computer can begin a new operation and is measured in megahertz (Mhz). The higher the processing time, the faster the computer.

A printer is a necessity. Print quality ranges from dot matrix at the low end to ink-jet and laser printers at the high end. Color ink-jet or laser printers are also available. An ink-jet or laser printer is strongly recommended. It is important to make sure that a printer will support the software programs (such as Postscript® graphics programs) to be used. The technology of printers is changing *very* rapidly, and like computers and software, printer prices have dropped dramatically and are continuing to drop.

Modems (an abbreviation of "modulation emulators") allow computers to exchange information over telephone lines. With a modem, computers can be connected to networks such as CompuServe®, America OnLine®, Delphi℠, and the Internet. Modems are available in different baud rates, depending on how fast they transmit information over the telephone line. The higher the baud rate, the shorter the connect time will be — which can save telephone charges.

Some modems have built-in facsimile capability, allowing the user to send messages over existing telephone lines. In other words, a facsimile machine does not need to be connected to an information network.

Hand-held or desktop scanners allow the user to electronically copy text and visuals. The text and visuals can then be imported into word processing and graphics packages. It is possible to resize and edit the scanned material. Scanners are very useful, and fire and life safety educators who use them should follow copyright laws.

CD-ROMs combine compact disk and computer technology. Compact disks hold enormous amounts of information — an entire encyclopedia, for example — and can be inserted much like the old-style computer cassettes. Their ability to hold so much information is especially helpful with computer electronics, which use large amounts of space.

Finally, some computers combine the computer, monitor, modem or fax-modem, and even a CD-ROM into one piece of hardware.

Computer Software

There are five primary kinds of computer software: word processors, spreadsheets, databases, and graphics and presentation programs. More and more computers are sold with a package of these programs already installed. Programs are available for both MS-DOS® and Macintosh® machines.

WORD PROCESSORS

Word processors were among the first computer programs for the consumer and are still the programs most critical to have. Modern word processors allow fire and life safety educators to justify or align type, to use boldface and italics, and to choose a font (typeface) from a large selection. The trade names include Microsoft®, Word and WordPerfect®, among many others.

Fire and life safety educators use word processors for letters, memos, and reports, as well as for creating simple handouts.

SPREADSHEETS

Spreadsheets are the basic computer tool for dealing with numbers. With spreadsheets, fire and life safety educators can develop budgets, monitor the number of presentations delivered, and keep the inventory of materials current. Many spreadsheets transform rows and columns of numbers into charts and graphs. These then can be imported into word processing or graphics programs.

DATABASES

Databases are electronic filing cabinets. The user creates forms to record information (such as the title of presentation, date and place, number in the audience, handouts or audiovisual materials used, and the name of the educator making the presentation). After the data is entered, the computer will sort the information from all the forms in the database. The result is a report that the fire and life safety education manager can use to document activity, plan future schedules, monitor inventory, etc.

Databases also can be used to develop mailing lists, organize class records and reports, track incident reports, organize libraries, and customize telephone and fax lists.

GRAPHICS AND PRESENTATION PROGRAMS

Graphics programs combine text and art, transforming text and images into materials that look professionally produced. The three basic kinds of graphics programs are paint and draw programs, desktop publishing programs, and presentation programs (software packages to create audiovisuals). Electronic clip art — even fire service clip art — can be imported into these programs. See *Resource Booklet* in the **Fire and Life Safety Educator's Resource Kit**.

Clip art is a collection of simple images that can be used over and over to illustrate handouts and audiovisuals (Figure 3.22). When clip art was available only in books, fire and life safety educators would literally snip it out and paste it in. Electronic clip art works the same way — but with the added advantages of being able to resize it or rotate it.

Desktop publishing software is electronic layout. Using this software, educators can arrange text and illustrations, create headlines, and add rule lines and boxes. In other words, desktop publishing lets fire and life safety educators

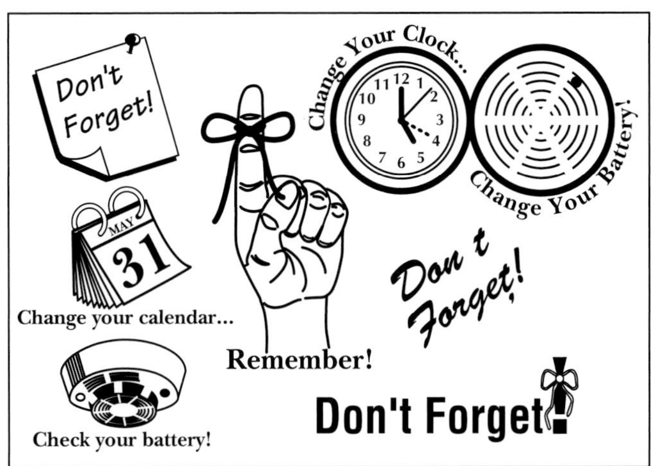
Don't Forget!
Change Your Clock...
Change Your Battery!
MAY
31
Change your calendar...
Don't Forget!
Remember!
Check your battery!
Don't Forget!

Figure 3.22 Clip art is a collection of simple images that can be used over and over to illustrate handouts and audiovisuals.

become their own designers. Templates (sample layouts) are available for common publications, such as newsletters and brochures.

Presentation programs create audiovisuals, primarily paper masters that can become slides or overhead transparencies. Some presentation programs project "slide shows" directly onto the computer screen (Figure 3.23). Presentation programs typically automatically number the overheads or slides as well as create instructor notes and handout pages (two to six reduced versions of the overhead or slide per page). Some presentation packages include clip art.

Many computers are sold "bundled" with a word processor, a spreadsheet, a database, and a presentation program. Electronic clip art must usually be purchased separately.

Communicating Via Computers

Communication is the latest application of computer technology. A computer and a modem put computer users in touch with each other worldwide. Presently, computers offer communication in two ways: by facsimile and via networks. Each method requires specialized software.

Facsimile by computer is very straightforward. A message is typed on the keyboard, the computer cable is plugged into a standard telephone line, and the facsimile is electronically transmitted to a receiver. There is no charge for local calls, and long-distance charges apply.

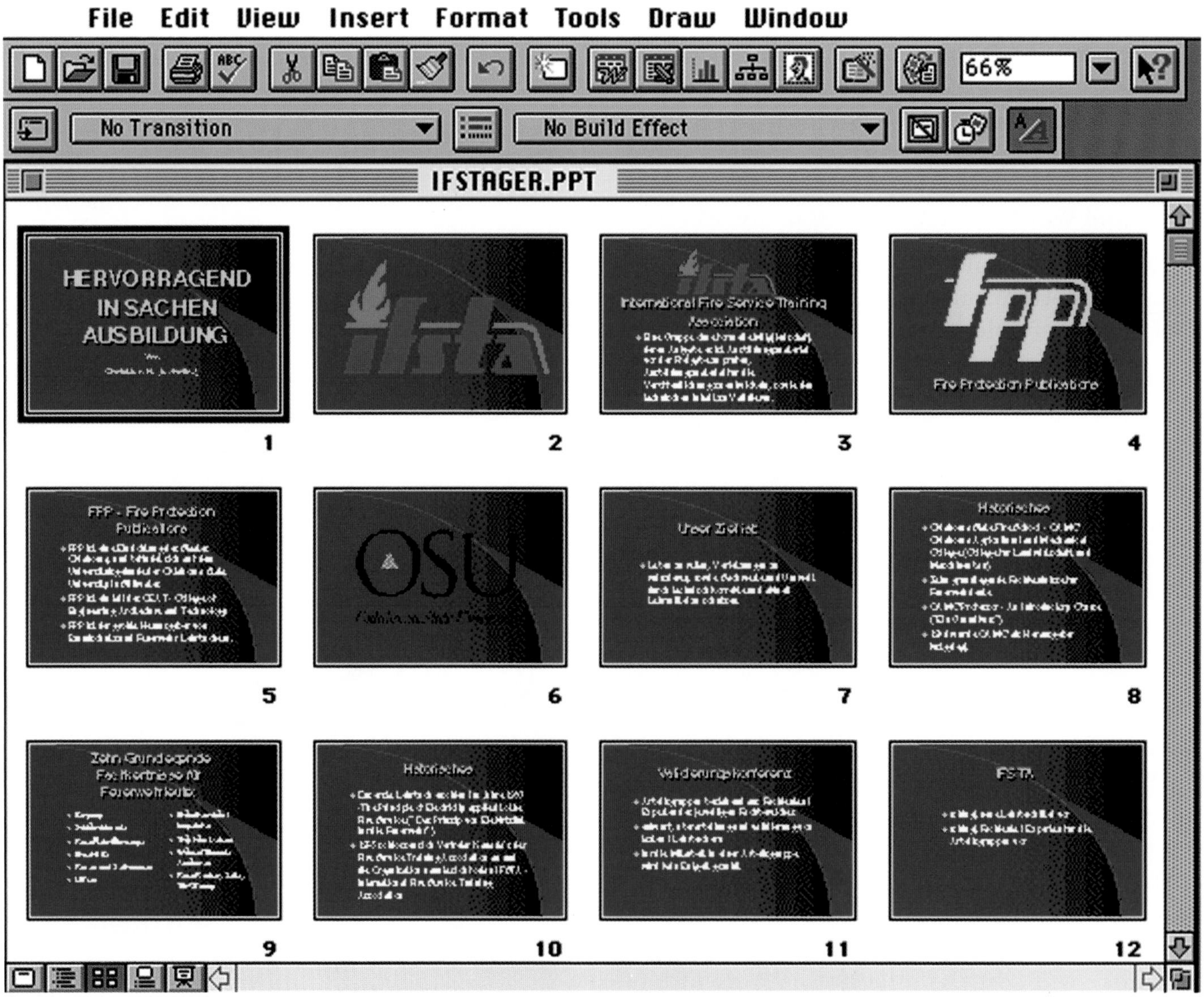

Figure 3.23 Some presentation programs create presentations that are shown directly on the computer screen.

Modems basically work the same way. Modems, however, connect users to computer networks. The computer networks charge users a small monthly membership fee and fees for connect time. Telephone charges also apply.

Network members each have a unique address so that users can electronically "talk" to each other. In addition, networks offer electronic bulletin boards that are often devoted to specialized subjects, including fire safety, education, public safety, health, travel, etc. Through these electronic bulletin boards, users can post messages, and then other people on the bulletin board can respond.

Two of the many electronic bulletin boards of interest to fire and life safety educators are ICHIEFS (operated by the International Association of Fire Chiefs) and CompuServe®'s Fire-Net®.

ICHIEFS includes a folder/directory for the National Fire Protection Association, which includes the tables of contents for *Fire Technology* and the *NFPA Journal*® (very useful for research), NFPA news releases, summaries of fire investigations, and news from the Association's Public Education and Public Fire Protection Divisions as well as from the Fire Marshal's Association of North America.

Fire-Net® is part of Safetynet™, one of several professional forums (also called *special interest* groups) within CompuServe®. CompuServe® membership includes a subscription to that network's monthly magazine.

More information, including fee and start-up information, is available from IAFC and CompuServe®.

CONCLUSION

Whether or not they are called "managers," fire and life safety educators are accountable for how they allocate people, time, money, and materials. Allocations are really decisions — and decisions depend on information. Decisions must be made whether or not computers are available, but computer technology can help educators access information for decision making.

FOR MORE INFORMATION

IFSTA **Fire Department Company Officer**, 2nd ed., 1989.

John A. Granito, "From Hoseline to Online," *NFPA Journal*®, January/February 1995, pp. 76-86.

James O'Toole, *Making America Work: Productivity and Responsibility*, Continuum, New York, 1981.

Thomas J. Peters and Robert Waterman, *In Search of Excellence: Lessons from America's Best-Run Companies*, Harper & Row, Publishers, New York, 1982.

Thomas J. Peters and Nancy Austin, *Passion for Excellence: The Leadership Difference*, Random House, New York, 1985.

Dr. Nancy Grant and Dr. David Hoover, *Fire Service Administration*, National Fire Protection Association, Quincy, MA, 1994.

Kenneth Blanchard and Spencer Johnson, *The One Minute Manager*, Berkley Books.

Harry C. Carter and Erwin Rausch, *Management in the Fire Service*, 2nd ed., National Fire Protection Association, Quincy, MA, 1994.

Chapter 3 Notes

1. For a detailed description of those activities, see Chapter 6, "Elements of Management," in IFSTA **Fire Department Company Officer**, 2nd ed.

2. Lester R. Bittel and John W. Newstrom, *What Every Supervisor Should Know*, 6th ed., McGraw-Hill, Inc., 1990, p. 268.

3. Excerpted by permission of the publisher, from *The Successful New Manager*, by Joseph T. Straub, p. 26. ©1994 AMACOM, a division of American Management Association. All rights reserved.

4. Excerpted by permission of the publisher, from *The Successful New Manager*, by Joseph T. Straub, pp. 18-19. ©1994 AMACOM, a division of American Management Association. All rights reserved.

Chapter 3 Review

Directions

The following activities are designed to help you comprehend and apply the information in Chapter 3 of **Fire and Life Safety Educator**, second edition. To receive the maximum learning experience from these activities, it is recommended that you use the following procedure:

1. Read the chapter, underlining or highlighting important terms, topics, and subject matter. Read the sidebar material, study the photographs and illustrations, and read the captions with each.
2. Review the list of vocabulary words to ensure that you know the chapter-related meaning of each. If you are unsure of the meaning of a vocabulary word, look up the word in the glossary or a dictionary, and then study its context in the chapter.
3. On a separate sheet of paper, complete all assigned or selected application and review activities before checking your answers.
4. After you have finished, check your answers against those on the pages referenced in parentheses.
5. Correct any incorrect answers, and review material that was answered incorrectly.

Vocabulary

Be sure that you know the chapter-related meanings of the following words:

- leadership *(62)*
- delegation *(62)*
- autocratic *(62)*
- dictatorial *(64)*
- controls (n.) *(64)*
- boilerplate *(65)*
- budget *(67)*
- prioritizing *(66)*
- expenditures *(67)*
- decentralization *(69)*
- inventory *(70)*
- font *(73)*

Application of Knowledge

1. Read your department's policies and procedures manual to find out its SOPs for personal use of equipment and for use of personal equipment.
2. Use each of the following types of computer software to create a work-related product. If you do not know how to use any one of these software programs, ask for access and training.
   - word processor
   - spreadsheet
   - database
   - graphics
   - presentation program

Review Activities

1. Distinguish among the terms *management, manager,* and *supervisor. (61,62)*
2. Explain the main characteristics of each of the following leadership styles: *(62)*
   - autocratic leadership
   - laissez-faire leadership
   - democratic leadership
3. How does one choose the "right" leadership style? Describe situations appropriate to the different leadership styles explained in Activity 2. *(62)*
4. Explain the main characteristics of each of the following leadership styles: *(63)*
   - bureaucratic leader
   - middle-of the road leader
   - single-issue leader
   - dual-issue leader
5. List the three "leadership mines" that modern-day managers try to avoid. *(63, 64)*
6. List examples of typical controls used by fire and life safety education managers. *(64)*
7. List characteristics of the best controls. *(65)*
8. Explain how managing time is closely related to managing money. *(65)*

9. List well-known techniques for managing one's own time. *(65, 66)*
10. List specialized time management techniques used by fire and life safety educators to manage their own time. *(66)*
11. Describe techniques that may be used by fire and life safety managers to control the way their supervised staff uses its time. *(66, 67)*
12. List actions the fire and life safety manager may take on finding that a supervised staff member is not managing his or her time wisely. *(67)*
13. Describe techniques that may be used by fire and life safety managers to control the way people whom they do not supervise use their time. *(67)*
14. List actions the fire and life safety manager can take to correct time management problems of unsupervised workers. *(67)*
15. Name the two principal skills involved in managing money for fire and life safety education. *(67)*
16. Explain the differences between budgeting and managing money. *(67)*
17. List general guidelines managers should follow when planning next year's budget. *(68)*
18. Explain why the fire and life safety manager should keep an expense log. *(69)*
19. List techniques for keeping expense logs useful. *(69)*
20. Distinguish between equipment and consumable materials. *(69, 70)*
21. State the purpose of an equipment and consumable materials inventory. *(70)*
22. List details that should be recorded on an inventory. *(70)*
23. Identify the following items associated with computers:
    - hardware *(71, 72)*
    - software *(71, 73)*
    - MS-DOS® *(72)*
    - Macintosh® *(72)*
    - monitor *(72)*
    - scanner *(72)*
    - CD-ROM *(71, 72)*
    - modem *(72)*
    - megabyte *(72)*
    - memory *(72)*
    - RAM *(72)*
    - gigabyte *(72)*
    - clock speed *(72)*
    - megahertz *(72)*
    - baud rate *(72)*
    - network *(72)*
    - facsimile *(74)*
    - E-mail *(66)*
    - bundled *(74)*
24. List guidelines to consider when selecting computer hardware and software. *(71)*
25. Compare and contrast the following types of computer printers: *(72)*
    - dot matrix
    - ink jet
    - laser
26. Describe each of the following kinds of computer software:
    - word processor *(73)*
    - spreadsheet *(73)*
    - database *(73)*
    - graphics *(73)*
    - presentation program *(73, 74)*
27. Compare and contrast the three basic graphics programs:
    - clip art *(73)*
    - desktop publishing *(73)*
    - presentation programs *(74)*
28. Briefly distinguish between ICHIEFS and Fire-Net® bulletin boards. *(75)*

Questions and Notes

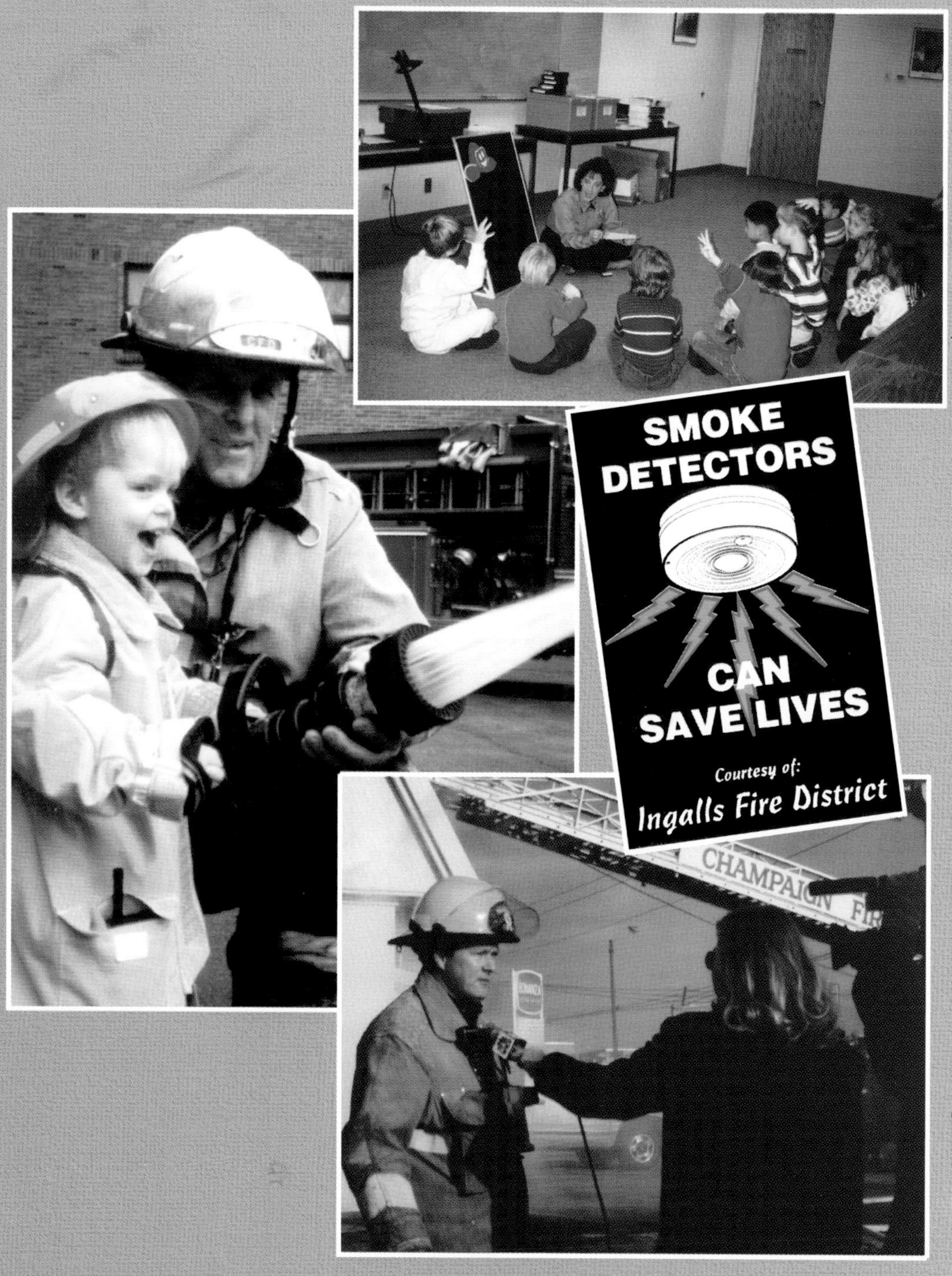
SMOKE
DETECTORS
CAN
SAVE LIVES
Courtesy of:
Ingalls Fire District
CHAMPAIGN

Managing Fire and Life Safety Personnel

4

LEARNING OBJECTIVES

This chapter provides information that addresses the following objectives of NFPA 1035, *Standard for Professional Qualifications for Public Fire and Life Safety Educator* (1993 edition):

Public Fire and Life Safety Educator I

3-2.3 Maintain a work schedule, given a list of events, program requests, preprogram requirements, and time allotments, so that all activities are scheduled and completed without conflict.

3-2.3.1 *Prerequisite Skills:* Time management, scheduling, organizing, and planning.

Public Fire and Life Safety Educator II

4-3.4 Prepare a plan for the use of human or material resources, given policies on soliciting, previous solicitation efforts, and specific program needs, so that resources are identified and program needs are addressed.

Public Fire and Life Safety Educator III

5-2.3 Evaluate subordinate performance, given written performance criteria, so that the employee is evaluated objectively.

5-2.3.1 *Prerequisite Knowledge:* Organizational personnel policies; local, state, and federal employment regulations; and personnel evaluation techniques.

5-4.3 Create a training program for public fire and life safety educators, given identified job performance requirements, so that job requirements are met.

5-4.4 Create an awareness program for the internal organization, given identified public fire and life safety education goals and policies, so that all members are informed of the role of public fire and life safety education in the community and the organization.

Chapter 4
Managing Fire and Life Safety Personnel

INTRODUCTION

As introduced in Chapter 3, "Managing Fire and Life Safety Resources," management is sometimes called "the art of accomplishing organizational objectives through and with people." In another view of management, managers are responsible for using the scarce resources of people, time, money, and materials as effectively as possible.

This chapter concentrates on managing the scarce resource of people. Topics covered include motivating people in the workplace, position descriptions and the fire and life safety educator, the employment interview, managing performance, discipline, and legal aspects of personnel management. For the most part, these topics deal with how fire and life safety educators manage employees under their direct supervision. Many of the same techniques can be used to manage the efforts of fire and life safety volunteers. As defined in Chapter 13, "Learning Fire and Life Safety Educational Theory," a volunteer is not necessarily a volunteer firefighter. A *volunteer* is anyone — inside or outside the fire department — who helps with fire and life safety education programs.

Personnel management is a complex subject, and the topics covered here are only a beginning. This chapter is designed to introduce key personnel management subjects and apply them to fire and life safety education. More information is available through books at the local bookstore or library, introductory courses at the local community college or library, or even "telecourses" offered through some public television stations.

Motivation

"Motivation causes employees to invest more of themselves in their jobs than they are required to do. Motivated people reach beyond the boundaries of their job description and push the limits of their abilities, not because they have to but because they want to. They go the extra mile to make sure that the people they serve, whether colleagues or customers, are fully satisfied. Motivated people not only do things right; they also do the right thing, and do it willingly."

Excerpted by permission of the publisher, from *The Successful New Manager*, by Joseph T. Straub, p. 71.

MOTIVATING PEOPLE IN THE WORKPLACE

Motivating people to achieve their best is a priority for all managers. New managers are especially concerned with motivation. Motivation is "what makes people tick," and a few simple concepts provide a good basis for understanding this complicated aspect of human behavior.

Maslow's Hierarchy of Needs

One of the earliest — and still very influential — concepts related to motivation is the 1954 book *Motivation and Personality* by Abraham Maslow. According to this theory, people have five kinds of needs that motivate their behavior. These needs are usually shown as a triangle, with the most critical needs at the bottom (Figure 4.1). The needs at the bottom of the triangle must be satisfied before people can turn attention to the less important needs that are higher up the triangle.

The most basic needs are *physiological:* food, water, and shelter. While these needs are usu-

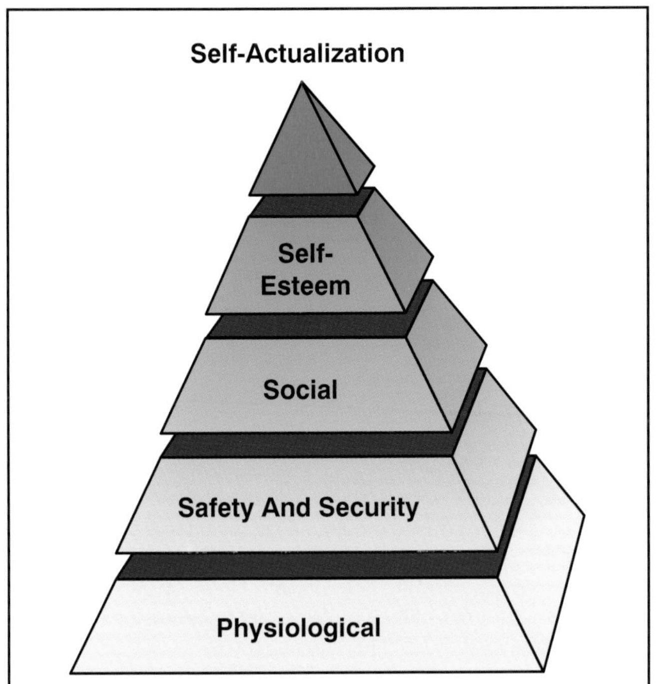

Figure 4.1 Maslow originated the Hierarchy of Needs. Generally, individuals strive for the higher needs after the lower needs have been secured.

ally satisfied before an employee arrives for work in the morning, there are lessons here for managers. For example, fire and life safety educators, no matter how committed they are to their work, still need a break for lunch and a chance to rest for a few minutes after a presentation.

Safety and security needs are similar to physiological needs. Firefighters and emergency medical technicians (EMTs) work to fulfill safety and security needs when they use a self-contained breathing apparatus in a fire or use gloves in a medical emergency. Using seat belts in a fire education van and scheduling two people for presentations in crime-prone neighborhoods are other examples of acting on safety and security needs.

People have a need for *belonging and group activity*. Group projects help fulfill this need. Badges, patches, T-shirts, or hats that say "Fire and Life Safety Education Unit" would also foster a sense of belonging. Volunteering for fire and life safety education projects is one way people act on their need for belonging and group activity.

People need more than to just belong to a group — they need *esteem and status* from the group. Rewarding good effort through plaques, certificates, or even recognition dinners provides esteem and status for fire and life safety educators.

The highest need is *self-realization and fulfillment*. The Army recruiting slogan "Be all you can be" captures this need perfectly! For the fire and life safety educator, this need may translate to feelings such as "I want this presentation to be the best one ever" or "This presentation wasn't quite right, but I'm going to fix it for the next time."

Job Satisfaction

Maslow's hierarchy does not mention several items that many people associate with motivation at work: fringe benefits, vacation, or even salary. However, a researcher named Frederick Herzberg conducted extensive interviews about people's attitudes toward their work.

According to Herzberg's interviews, the nature of the work itself, responsibility for a job, achievement in a job, recognition of good work, and advancement provided job satisfaction. These factors are motivators (Figure 4.2).

Other factors — fringe benefits and vacation, for example — Herzberg called "hygiene factors." Hygiene factors did not increase job satisfaction, although their absence could detract from job motivation. Salary was negative to neutral in providing job satisfaction. In other words, work motivates the worker.

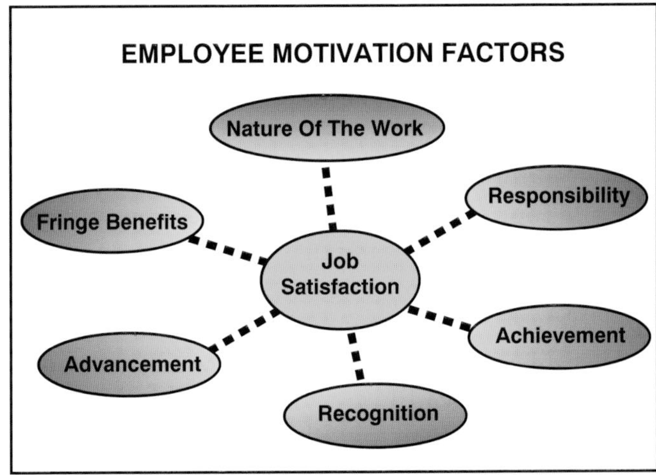

Figure 4.2 Frederick Herzberg determined that an employee's job satisfaction was affected by these motivating factors.

Theory X and Theory Y

Douglas McGregor had a very different view of how managers motivate. According to McGregor, managers saw employees in one of two ways, called *Theory X and Theory Y.* Theory X views employees as hating work, needing to be pushed and directed, avoiding responsibility, and having little ambition (Figure 4.3). (**NOTE:** For example, Captain Bligh in *The Mutiny on the Bounty* was a Theory X manager. As he said, "The floggings will continue until morale improves.")

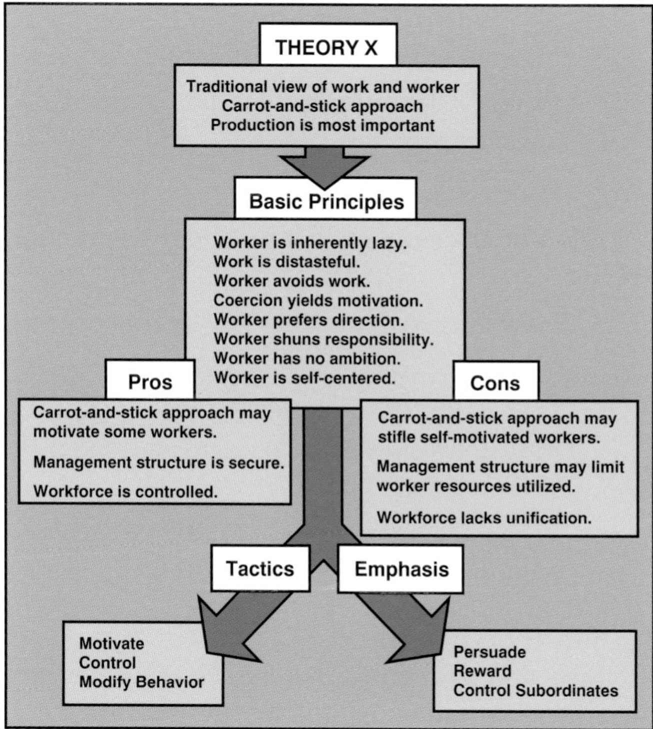

Figure 4.3 Theory X views employees as hating work, avoiding responsibility, and having little ambition.

Theory Y, on the other hand, views work as a natural human activity (Figure 4.4). Control and force are not the only way to get people to work, and people will accept and look for responsibility (in some circumstances). Authoritarian management uses only part of an employee's abilities in the Theory Y view.

For example, a Theory X fire and life safety education manager believes that employees would hate the extra effort of developing a new presentation. That manager believes that fire and life safety educators would not develop new presentations until they were told to and would want very specific directions about the content and format for the new presentation.

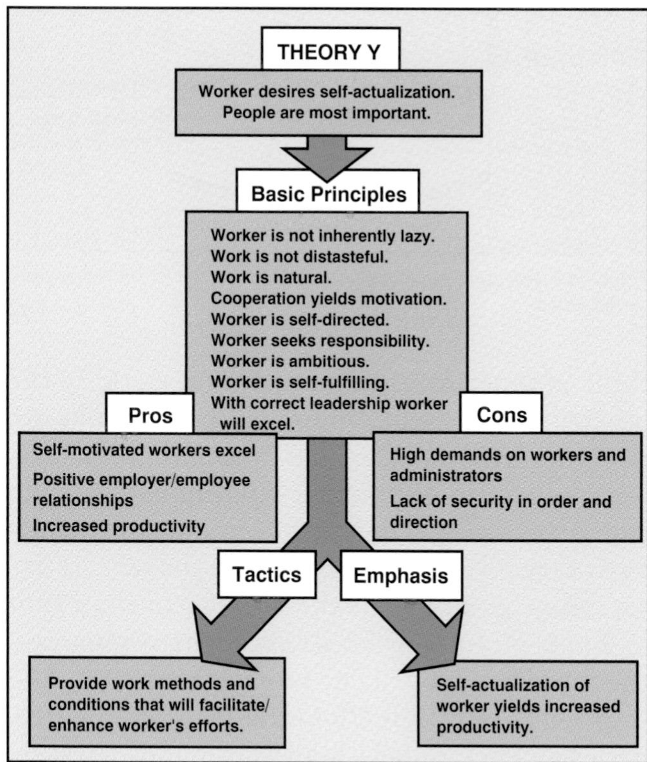

Figure 4.4 Theory Y views employees as willing to look for and accept responsibility.

The Theory Y fire and life safety education manager would have a very different view of the same situation. To the Theory Y manager, developing a new presentation would be an opportunity that employees would accept — and welcome. Compared to the Theory X manager, the Theory Y manager would tend to give less direction, have fewer checkpoints, and less frequent technical review of the new presentation.

Many effective managers use Theory X in some situations and Theory Y in other situations, achieving a balance of techniques.

Expectations as Motivators

Expectations by managers and by workers can be powerful motivators. If a manager expects good performance, employees perform well. If a manager expects poor performance, employees perform poorly. Treating employees indifferently often signals an expectation of poor performance (Figure 4.5).

In 1982, Thomas J. Peters and Robert H. Waterman, Jr., released *In Search of Excellence: Lessons from America's Best-Run Companies.* According to this widely read book, people like to

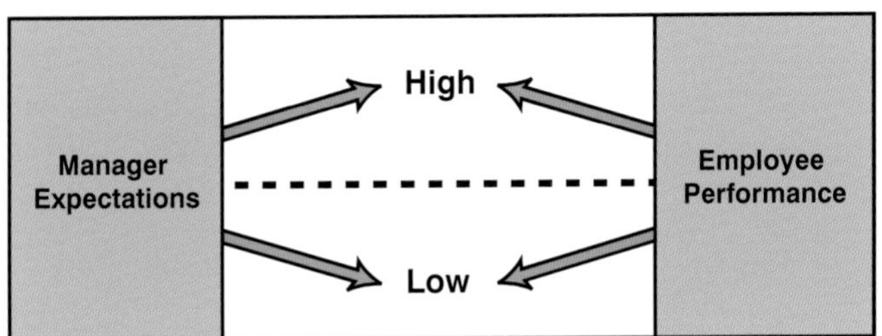

Figure 4.5 Manager expectations have a direct effect on employee's performance.

think of themselves as "winners" at work. In the best run companies, "most of their people are made to feel that they are winners...their systems reinforce degrees of winning rather than degrees of losing. Their people by and large make their targets and quotas, because the targets are set (often by the people themselves) to allow that to happen. In the not-so-excellent companies, the reverse is true...[The workers] resent it, and that leads to dysfunctional, unpredictable, frenetic behavior. Label a man a loser and he'll start acting like one."[1]

Consider how a fire and life safety educator would react to these two conversations with a manager:

Conversation 1:

"My budget request says that you will give a presentation in every classroom in town this year. *And,* all the civic clubs too! But don't worry about it. Between you and me, you're never going to get all those presentations done. Just do as many as you can."

Conversation 2:

"I was really impressed to see your plans in your budget request. Making presentations to every classroom and to all the civic clubs is pretty ambitious. You're the one who can make it happen! And, thanks for taking on the extra responsibility."

Expectations are central to a *goal-setting theory of motivation* developed by Craig Pinder. Higher goals, he says, result in higher performance. Clear goals tell people exactly what is expected, but ambiguous goals frustrate workers.

Expectations and goals can become very real! This is sometimes called a "self-fulfilling prophecy" or a *Pygmalion theory.* Telling an audience, for example, "You probably won't understand this presentation" almost assures that few people will listen. On the other hand, telling an audience "You'll like learning this because we're going to make it fun" sets a positive expectation and encourages learning.

"What's in it for Me?"

Another form of the self-fulfilling prophecy is the *expectancy theory* developed by Victor Vroom. People are motivated to work by answers to three questions:

- How easy is the work to accomplish?
- What is the reward for doing the work successfully?
- How likely is success?

Fire and life safety educators might ask themselves:

- How long will it take to revise this presentation?
- Is this part of the expectations for my next appraisal period?" "Will my name go on the new material?
- What are my chances of getting the revision done before school starts?

Putting Theory to Work

Fire and life safety educators can use very specific techniques for putting motivation theories to work. The American Management Association recommends five tools for the "motivator's tool kit" (Figure 4.6). These tools reflect the ideas of McGregor and Herzberg and are these[2]:

- Delegate authority
- Give praise for work well done
- Enlarge the job
- Use participative management
- Rotate jobs

AT&T — one of the largest employers in the United States — has identified six factors of job design that increase motivation at work. These are the following[3]:

- A whole job from beginning to end
- Regular contact with users or clients

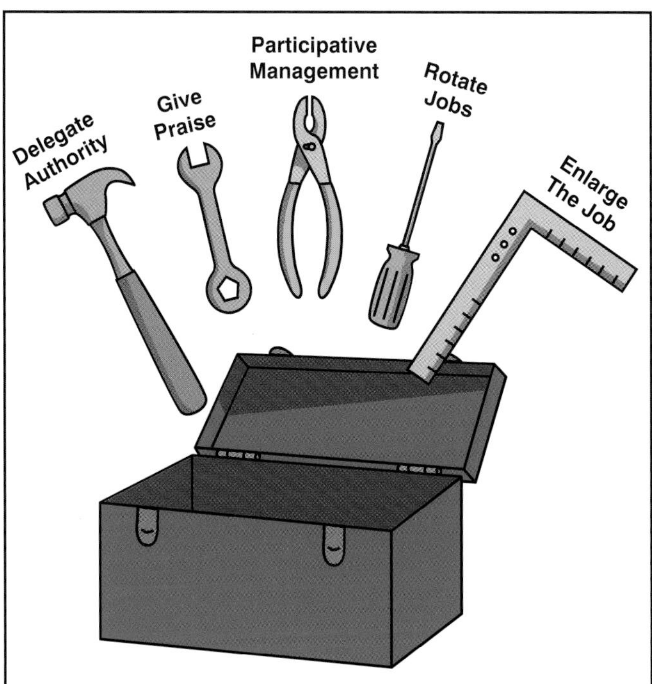

Figure 4.6 Fire and life safety educators can use tools from the "motivator's tool kit" to put motivation theories to work.

- Use of a variety of tasks and skills
- Freedom for self-direction
- Direct feedback from the work itself
- A chance for self-development

In assigning major revisions to several fire and life safety education presentations, the manager could use the insights from AT&T by saying:

> "You'll be responsible for this from start to finish — from the ideas for content to the production of the handouts and slides. If you want to interview some of the teachers who have been to these presentations in the past, that's fine with me. You'll need to use your organizing and creative skills at the same time for the revisions, but I'll leave it to you to sort out the details of scheduling and budget — just give me a proposed work plan by the beginning of next month. You're a pretty tough critic, so it's important that you're happy with the end product. This will give you a great chance to see how the city AV shop works!"

POSITION DESCRIPTIONS AND THE FIRE AND LIFE SAFETY EDUCATOR

Right after going into the Oval Office for the first time after his inauguration, President John F. Kennedy asked jokingly, "Now that we're here, what do we do all day?" A good position description can answer that question for the fire and life safety educator.

Position descriptions come in a variety of formats, but all are designed to spell out the expectations of the job, the activities that are needed to meet those expectations, and the qualifications needed to fill the job. Position descriptions are the basis for hiring decisions. An effective position description is also a useful tool in measuring job performance (Figure 4.7).

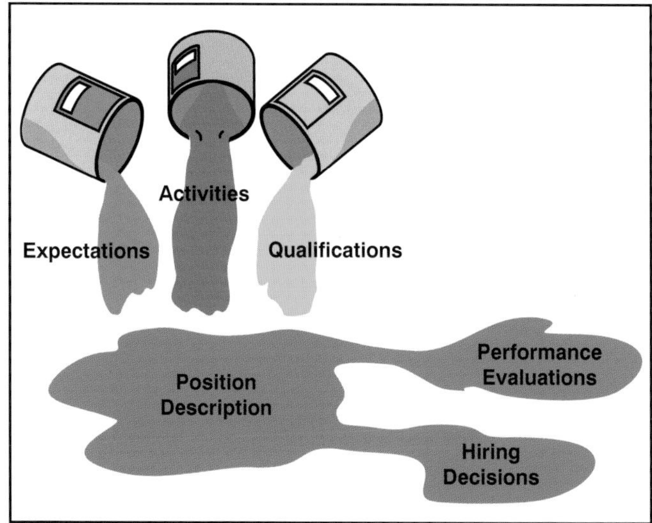

Figure 4.7 Effective position descriptions contain job expectations, job activities, and required qualifications for a job. Position descriptions are the basis for hiring decisions and job performance evaluation.

Position descriptions may be extremely detailed. The Fire and Rescue Training Institute at the University of Missouri, for example, uses a format that includes a brief mission statement, general description, major duties and responsibilities, knowledge required, supervisory control guidelines used, complexity, scope and effect, type and purpose of personal contacts, physical demand, work environment, and education and experience. A typical Missouri Fire and Rescue Institute position description is three single-spaced pages. Figure 4.8 is a sample position description for a fire and life safety educator, using the Missouri Fire and Rescue Training Institute format.

Because it is based on NFPA 1035, *Public Fire and Life Safety Educator,* the sample job description shown in Figure 4.8 is essentially a "results-oriented job description."[4] This type of

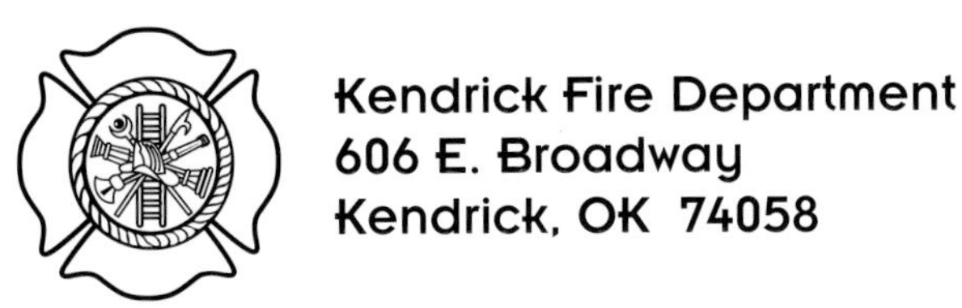

Fire and Life Safety Educator I
Position Description

The Kendrick Fire Department provides fire and life safety services, including injury prevention programs, inspection and plans review services, and response to fires, medical and other emergencies.

Position Description

The Fire and Life Safety Educator I will coordinate and deliver existing educational programs and information. Collateral responsibilities include maintaining an accurate inventory of educational materials, keeping records of program delivery, and maintaining audiovisual equipment and teaching aids.

Major Duties and Responsibilities

The Fire and Life Safety Educator I will carry out the following activities, based on NFPA 1035, *Professional Qualifications for Public Fire and Life Safety Educator,* 1993 edition.

1. Select instructional materials, given a subject, program objective, the intended audience, and related resources, so that the materials are appropriate to the audience and program objectives.
2. Present a prepared program, given lesson content, time allotments, and identified audience, so that the program objectives are met.
3. Use multiple presentation methods when presenting prepared programs, given program objectives, time allotments, and a specified audience, so that the chosen presentation methods are used.
4. Notify the public, given a scheduled event, so that the location, date, time, topic, and sponsoring agency are included.
5. Document public fire and life safety educational programs, given appropriate forms or formats, so that all programs are recorded and each element of the form or format is addressed.
6. Maintain a work schedule, given a list of events, program requests, preprogram requirements, and time allotments, so that all activities are scheduled and completed without conflict.
7. Distribute educational information, given material, specified audience, and time frame, so that information reaches the audience within the specified time frame.

Knowledge Required

1. As specified in NFPA 1035, required minimum knowledge includes fire behavior; organizational structure, function, and operation; human behavior during fire; injury causes/prevention; escape planning; hazard identification and correction; basic fire protection systems/devices; emergency reporting; and firefighter personal protection equipment.
2. As specified in NFPA 1035, required knowledge includes types of educational programs, classifications for programs, types of documentation methods and authority having jurisdiction preferred methods, the purpose of the forms or formats, and implications of not appropriately documenting programs.
3. As specified in NFPA 1035, required knowledge includes basic learning characteristics of preschool children, elementary school-age children, secondary school-age children, adults, and senior adults.
4. As specified in NFPA 1035, knowledge of local media resources and legal requirements for the distribution and posting of materials are also required.

Figure 4.8 A sample Fire and Life Safety Educator I position description prepared from information in NFPA 1035. *Reprinted with permission from NFPA 1035,* Professional Qualifications for Public Fire and Life Safety Educator, *Copyright© 1993, National Fire Protection Association, Quincy, MA 02269. This reprinted material is not the complete and official position of the National Fire Protection Association, on the referenced subject which is represented only by the standard in its entirety.*

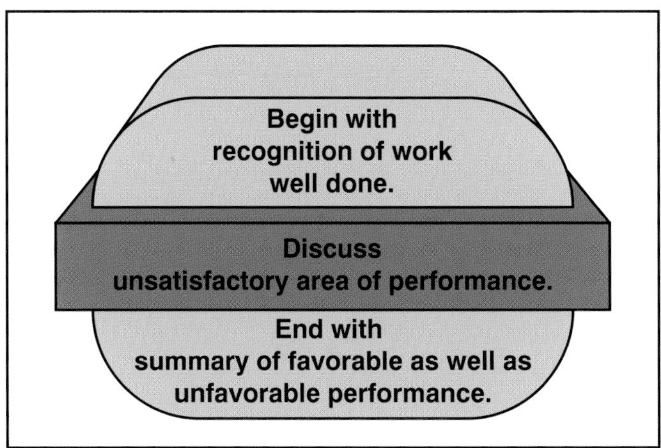
Begin with
recognition of work
well done.
Discuss
unsatisfactory area of performance.
End with
summary of favorable as well as
unfavorable performance.

Figure 4.9 Some managers find the "sandwich technique" useful when conducting performance appraisal interviews. *From* What Every Supervisor Should Know, *6th ed., by Lester R. Bittel and John W. Newstrom, McGraw-Hill, 1990. Reproduced with permission of The McGraw-Hill Companies.*

"I'm very happy that the new materials for the school program were ready to start the new school year. It was important to start the year with those new materials. On the other hand, not having the brochure on carbon monoxide poisoning ready for the Home Show was a low point in this year's performance. For this coming year, I know that you'll alert me if you see trouble with the schedule or need help."

DISCIPLINE

Performance appraisal happens whether performance has been excellent or poor. Disciplinary action, on the other hand, comes about as a result of problems. In fact, discipline usually occurs after specific kinds of problems: a pattern of unsatisfactory performance (which may or may not be related to personal problems), rules violations, or illegal or dishonest acts. Authorities having jurisdiction often have very detailed guidelines of which kind of problem leads to what kind of disciplinary action.

Discipline is not the same as punishment. Discipline also corrects unsatisfactory performance or behavior, and it is a fundamental tool of personnel management.[6]

Most jurisdictions use a system of *progressive* discipline, consisting of the following steps:

Step 1: Oral reprimand

Step 2: Written reprimand

Step 3: Transfer

Step 4: Suspension

Step 5: Demotion

Step 6: Termination

Any formal disciplinary action is serious. Fire and life safety education managers should always check with their personnel department before beginning progressive discipline. (**NOTE:** For a description of each step of progressive discipline, see IFSTA **Fire Department Company Officer**, 2nd ed.)

LEGAL ASPECTS OF PERSONNEL MANAGEMENT

Fire and life safety educators usually are not personnel specialists and usually are not lawyers, either. While the legal counsel is the authority on legal matters, anyone who manages people needs to be aware of the laws that govern relationships between people and their employers. Two kinds of laws are of particular interest: Equal Employment Opportunity (EEO) laws and the Americans with Disabilities Act (ADA).

Equal Employment Opportunity Laws

Regardless of their race, color, nationality, origin, sex, handicap, or age, job applicants and employees have specific rights and privileges that are protected by law. U.S. Supreme Court decisions that weaken affirmative action programs do not affect the basic rights and privileges of applicants and employees.

Equal Employment Opportunity (EEO) laws are often said to be for "minorities." However, as the population changes (see Chapter 8, "Knowing Your Audience"), saying that EEO laws apply to *protected groups* is more correct. Protected groups are those who have experienced past workplace discrimination, including certain ethnic groups (blacks, Hispanics, Asians, and Native Americans), women, disadvantaged young people, Vietnam era veterans, and people over age 40. Table 4.3 summarizes the major federal EEO laws.

Americans With Disabilities Act

The 1992 Americans with Disabilities Act (ADA) touches the lives of people with disabili-

TABLE 4.3
Summary Of Major Federal EEO Laws

Law	Description
Equal Pay Act of 1993	Requires equal pay for men and women doing the same job.
Titles VI and VII, 1964 Civil Rights Act, as amended by the 1972 Equal Employment Act	Prohibits job discrimination in all employment practices (recruiting, selecting, compensating, classifying, assigning, promoting, disciplining, terminating, and setting eligibility for union membership) based on race, color, sex, religion, or national origin.
Executive Order 11246, as amended by Executive Order 11375 of 1967	Prohibits employment discrimination by organizations having federal contracts of $10,000 or more. Requires affirmative action programs where necessary.
1975 amendments to the Age Discrimination in Employment Act (1967)	Prohibits hiring or employment discrimination of workers over 40 years of age, unless a bona fide occupational qualification (BFOQ) can be established.
1973 Rehabilitation Act and Executive Order 11914 of 1974	Prohibits discrimination of physically or mentally handicapped applicants and employees by federal contractors.
Vietnam Era Veterans Readjustment Assistance Act of 1974	Prohibits federal contractors from discriminating against disabled veterans and Vietnam era veterans. Requires affirmative action in employing veterans.
Americans with Disabilities Act of 1992	Prohibits job discrimination against disabled people. Requires businesses with 25 or more employees to provide "reasonable accommodations" for qualified disabled job applicants and employees.

ties in many ways, including their employment. First, the Act defines a disabled person as one who has a physical or mental impairment that limits one or more "life activities," has a record of such impairment, and is regarded as having the impairment. (**NOTE:** This definition is very much in line with the 1973 Rehabilitation Act.)

The ADA then goes on to prohibit certain questions of job applicants and require employers to do certain things for employees. The list of banned questions includes medical history, workers' compensation or health insurance claims, absenteeism due to illness, past treatment for alcoholism, and mental illness. Employers must make "reasonable accommodations" for disabled workers; these accommodations include acquiring or modifying work equipment, providing qualified readers or interpreters, adjusting work schedules, making existing facilities (restrooms, telephones, and drinking fountains, for example) accessible. The accommodations are required for "qualified" disabled workers (those who can perform the "essential functions" of a job).[7]

Legal Aspects and the Future

Of course, jurisdictions may have their own laws or policies. Legislatures are always making new laws, and courts are always interpreting old ones. Like anyone who manages people, fire and life safety educators need to stay current on the changing legal aspects of personnel management, as well as the jurisdiction's own policies and procedures.

CONCLUSION

Fire and life safety educators — whether or not they hold a management title — are often responsible for managing people, time, money, and materials. Personnel management is especially complex, particularly given the legal aspects of managing people at work.

Key skills for the fire and life safety personnel manager are motivating workers, setting expectations (through results-oriented position descriptions and performance agreements), managing performance, and taking disciplinary action when necessary.

Personnel management has a very specific objective: better performance by fire and life safety educators. Seen another way, effective personnel management lets fire and life safety educators do their best — with increased public safety as the ultimate result.

FOR MORE INFORMATION

IFSTA **Fire Department Company Officer**, 2nd ed., 1989. The chapters on "The Company as a Group," "Leadership as a Group Influence," and "Career Counseling" are especially relevant to this chapter.

Harry R. Carter and Erwin Rausch, *Management in the Fire Service*, 2nd ed., National Fire Protection Association, Quincy, MA, 1994.

Pam Powell, *Managing People: Fire Service Personnel Strategies*, National Fire Protection Association, Quincy, MA, 1984.

Chapter 4 Notes

1. Thomas J. Peters and Robert H. Waterman, Jr., *In Search of Excellence: Lessons from America's Best Run Companies*, Harper and Row, New York, 1982, p. 57.

2. Excerpted by permission of the publisher, from *The Successful New Manager*, by Joseph T. Straub, pp. 74-76. ©1994 AMACOM, a division of American Management Association. All rights reserved.

3. Lester R. Bittel and John W. Newstrom, *What Every Supervisor Should Know*, 6th ed., McGraw-Hill, 1990, pp. 256-257. Reproduced with the permission of The McGraw-Hill Companies.

4. For a fuller discussion of results-oriented job descriptions, see Nancy Grant and David Hoover, *Fire Service Administration*, National Fire Protection Association, Quincy, MA, 1994, pp. 126-130.

5. Lester R. Bittel and John W. Newstrom, *What Every Supervisor Should Know*, 6th ed., McGraw-Hill, 1990, pp. 199-204. Reproduced with the permission of The McGraw-Hill Companies.

6. For a good discussion of the importance of discipline, see Grant and Hoover, pp. 179-197.

7. "Disability Act Helps, But Not Much," *Wall Street Journal*, July 19, 1993, p. B1.

Chapter 4 Review

Directions

The following activities are designed to help you comprehend and apply the information in Chapter 4 of **Fire and Life Safety Educator**, second edition. To receive the maximum learning experience from these activities, it is recommended that you use the following procedure:

1. Read the chapter, underlining or highlighting important terms, topics, and subject matter. Read the sidebar material, study the photographs and illustrations, and read the captions with each.
2. Review the list of vocabulary words to ensure that you know the chapter-related meaning of each. If you are unsure of the meaning of a vocabulary word, look up the word in the glossary or a dictionary, and then study its context in the chapter.
3. On a separate sheet of paper, complete all assigned or selected application and review activities before checking your answers.
4. After you have finished, check your answers against those on the pages referenced in parentheses.
5. Correct any incorrect answers, and review material that was answered incorrectly.

Vocabulary

Be sure that you know the chapter-related meanings of the following words and abbreviations:

- ADA *(91)*
- EEO *(91)*
- motivation *(81)*
- sandwich technique *(90)*

Application of Knowledge

1. Using NFPA 1035 definitions for Public Fire and Life Safety Educator I and II, outline what expectations you as a Public Fire and Life Safety Educator III would have in regard to job performances of Public Fire and Life Safety Educators I and II.

   NOTE: If you need to review the NFPA 1035 definitions, refer to Chapter 1 of this manual, page *12.*

2. Assume you are a Fire and Life Safety Educator III. Using the information on employment interview techniques, outline a list of questions you would ask a candidate applying for the position of Public Fire and Life Safety Educator I. Be sure to keep all questions strictly job-related.

Review Activities

1. List in order from most to least critical Maslow's hierarchy of needs. Briefly explain each level. *(81, 82)*
2. Contrast McGregor's Theory X and Theory Y as they pertain to employee management. *(83)*
3. Explain how managers' high expectations motivate employees. *(83, 84)*
4. Discuss the expectancy theory developed by Victor Vroom. *(84)*
5. List the five tools the American Management Association recommends for increasing employee motivation. *(84)*
6. List the six factors of job design identified by AT &T that increase motivation at work.*(84, 85)*
7. Define the term *position description* and explain its value in hiring or measuring job performance. *(85)*
8. List accepted employment interview techniques. *(88)*
9. List topics that should be avoided during employment interviews because of legal reasons. Explain why these topics should be avoided. *(88, 89)*
10. State the three principal guidelines that managers should follow during appraisal interviews. *(89)*
11. List tips for handling appraisal interviews. *(90)*
12. Discuss several types of job performance problems requiring employee disciplinary action. *(91)*
13. Explain how discipline differs from punishment. *(91)*
14. List the progressive discipline steps used to correct unsatisfactory job performance. *(91)*
15. Explain the importance of the following laws in the workplace:
    - Equal Employment Opportunity *(91)*
    - Americans with Disabilities Act *(91)*

Questions and Notes

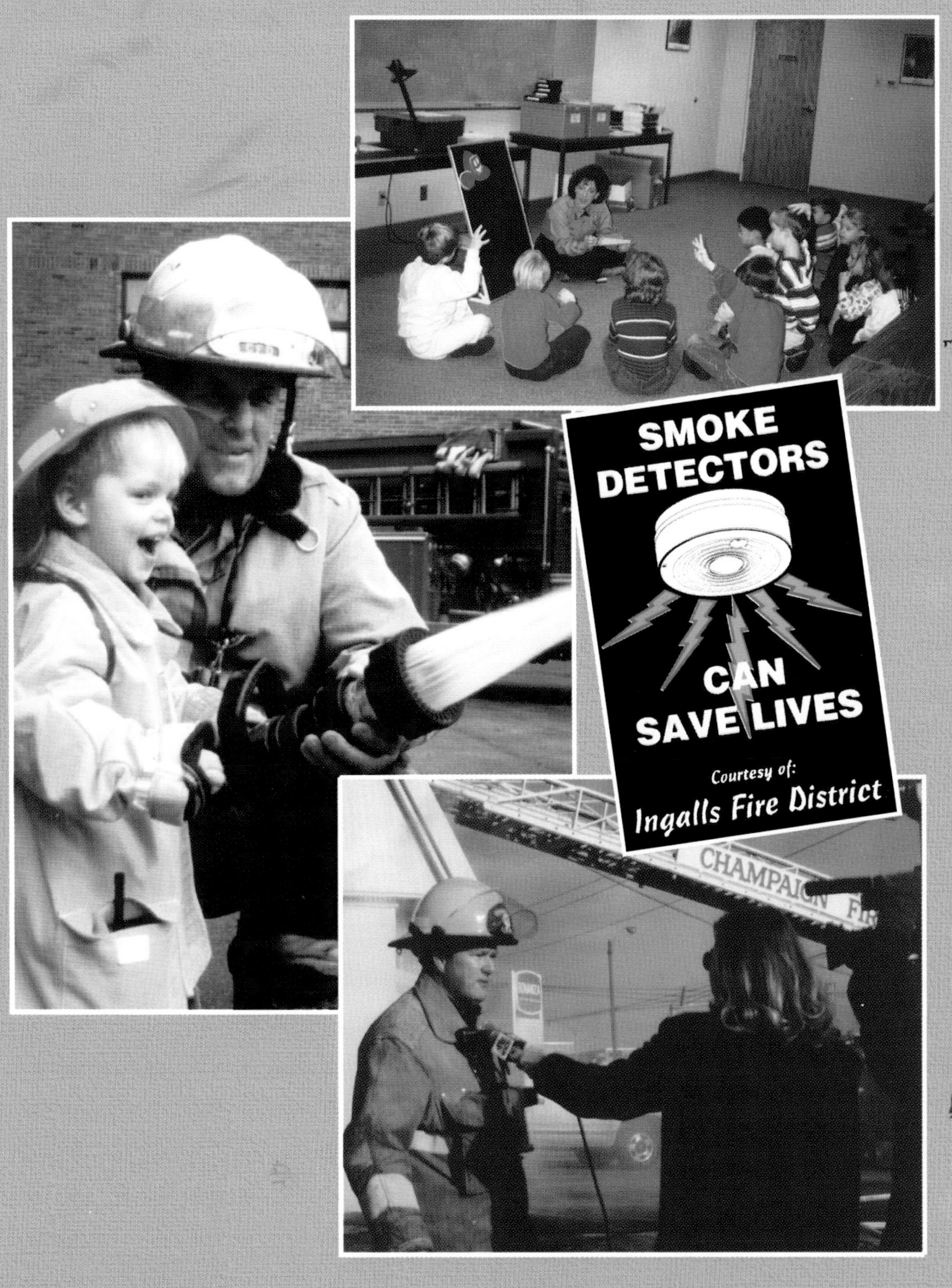
SMOKE
DETECTORS
CAN
SAVE LIVES
Courtesy of:
Ingalls Fire District
CHAMPAIGN

Working Within the Legislative Process

5

LEARNING OBJECTIVES

This chapter provides information that addresses the following objectives of NFPA 1035, *Standard for Professional Qualifications for Public Fire and Life Safety Educator* (1993 edition):

Public Fire and Life Safety Educator III

5-3.1.1 *Prerequisite Knowledge:* Familiarity with public fire and life safety education issues, program administration issues, political issues in public fire and life safety education, and cost/benefit analysis methods.

5-3.3 Develop a public policy recommendation, given an issue, so that solutions are identified, justification addressed, and impact stated.

5-3.3.1 *Prerequisite Knowledge:* Procedures for legislative implementation at the local, state, and national level.

5-4.5 Create a comprehensive public fire and life safety education report for policy makers, given relevant information, so that program goals, objectives, activities, impact, and outcomes are clearly described, evaluated, and summarized.

Chapter 5

Working Within the Legislative Process

INTRODUCTION

Fire and life safety is a public issue for two reasons. First, the need for fire and life safety affects people throughout any community. (NOTE: The "community" could be a city or town, state or province, or nation.) Second, public funds, whether raised through taxes or contributions, pay for fire and life safety education programs in many cases.

For these reasons, fire and life safety educators are affected by the legislative process. From time to time, educators are more directly involved with this process. This involvement may be providing information to citizens and legislators, drafting legislation, or testifying.

This chapter focuses on appropriate ways for fire and life safety educators to work within the legislative process. Lobbying and the differences between policy and politics are addressed, along with techniques for building public support and working with elected officials.

POLICY OR POLITICS?

Fire and life safety programs are part of a community's *public policy*, an overall plan that embraces a community's goals and acceptable procedures. Public policy often involves making tough decisions about public needs and public money. For example:

- Is the community willing to accept the risk of unsprinklered day-care centers?
- Is the community willing to accept the risk of reduced fire department staffing, closed fire stations, or increased emergency response time?
- How much is the community willing to pay to reduce its risks to fire and life safety?
- How will the community pay to reduce its fire and life safety risks? By increasing revenue? (If so, how?) By cutting other expenses? (If so, which ones?)

These decisions are not the fire and life safety educators' decisions to make. Usually, high-level government officials (such as the city manager or fire chief) or other elected representatives (such as the mayor) make public policy decisions. Many times, the decisions happen in the context of budgets, staffing plans, and organizational charts. In other words, the fire and life safety education program's budget, staffing level, and position in the fire department hierarchy, or even the passage of a sales tax to support safety programs define — at least partially — the community's policy on fire and life safety.

Occasionally, the public will make public policy decisions directly, as when voters decide a referendum question. More often, the public influences the decision-makers — by calling and writing, by attending town meetings and budget hearings, and by testifying. For some issues, the public will naturally turn to the fire and life safety educator for information or for support. Providing information and support are very appropriate, as long as the fire and life safety educator identifies the position of management and has the authority to act as a spokesperson *beforehand*.

Policy questions may seem very "political," but the term *politics* usually refers to elective politics. It is not appropriate to mix personal political views and safety legislative business. Elective or party politics is no place for the fire and life safety educator.

WHAT IS LOBBYING?

In everyday use, *lobbying* means educating a person or an organization about your position on an issue or even urging the person or organization to adopt your position. Lobbying also has a legal definition, which is:

> All attempts including personal solicitation to induce legislators to vote in a certain way or to introduce legislation. It includes scrutiny of all pending bills which affect one's interest or the interests of one's clients, with a view towards influencing the passage or defeat of such legislation...Federal, and most state, statutes require that lobbyists be registered.[1]

The message is clear: Their work may place fire and life safety educators on the fringe of lobbying. Fire and life safety educators should always know and follow their jurisdiction's regulations on lobbying.

In many communities, fire and life safety educators are technical resources for legislation on topics ranging from smoke detectors to residential sprinklers to fireworks to bicycle helmets to child safety seats. In other places, the educators are active advocates for legislation on those topics. Both types of activity are appropriate so long as the following conditions are met:

- The fire and life safety educator provides accurate, complete, and current information. For instance, when describing the lifesaving value of smoke detectors, the educator must also discuss the need to maintain the detectors. If the topic is residential sprinklers, the educator needs up-to-date information on installation costs and possible savings on insurance. When giving information in support of fireworks legislation, the educator needs to be prepared to discuss the amount of revenue generated through sales tax, for example, compared to the costs of personal injury, lost acreage, and so forth.
- The fire and life safety educator's management knows about and approves the activity beforehand.
- The activity follows the jurisdiction's regulations on lobbying.

BUILDING PUBLIC SUPPORT

More and more fire and life safety educators have heard the fire chief say, "We have got to get legislation on the books. I want you to make sure it happens." From that moment, the educator must begin to build public support for legislation — legislation that may not even have been drafted yet.

Recently, residential sprinklers have been the topic of local legislation (Figure 5.1). *Strategies for Residential Fire Sprinklers: A Checklist for Community Action* includes guidelines for gaining support for residential sprinklers; many of the ideas apply to other fire and life safety topics. According to that booklet:

> The idea of residential sprinkler legislation will not sell itself in the community. Even if legislative decision-makers are personally convinced that residential sprinklers are needed, their vote will depend upon sentiment in the community and among the builders. *In other words, to convince the City Council, activists for residential sprinklers must first convince community leaders and builders.* Convincing

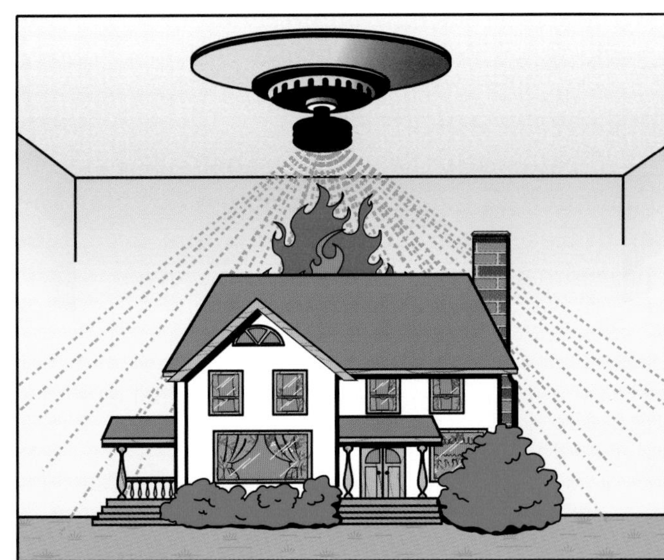

Figure 5.1 The fire and life safety educator must build public support for legislation, such as legislation concerning residential sprinklers.

is not only a first activity; it is a constant activity.[2]

The *Strategies* book lists five steps for gaining community support for legislation. They are "Build In-House Support," "Recruit a Task Force," "Agree on a Legislative Strategy," "Work Effectively with the City Council," and "Agree on Implementation Plans."

Build In-House Support

It is frustrating but true: Gaining support from the fire department and other agencies may be difficult. As a result, the first step in any legislative effort is educating other people in the department and other agencies.

The fire service and other government departments must know about and support plans before going "outside" for community support. It is especially critical that various parts of the fire department — firefighters, fire prevention bureau, all education personnel, union leadership, and public information officer — support the plans early in the coalition-building process (Figure 5.2). The legislation also will need the support of the building official, public works department, and zoning department long before going to the city council.

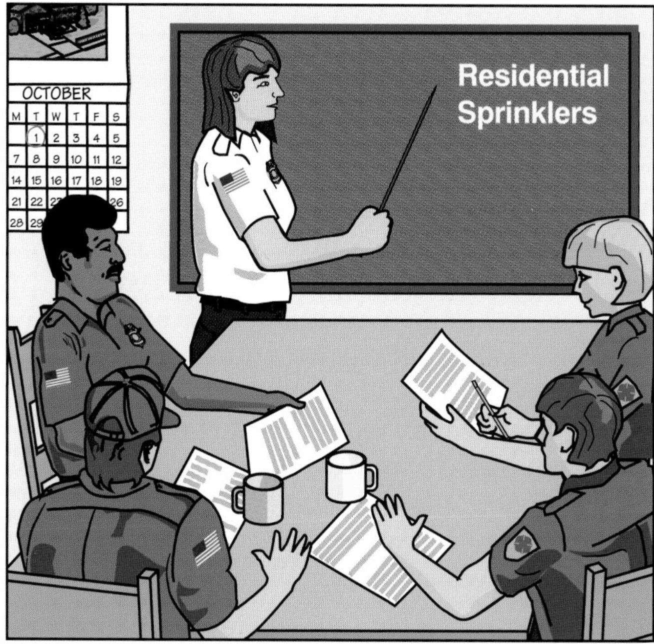

Figure 5.2 The educator must gain "in-house" support before going "outside" for community support.

Recruit a Task Force

Legislation balances the legitimate — but sometimes opposing — viewpoints of different groups. The task force is an informal group formed for a specific purpose; usually a task force will disband after its specific work is done. The task force is a useful way to bring those opposing views into balance (Figure 5.3). In addition, the task force is a fact-finding group. Task groups on residential sprinklers, for example, can be charged with answering questions such as these:

- How many new housing units will be built in 5 years? in 10 years?
- How many local companies are qualified to install residential sprinklers? Who determines what the qualifications should be?
- How much do local builders estimate that a sprinkler system will add to the cost of a home? How do those estimates compare with costs in other communities?
- What companies offer insurance discounts? how much of a discount?
- Will the water company or public works department charge special hookup or monthly fees? how much?
- Do nearby jurisdictions have legislation pending? in place?
- What have other communities done?

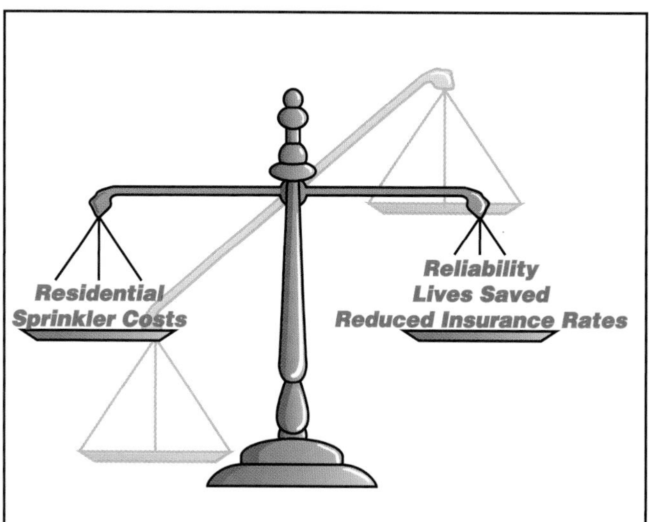

Figure 5.3 A task force can be used to bring opposing viewpoints concerning legislation into balance.

In the area of child passenger safety seats, questions include the following:

- What are the injury rates? in cars? in vans? in other vehicles? What ages are affected?
- What are the costs of the injuries?
- Has similar legislation been attempted somewhere else?
- How much will it cost to enforce a law on child passenger safety seats?

In the area of fireworks, questions would include the following:

- Which groups support a ban? Which groups oppose one?
- How much sales revenue is generated? How much tax revenue is generated?
- How widespread is the use of fireworks?
- How many injuries happen? What kinds of injuries occur? How much do the injuries cost? hospitalization? medical bills? medication? lost wages?
- What is the injury experience of states that do not permit fireworks?
- What are transportation and storage issues?
- How would enforcement work? Who would do the enforcement? How much would it cost?
- In what areas do most injuries occur?

To answer questions such as these, a good task force needs both advocates and adversaries. A task force of friends and foes of legislation allows different facts to come out. Different views will be heard. Disagreements can be worked out at the task force level, before going to the public.

Agree on a Legislative Strategy

The facts and views that a task force discovers will lead to a legislative strategy. A *legislative strategy* is "the task force's idea for which kind of legislation offers the most protection — and also has the best chance of adoption. In other words, *the legislative strategy is a compromise between what some parties want and what all parties can live with*"[3] (Figure 5.4).

There are many areas for negotiation in developing a legislative strategy. For example, areas for negotiation include the kind of housing to be covered in residential sprinkler legislation (new or existing housing? single-family or apartment? manufactured housing?), the effective date (now or three years from now? one date for all occupancies or one effective date for each type of occupancy?), and any other protection that will not be required if sprinklers are in place.

Fire and life safety educators are used to being strong advocates. The idea of negotiating safety may make them uncomfortable. However, give-and-take is a legislative reality. *The goal is to find the best legislation that can be passed.* In the interests of getting legislation passed soon, some issues may simply have to wait for another time. For example, Oklahoma's first passenger seat belt law applied only to passenger vehicles. Later, however, the law was expanded to include pickup trucks.

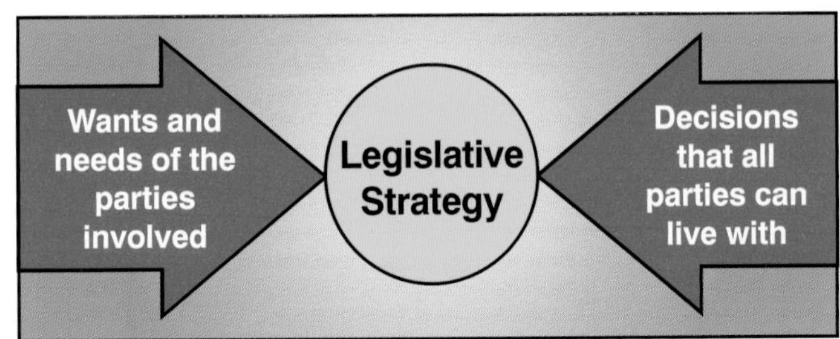

Figure 5.4 After the task force gathers the needed information, it develops the legislative strategy.

Agree on Implementation Plans

In the area of safety legislation, *implementation* is another way of saying "quality control." In other words, implementation is activity by the fire department and others to make sure that the sprinkler systems will meet standards, that fireworks regulations are enforced, etc. Some legislation will include specific implementation plans; other will not. The important thing is to have all implementation plans in place well before the legislation's effective date.

The media can play a key role in implementation plans. For example, feature segments on television news programs can highlight the upcoming effective date of a ban on certain kinds of fireworks. This kind of public awareness makes enforcement much easier!

WORKING WITH ELECTED OFFICIALS

At one time or another, many fire and life safety educators will find themselves working with elected officials. The activity may range from testifying before the city council about the fire department budget, to meeting with state or provincial legislators about pending legislation, to writing to a U.S. representative, senator, or Canadian member of Parliament about federal legislation or regulation. The basic techniques for working with elected officials apply at any level of government and on any topic.

Whatever their party or philosophy, elected officials have two qualities that fire and life safety educators need to work with.

First, elected officials are political people. They decide issues based on what their constituents want. That is what elected government is all about! For every issue, elected officials will want to know answers to the following questions:

- How does this affect my constituents?
- What do my constituents feel about this?
- Who supports this issue and why? Who opposes this issue and why?
- What will I gain or lose by supporting this issue? by opposing it?

In short, fire educators and legislators decide issues very differently. To the educator, public safety is the deciding factor. To the legislator, public perception is all-important. For this reason, building public support is critical.

Second, elected officials are extremely busy. Their time is fragmented. They have to know about and make decisions about a very wide variety of topics. Informing them about an issue and gaining their support is often a matter of presenting information as quickly and clearly as possible. As soon as the information is presented, the legislator will want to know exactly what the educator wants. Does the educator want a meeting with the legislator? help in arranging a meeting with someone else? help in introducing or cosponsoring a bill? *The educator must be prepared to explain the issue and ask for specific help in as few words as possible.*

NOTE: As used here, "elected officials" could serve on any level of government and could be legislators or senior administrators (such as the mayor). For simplicity, this chapter uses "legislators" to refer to all elected officials.

What determines how to work with elected officials? The educator's own experience, how well the educator and legislator know each other, the political climate in the community, and the jurisdiction's rules about lobbying are just a few of the determining factors. Regardless of these factors, seven general guidelines apply (Figure 5.5).

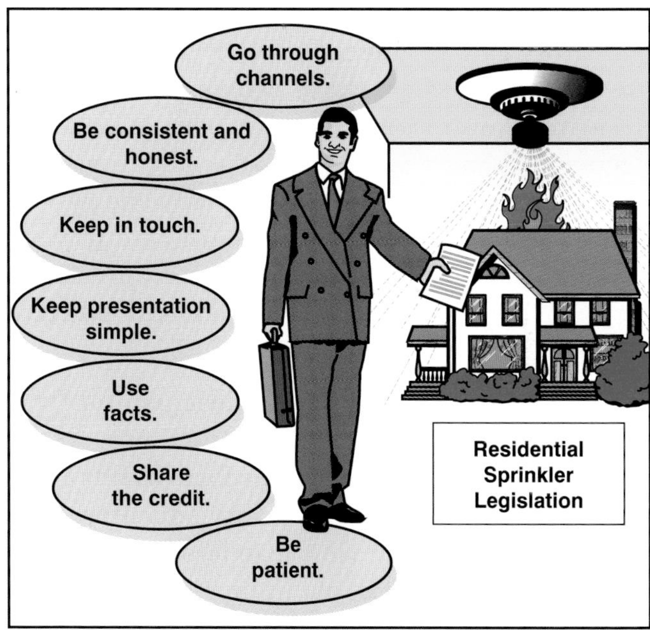
Go through channels.
Be consistent and honest.
Keep in touch.
Keep presentation simple.
Use facts.
Share the credit.
Be patient.
Residential Sprinkler Legislation

Figure 5.5 Guidelines for working with elected officials.

Go Through Channels

Working with powerful elected legislators sounds very exciting — and it can be! The chance to be part of the action, part of an inner circle, and even part of the behind-the-scenes maneuvering is attractive. However, the only way to be part of the legislative process is to go through channels. Quite simply, fire and life safety educators who do not work through channels risk losing a good working relationship with their management long after a bill is passed or defeated.

Educators should keep their management fully informed about contacts with legislators or legislative staff. It is a good practice to report all contacts.

Large fire service organizations (a large urban department or state agency) may have one person who handles legislative matters. In addition to going through management channels, fire and life safety educators should work with these legislative experts.

Be Consistent and Honest

Legislators are not safety experts. As a result, they need information presented consistently so that they can understand it clearly. For example, the distinction between the number of fire deaths and the rate of fire deaths per 100 people may not be clear to the legislator. Fire educators can help legislators by saying things such as, "Last year, three people died in home fires in your district. That's about X per 100 people, or almost twice the national average. In Representative Smith's district, only one person died in a home fire. The fire death rate in your district is three times as high as in Representative Smith's. That's why we need your positive vote on the residential sprinkler bill."

Every story has two sides, and legislators will *always* hear the other side of the story. Being honest about opposing views or facts builds credibility for the fire and life safety educator. Presenting the opposing view also lets that view be heard in the best possible light. For example:

> "You'll hear that residential sprinklers add to the cost of a home, and they do. Contractors in this town estimate that sprinklers will cost between 60 cents and a dollar per square foot. In other words, the home buyer would spend about as much on fire sprinklers as on an intercom system. Over the lifetime of the home, the reduced insurance rates will pay for the fire sprinklers."

Be in Touch Regularly

Legislators are busy, but they also crave information. Passing along information routinely satisfies their hunger for information and makes the educator (and fire and life safety issues) known to the legislator. Newspaper clippings or notes are good ways to stay in regular touch. For example, a clipping about a neighboring jurisdiction's new fireworks regulation, sent with a note about the number of fireworks injuries in the legislator's district, will get attention.

Keep Presentations Simple

Legislators often decide complex issues based on the information on one piece of paper. Sometimes, legislators read this information on the way to the vote. They do not have time to become experts, but they will rely on others to be technical resources for them.

Whether written or verbal, make material for legislators easy to understand. (**NOTE**: Try testing the material on a nonfire person, such as a neighbor.) Present technical information simply. Present all information consistently and honestly.

Use Facts to Make the Case

Fire and life safety educators believe in what they are doing and know that their work is critical to public safety. As a result, educators may rely on emotion to make their case. "You have to do this, or people will die!" is an example of relying on emotion.

Legislators use emotion, too, but will need solid facts. Providing solid facts about the safety impact of legislative decisions is an important part of the educator's job.

Share the Credit

Elected officials thrive on credit for helping their constituents. Their need for credit, in fact, may make them take *all* the credit. This is a political reality that fire and life safety educators simply must accept. Sharing the credit with legislators needs to happen privately and publicly. For example, a news photo of a legislator dedicating a new fire and life safety education van is a very public recognition of the legislator's assistance. Some educators make special efforts to share the credit with legislators — knowing that the elected officials will then be happy to support the *next* piece of safety legislation.

Be Patient

Fire and life safety educators are people in a hurry. The legislative process, on the other hand, seems painfully slow and deliberate. Legislation takes time. And all proposed legislation does not get enacted. A fire and life safety education bill might not get passed on the first few attempts. However, the issue will have gained some public support, and the educator will have gained valuable contacts and experience. The outcome may be better the next time.

CONCLUSION

Fire and life safety educators are persuasive people; they use their skills daily to persuade their audiences to change their behavior to be more safe. Their persuasive skills and work specialty sometimes move fire and life safety educators from the classroom to the hearing room. As they become involved in the political process, fire and life safety educators do the following:

- Recognize that high-level government officials or elected representatives make public policy decisions.
- Avoid partisan politics.
- Know and follow the jurisdiction's rules on lobbying.
- Know how to build public support.
- Work effectively with elected officials.

The legislative process is a new arena for most fire and life safety educators. Following the techniques and guidelines in this chapter increases the chances of getting safety legislation adopted.

Chapter 5 Notes

1. *Black's Law Dictionary*, West Publishing Company, St. Paul, MN, 1990, p. 938.
2. Pam Powell, *Strategies for Residential Sprinklers: A Checklist for Community Action*, Operation Life Safety/International Association of Fire Chiefs, Fairfax, VA, 1992, p. 9.
3. Powell, p. 18.

Chapter 6
Planning Fire and Life Safety Education

INTRODUCTION

Public educators almost always agree that there is never enough money and rarely enough time to deliver their programs. Because money and time are so scarce, public fire and life safety educators have become very skilled at finding new resources and at targeting their resources for maximum impact. In the language of public education, these skills are often called "planning" or "systematic planning."

Although planning is as old as public education, the roots of modern public fire and life safety education planning can be traced to 1979 when the U.S. Fire Administration (USFA) published *Public Fire Education Planning: A Five Step Process*.[1] The overall goal of the publication is to assist public fire and life safety educators in finding new resources and targeting these resources for maximum impact.

For more than a decade, public fire and life safety education planning has developed into the evolving field of public fire and life safety education. The National Fire Academy included the five-step process in its earliest public fire and life safety education curricula, reaching large numbers of fire service personnel. The Academy's newest public education course, titled "Presenting Effective Public Education Programs," includes basic education principles and presentation skills. The first edition of IFSTA 606, **Public Fire Education**,[2] devoted its first chapter to the five-step process. The five-step process was discussed and illustrated in "The Need to Know" chapter of the fifteenth edition of *Fire Protection Handbook*.[3] NFPA 1035, *Standard for Professional Qualifications for Public Fire and Life Safety Educator*, includes planning as a professional qualification for public fire and life safety educators in the fire service. *Introduction to Fire Prevention*[4] discusses the systematic planning process.

In recent years, there have been some significant refinements to public fire and life safety education planning. For example, the *Fire Education Evaluation Guide*[5] and *Proving Public Fire Education Works*[6] have advanced the public educator's understanding of how to assess program impact. As part of its two-week course, "Developing Fire and Life Safety Strategies," the National Fire Academy teaches participants the planning, implementation, and evaluation strategies necessary to make public education decisions.

This chapter discusses the five-step planning process and the decisions and tasks involved with each step. The last sections show how the five-step process was applied in various public education programs.

THE FIVE-STEP PLANNING PROCESS: OVERVIEW

Public Fire Education Planning: A Five Step Process presents a systematic planning and action process composed of five steps (Figure 6.1):

- **Identification** of major fire problems
- **Selection** of the most cost-effective objectives for the education program

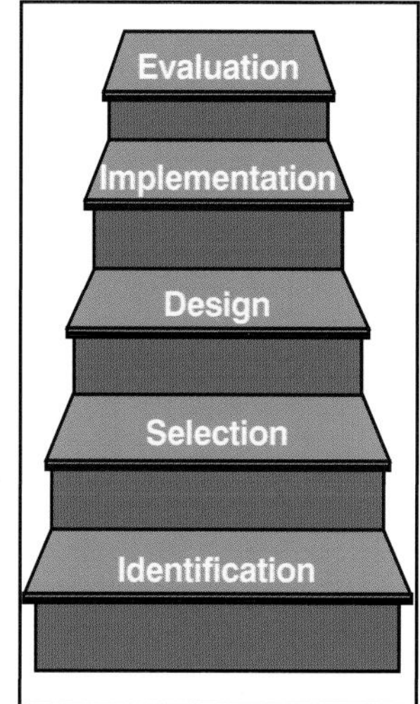

Figure 6.1 The five-step planning process.

- **Design** of the program itself
- **Implementation** of the program plan
- **Evaluation** of the fire safety program to determine impact

These steps — or similar steps with different names — are not limited to public fire and life safety education planning; they are also well recognized in other safety education disciplines.[7]

In the five-step planning process, each step consists of several fact-finding activities and a decision (Figure 6.2). The fact-finding activities involve answering a series of questions about the local jurisdiction. A suggested "to do" list is

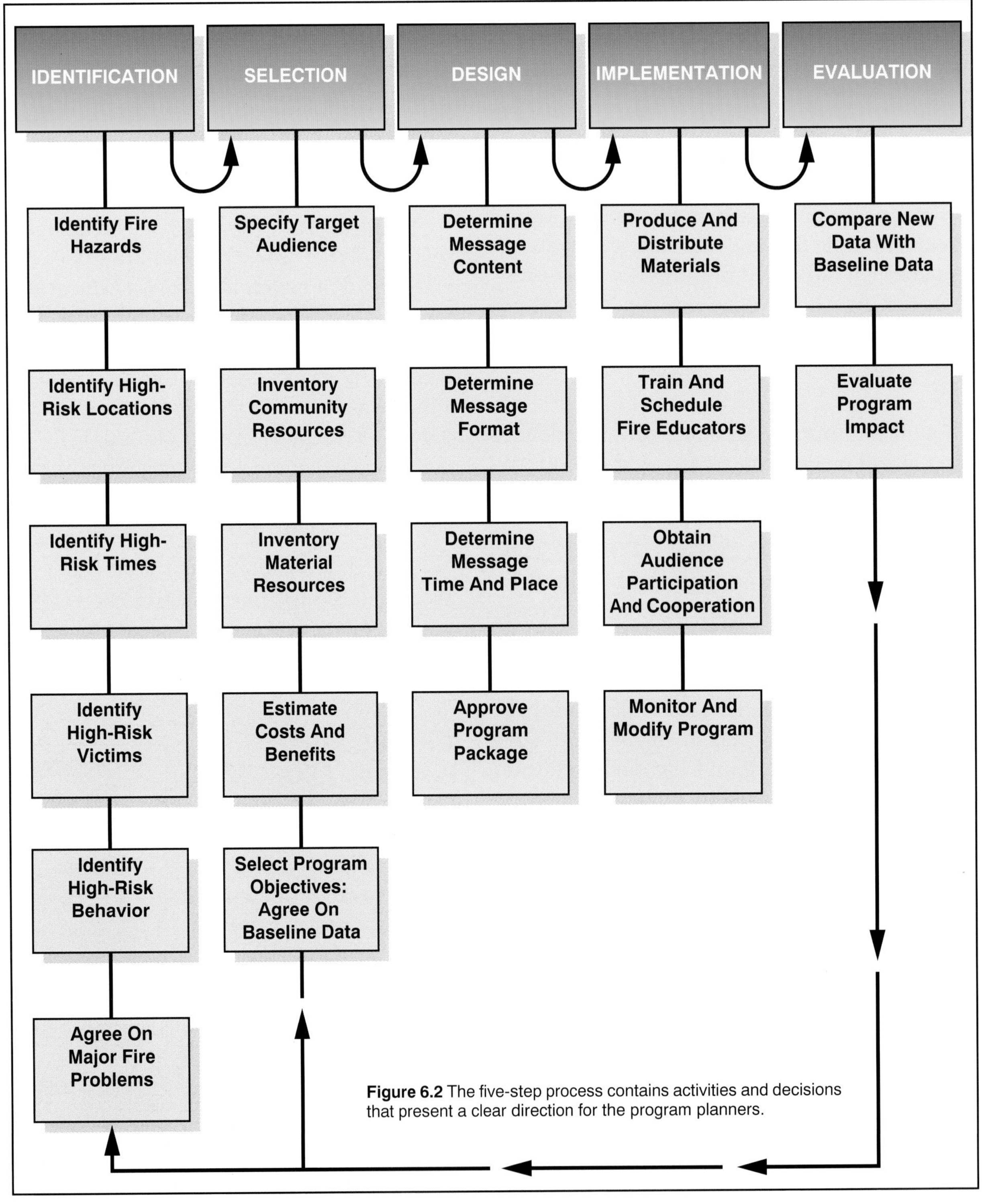

Figure 6.2 The five-step process contains activities and decisions that present a clear direction for the program planners.

included for each activity. Experienced users of the five-step planning process advise "first-timers" to be flexible with the "to do" list — the list illustrates the kind of tasks that will need doing, not a hard and fast checklist. The five-step method can be used for planning any of the various types of fire and life safety education programs. However, for the purposes of this discussion, the examples focus on fire and burn prevention themes.

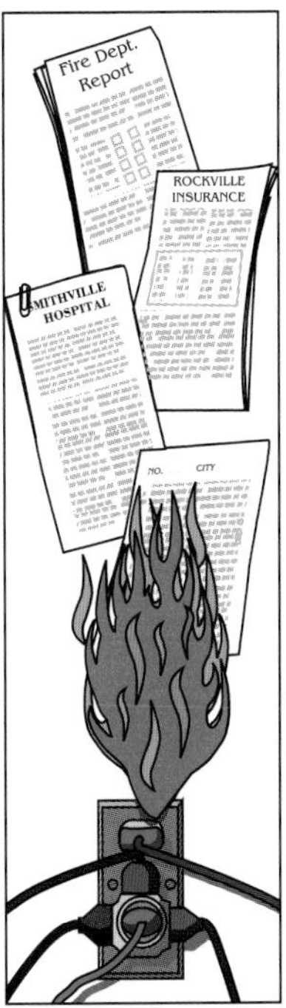

Figure 6.3 A successful public fire education program begins with identifying the most important local fire problems.

Identification

Identifying major local fire and life safety problems and concerns is the objective of Identification. The following are some of the questions asked during the identification process:

- **What are the major fire and burn hazards** (Figure 6.3)**?**
  - — Locate records showing causes of fires and burns.
  - — Select most frequent causes of fires and burns.
  - — Determine local patterns of fires and burns.
- **Where are the high-risk locations** (Figure 6.4)**?**
  - — Locate neighborhoods or building occupancy types with high fire and burn risks.
  - — Discover what is causing the risks to be above-average.
  - — Plan to concentrate programs and personnel in high-risk locations.
- **When are the high-risk times** (Figure 6.5)**?**
  - — Identify times of day, week, or year with the highest incidence of fire loss or burn injuries.
  - — Identify types of fires occurring at these times.
  - — Plan to concentrate fire safety messages at these times.

Figure 6.4 Those neighborhoods or building types determined as having the highest rate of fires are identified on a map.

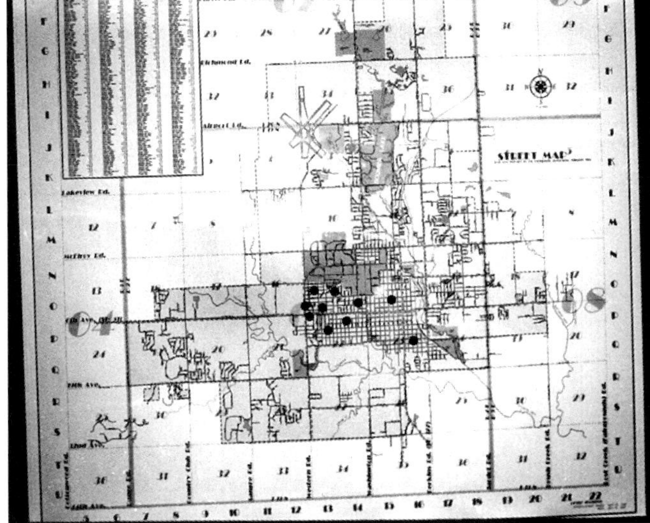

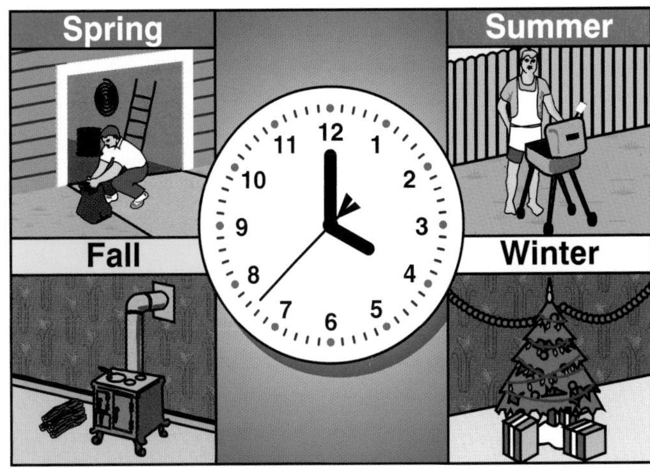

Figure 6.5 Identify high-risk times, and organize programs that alert people to the times of high fire danger.

- **Who are the high-risk victims** (Figure 6.6)**?**
  - — Identify groups with high fire death and injury rates.
  - — Determine why they have a high fire rate.
  - — Involve these groups in the fire education effort.
- **What is the high-risk behavior** (Figure 6.7)**?**
  - — Determine which behaviors — acts or omissions — cause fires and burn injuries.
  - — Decide how the behaviors can be changed.
  - — Teach the people exactly what to do.

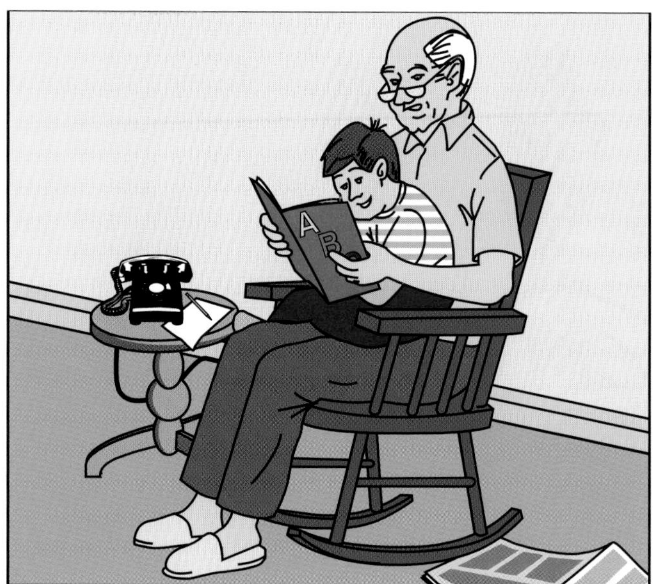

Figure 6.6 Identify high-risk victims, and direct fire and life safety education toward them.

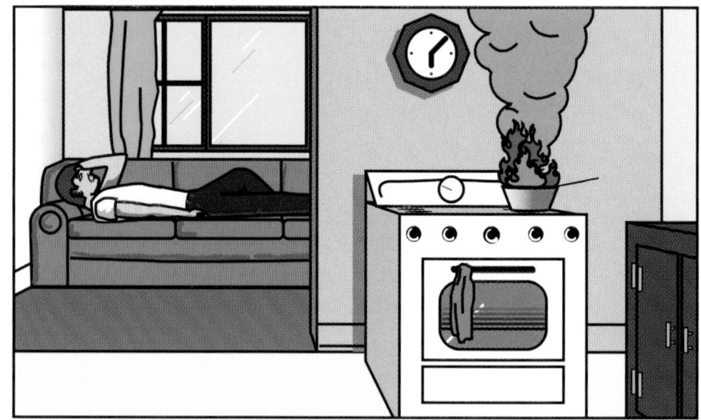

Figure 6.7 Identify behavior patterns that may lead to a fire, and design intervention programs to change these behaviors.

What's the Difference Between a *Hazard* and a *Risk*?

In everyday speech, the terms *hazard* and *risk* are often used interchangeably. Technically, however, hazards and risks describe two different things.

The term *hazard* usually refers to the source of a risk. A *risk*, on the other hand, is the likelihood of suffering harm from a hazard.* Risk can also be thought of as the potential for failure or loss. In other words, *risk* is the exposure to the hazard, and a *hazard* is a condition, substance, or device that can directly cause an injury or loss.

Examples of fire-related hazards include ignition sources (such as smoking materials or electrical wiring) or behaviors (such as children playing with smoking materials or persons overloading electrical outlets).

Fire risk is often expressed as the number of incidents, injuries, or deaths per capita (for each unit of the population). Depending upon the source of information, the per capita unit may be 1,000 people — or a million people. It pays to be clear as to what per capita means in each statistical table or report; that way, the public fire and life safety educator can avoid comparing apples to oranges!

Education programs — no matter how good they are — cannot change hazards that are substances or devices. For example, education simply cannot change the temperature of a cigarette lighter or the flammability of gasoline. (**NOTE:** Technology may change substances or devices.) Education can, however, change some conditions or behaviors, such as smoking and drinking at the same time. Other conditions — age or disability, for example — are unchangeable. In those cases, the educator will develop programs to reduce the risk, the exposure to the hazard. For example, a program to teach nursing home caregivers to supervise residents' smoking helps reduce risk (likelihood of suffering harm from a hazard, potential for failure or loss, or exposure to a hazard) even though the hazards (sources of risk or the condition, substance, or device) are unchanged.

*These definitions are taken from *Risk Analysis: A Guide to Principles and Methods for Analyzing Health and Environmental Risks* by John J. Cohrssen and Vincent T. Covello. *Risk Analysis* was published in 1989 by the Council on Environmental Quality, Executive Office of the President, and is available from the National Technical Information Service, U.S. Department of Commerce, 5285 Port Royal Road, Springfield, VA 22161, as NTIS Order Number PB 89-137772.

Gradually, a picture or scenario of a community's biggest fire and life safety problems will begin to emerge. In some cases, answers to two or three of the questions may combine to form a scenario (such as "inoperable smoke detectors in single-family homes" or "burn injuries from scalds to residents of the Pine Meadow Retirement Apartments"). In other cases, a single issue (juvenile firesetting, for example) will emerge as "the" problem.

Pinpointing fire and life safety problems to be attacked is the critical first step in developing a targeted training program. The answers lead to a decision: Agree on the major fire or burn or life safety problem to be reduced through education.

Selection

The objective of Selection is to choose the most cost-effective or achievable objectives for the fire education program. Knowing resources is key to being realistic about what an education program can accomplish. As a result, the questions in the Selection step focus on resources. In many ways, the Selection step comes close to a primer on finding new resources — funding, materials, and talented people — for public fire and life safety education.

Following are some of the questions and sample tasks considered in the selection step of planning:

- **Who are your potential audiences?**
  - — Refer to the high-risk victims listed in Identification.
  - — Identify those who influence the high-risk victims.
  - — Select the audience on which the educator will have the greatest potential impact.
- **What are your community resources for fire and life safety education?**
  - — Identify influential people in the community.
  - — List all local media and civic organizations.
  - — Make personal contact with key people and groups.
- **What materials can you use** (Figure 6.8)**?**
  - — Ask local businesses and organizations what materials, equipment, or skills they could donate to your program.
  - — Determine availability and cost of fire education materials.
  - — Review existing programs, and determine the advantages of purchasing educational materials versus making your own.
- **What are the potential costs and benefits of various training options** (Figure 6.9)**?**
  - — List alternative program objectives.
  - — Estimate costs of alternative program objectives.
  - — Estimate loss-reduction impact of each program objective. (How much reduced loss can *realistically* be expected?)

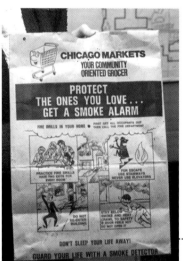

Figure 6.8 Local stores may donate their services or provide materials for fire prevention activities. *Courtesy of Glenn Rousey, Rock Island Fire Department, Rock Island, Illinois.*

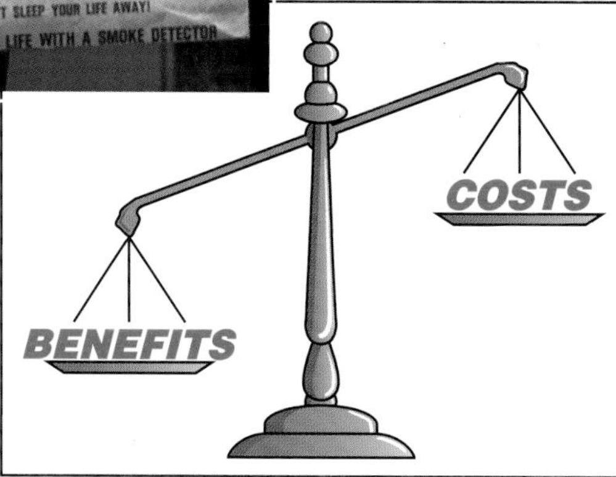

Figure 6.9 The benefits of meeting the program's objectives should outweigh the costs of implementation.

— Choose the most effective approach within limits of local resources.

By the end of the Selection step, the public fire and life safety educator will be able to reach a crucial decision — the specific objectives of the education program. The objectives should be clear, measurable, and attainable.

> **A Sample Objective**
>
> A good objective states what the student (audience member) is expected to learn and also how the student will be evaluated. The following is a psychomotor objective — that is, an objective dealing with learning a psychomotor skill or performance:
>
> At the conclusion of the presentation to the Kiwanis Club on residential fire safety and given a smoke detector for demonstration purposes (*conditions*), the Kiwanis participant will be able to change the smoke detector's battery (*performance or criterion*) so that the detector's alarm sounds when tested (*standard or criterion*).

In addition, answers from the questions in Selection will be used to complete the design, implementation, and evaluation steps. For example, information about major fire hazards and high-risk locations, times, victims, and behaviors will be very helpful when it is time to answer Design questions such as "What is your primary message?" In much the same way, insight about high-risk victims and potential audiences is critically important in deciding on the best formats, times, and places for education messages.

> **Program Design**
>
> The selection and design steps are so closely related that they tend to blend together. That is okay! The important thing is to make sure that the program design is based on specific objectives selected to solve the local problem.

Design

The Design step is the bridge between planning a fire education program and actually implementing it in the field. The objective of Design is to design and develop effective educational materials for the program. In other words, this is the time when the fire educator decides what to say and how to say it, based on message, audience, and resources.

Following are some of the questions asked during the Design step of planning (Figure 6.10):

- **What is the content of the fire and life safety education message?**
  — Direct messages toward specific hazards.
  — Appeal to positive motives.
  — Show the context of the problem and desired behavior.
- **What is the best format for the message?**
  — Match format to message.
  — Match format to audience.
  — Match format to resources.
- **What is the best time and place to deliver the message?**
  — Determine when the target audience will be most receptive to fire and life safety messages.
  — Schedule (both time and place) messages for maximum effect.

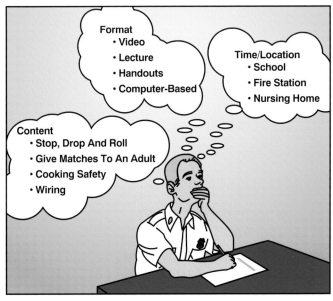

Figure 6.10 During the design phase, the educator decides what to say and how to say it and then puts the program into a package that can be used by everyone involved in the effort.

After answering these questions, the public fire and life safety educator is ready to actually design a program package and determine how to produce the program materials. Presenting the planned materials to a sample audience is a good "reality check" at this point. The decision at the end of the Design step is to approve an education program package.

Implementation

Implementation is the step in which the day-to-day job of public fire and life safety education happens. Most educators can expect to spend most of their time implementing (or "delivering") programs (Figure 6.11).

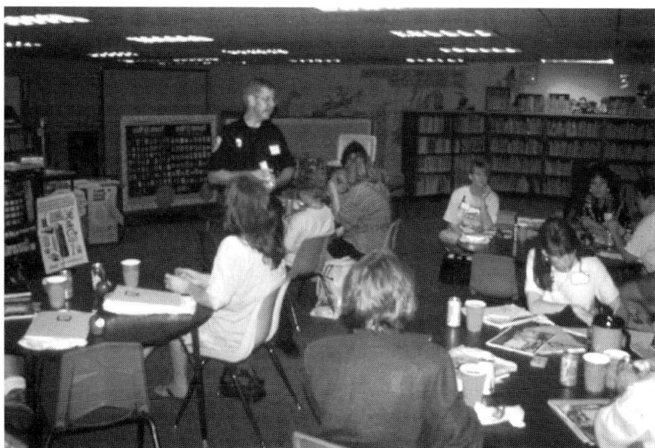

Figure 6.11 An educator makes a presentation — an important component of the program delivery.

The Implementation step of planning includes the following questions and tasks:

- **How will the target audience participate and cooperate in implementing the program?**
  - Involve target groups in implementing programs.
  - Tell target audiences what to expect.
  - Reinforce messages through endorsement by local opinion leaders.
- **How will fire educators be trained and scheduled?**
  - Organize fire service personnel and volunteers from outside the fire service.
  - Match community contacts with target audiences.
  - Train people for their education job.
- **How will materials be produced and distributed** (Figure 6.12)**?**
  - Assign production responsibilities.
  - Produce or purchase materials.
  - Distribute materials to target audiences.

To make sure that the education program plan that looked so good "on paper" works, the educator will need to observe day-to-day program operation. In this way, the public fire and life safety educator will be guided to the ultimate Implementation decision: Monitor and make ongoing refinements to the program as needed during its implementation.

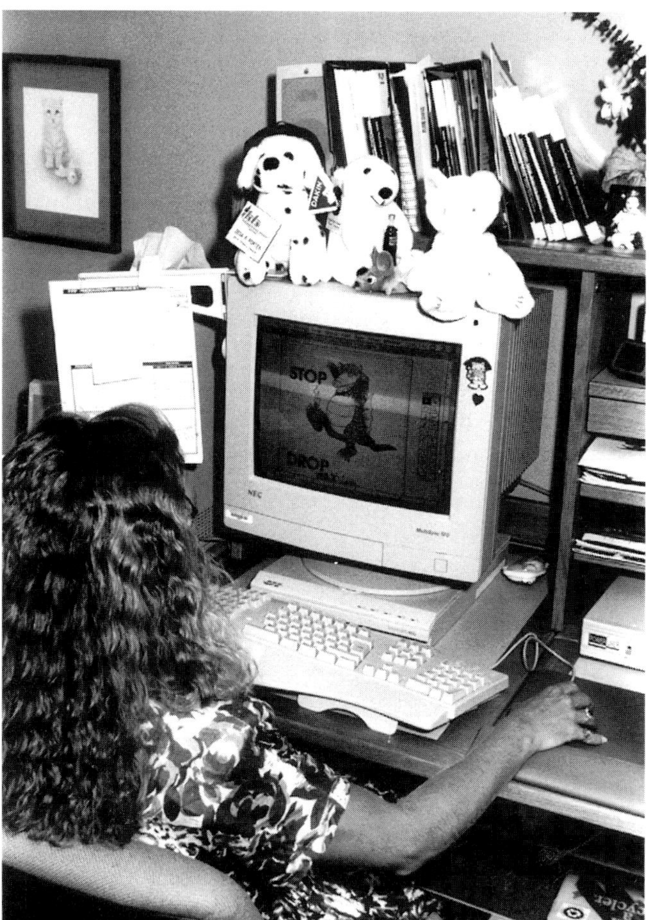

Figure 6.12 An educator creates educational materials for a fire and life safety education program.

Evaluation

Evaluation is public fire and life safety education's "bottom line," the point for measuring the impact of education programs and modifying programs as needed. The techniques of public education program evaluation have improved significantly since *Public Fire Education Planning: A Five Step Process* was published. These state-of-the-art techniques are covered in Chapter 11, "Evaluating Presentations and Programs."

FIRE AND LIFE SAFETY EDUCATION PLANNING IN ACTION

Fire departments (and other fire organizations) across North America now use some sort of "planning" as a tool for targeting scarce public fire and life safety education resources for maximum impact. In some cases, the fire educators use a formal planning approach such as the five-step planning process. In other cases, the educators adopt the concepts of planning and targeting resources even though they do not follow a step-by-step approach.

Two recent publications, *Public Fire Education Today: Fire Service Programs Across America*[8] and *Proving Public Fire Education Works*, are filled with examples of how local fire departments have targeted their resources for public fire and life safety education. The first three of the following four examples are taken from *Proving Public Fire Education Works*.[9]

Case Study 1 — Southeast Asian Fire Awareness Program (Portland, Maine)

Identification. Cambodian, Vietnamese, and other Southeast Asian people were often living communally with several families sharing one apartment in a neighborhood approximately 1 square mile in size. Though this group represented only 2 percent of the city's total population, they accounted for a disproportionately large share of the city's fire runs and more than half of the fire deaths.

Selection. In cooperation with the local Knights of Columbus, Portland obtained funding from the U.S. Fire Administration's National Community Volunteer Fire Prevention Program. The objective of the program was to decrease fire runs in the Southeast Asian neighborhood so that the neighborhood's run rate matched that of other neighborhoods in the city.

Design. The education program package consisted of two fire safety brochures in each of four languages (Cambodian, Vietnamese, Laotian, and English) and three television public service announcements (with English subtitles) in Cambodian and Vietnamese. The educational messages in the program package were refined through results of fire safety surveys, which were knowledge tests taken by 400 to 500 members of the target population.

Implementation. More than 4,000 brochures were distributed to the target population, according to fire department estimates. Actors for the public service announcements (PSAs) came from the target groups, an excellent example of gaining the participation of the target population. Thanks to the cooperation of local television stations, the PSAs were aired more than 100 times — in the daytime — during the summer, reaching an estimated 1,800 members of the Southeast Asian community.

Evaluation. Fire runs to the target neighborhood dropped from 316 the year before the program to 96 runs during the year of the program, a drop of more than 70 percent. This new run rate approximated the run rate in other Portland neighborhoods — fulfilling the objective set for the program.

There was a 95 percent confidence level that the decrease was *not* due to chance, according to fire department calculations. Although the number of runs rose to 111 the year after the program, that number is still far lower than the preprogram level.

Case Study 2 — "Fry It Safe" Program (Chesterfield County, Virginia)

Identification. Cooking was the number-one cause of structural fires countywide.

Selection. With free material provided by the Institute of Shortening and Edible Oils, the fire department intended to reach 500 middle school students in home economics classes.

Design. The education program package included handout sheets and a video called *Fry It Safe*, both provided by the Institute of Shortening and Edible Oils and covering cooking fire safety.

11. List questions that the public fire and life safety educator should ask when planning the implementation of the program. *(117)*

12. List two methods of answering each of the questions in Activity 11. *(117)*

13. Describe several ways that you could evaluate (at the conclusion of the program) whether or not your program objectives had been met. Glean some ideas about evaluation methods by examining those in the examples in the "Fire and Life Safety Education Planning in Action" section of the chapter. *(118-120)*

Questions and Notes

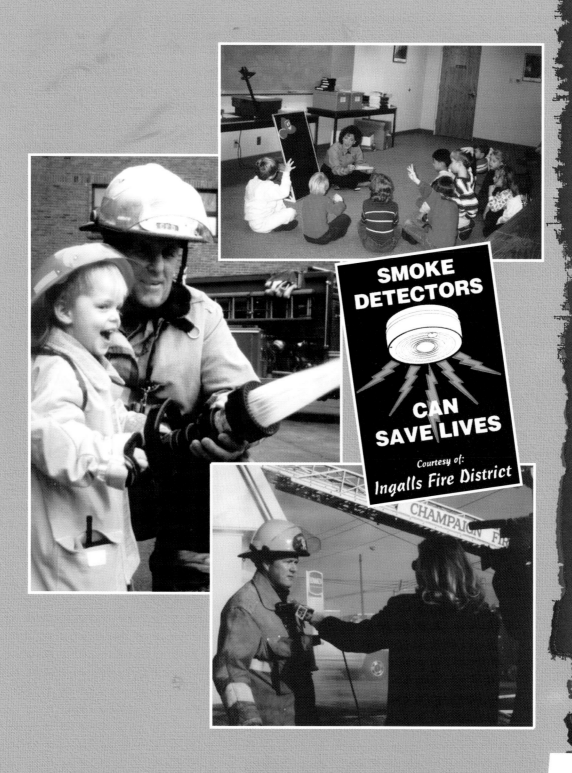

7 Using Data to Plan Programs

LEARNING OBJECTIVES

This chapter provides information that addresses the following objectives of NFPA 1035, *Standard for Professional Qualifications for Public Fire and Life Safety Educator* (1993 edition):

Public Fire and Life Safety Educator II

4-3.1 Establish public fire and life safety education program priorities, given relevant local loss and injury data, so that local public fire and life safety education needs are identified.

4-3.1.1 *Prerequisite Knowledge:* Content of reports and data.

4-3.1.2 *Prerequisite Skills:* Systematic data collection and analysis.

Public Fire and Life Safety Educator III

5-2.1 Create public fire and life safety education goals and objectives, given an organization's mission statement, available resources, and local loss statistics, so that the goals are consistent with the organization's mission and reflect the public's need for education.

5-2.1.1 *Prerequisite Skills:* Organizational planning, resource management, and data analysis.

5-3.2 Evaluate current and future trends, given trend data, so that current and anticipated fire and life safety issues are identified.

5-3.2.1 *Prerequisite Knowledge:* Demographics, cultural and value shifts, governmental regulations, environmental issues, and technological changes.

5-3.2.2 *Prerequisite Skills:* Trend analysis.

Chapter 7 Review

Directions

The following activities are designed to help you comprehend and apply the information in Chapter 7 of **Fire and Life Safety Educator**, second edition. To receive the maximum learning experience from these activities, it is recommended that you use the following procedure:

1. Read the chapter, underlining or highlighting important terms, topics, and subject matter. Read the sidebar material, study the photographs and illustrations, and read the captions with each.
2. Review the list of vocabulary words to ensure that you know the chapter-related meaning of each. If you are unsure of the meaning of a vocabulary word, look up the word in the glossary or a dictionary, and then study its context in the chapter.
3. On a separate sheet of paper, complete all assigned or selected application and review activities before checking your answers.
4. After you have finished, check your answers against those on the pages referenced in parentheses.
5. Correct any incorrect answers, and review material that was answered incorrectly.

Vocabulary

Be sure that you know the chapter-related meanings of the following words:

- acute *(132)*
- baseline data *(134)*
- catastrophic *(131)*
- database *(133)*
- data/datum (127)
- demographic *(127)*
- etiological/etiology *(132)*
- incendiary *(128)*
- optimum *(132)*
- random sample (127)
- statistics *(127)*
- stratified *(127)*
- tally *(128)*
- target audience *(127)*
- therapeutic *(132)*

Application of Knowledge

1. Obtain the latest September/October *NFPA Journal®* or a copy of *Fire Loss in Canada.* Read the fire loss articles and data, and then answer the following questions:
   - What category of fires caused the largest dollar losses?
   - What was the total monetary loss for direct property damage for the year?
   - What was the year's most costly fire?
   - Was the number of large-loss fires for the year higher or lower than the previous year's large-loss fires?
   - Was the number of civilian deaths higher or lower than the previous year?
   - What area of the country had the highest civilian deaths and injuries?
   - What area had the highest fire incident rates in the nation?
2. Obtain the latest November/December *NFPA Journal®* or a copy of *Fire Loss in Canada.* Read the articles and data about firefighter injuries, and then answer the following questions:
   - How many line-of-duty injuries occurred during the year in question? Was this an increase or a decrease over the previous year?
   - How many or what percent of the firefighter injuries occurred during fireground operations?
   - What area of the country had the highest firefighter injury rate?
   - Rank in order from most to least the major types of injuries sustained.
3. Read *America Burning* and/or *Injury in America.*
4. List local sources of data on fire and burn injury.

Review Activities

1. List the two categories of national data used in planning local public fire and life safety education programs. *(127)*

2. Name the three main national fire databases. *(127)*
3. Explain the types of information compiled in the annual NFPA survey. *(128)*
4. List the nine major property-use groups from which the NFPA collects data for its annual survey. *(128)*
5. Distinguish among rooming, boarding, and lodging houses. *(NFPA 901)*
6. Distinguish among apartments, tenements, and flats. *(NFPA 901)*
7. Describe the type of information collected by FIDO. *(130, 131)*
8. List several facts found in the book *Injury in America*. *(131, 132)*
9. List the objectives of the National Burn Information Exchange. *(132)*
10. Briefly describe four national sources of fire and burn data other than NFPA, FIDO, and NBIE. *(133)*
11. Compare and contrast statewide collections of fire and burn injury data. *(133)*
12. Explain how collected data may be compared for program evaluation. *(134, 135)*
13. Briefly identify each of the following abbreviations and acronyms.
    - ACFM&FC *(129)*
    - NFIRS *(127)*
    - FIDO *(127)*
    - NBIE *(132)*
    - NEISS *(133)*
    - NIOSH *(133)*
    - NHTSA *(133)*
    - FEMA *(127)*
    - USFA *(127)*
    - NFPA *(127)*
    - CPSC *(133)*
    - IAFF *(133)*
    - NTSB *(133)*

Questions and Notes

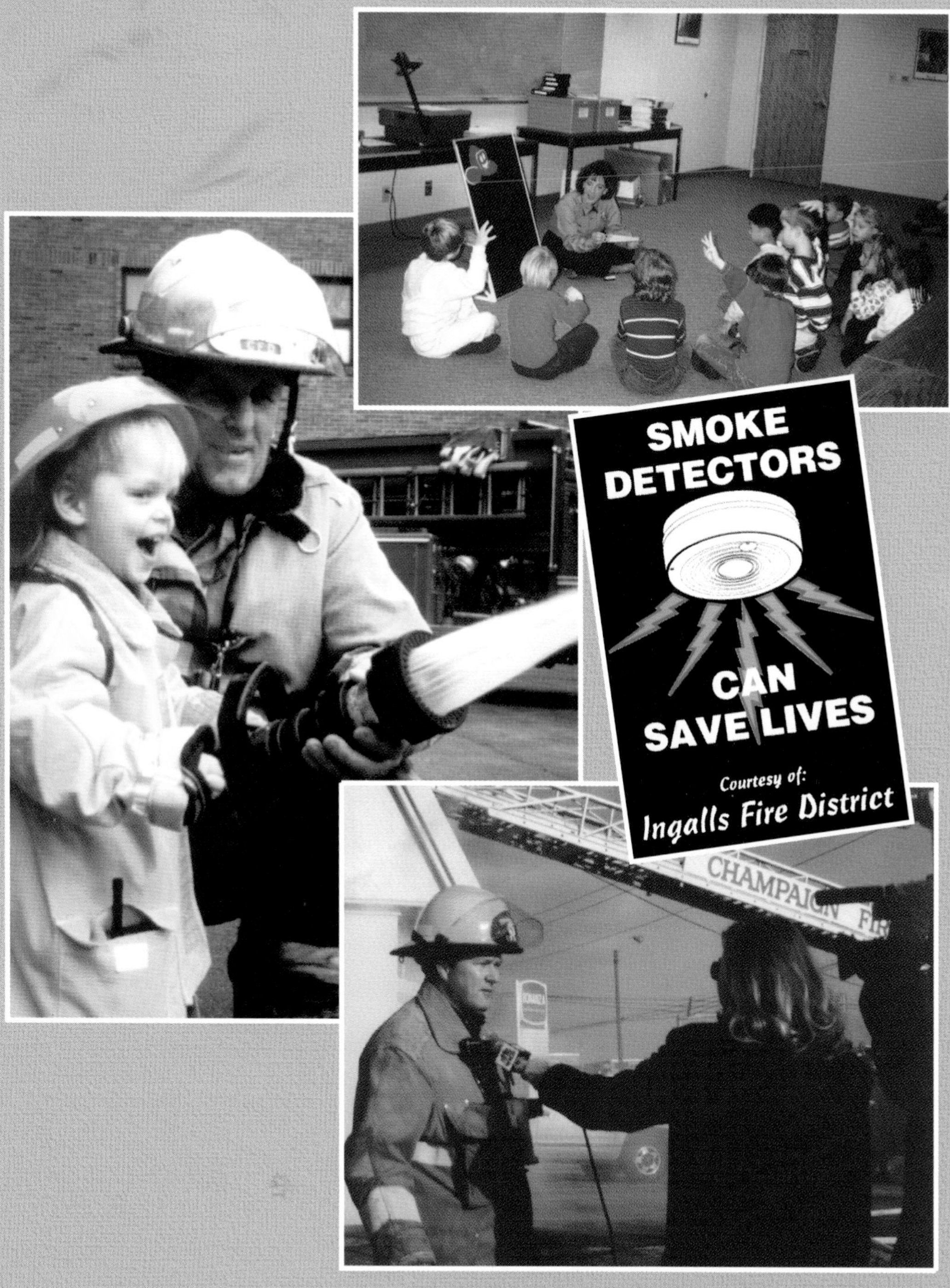
SMOKE
DETECTORS
CAN
SAVE LIVES
Courtesy of:
Ingalls Fire District
CHAMPAIGN

8 Knowing Your Audience

LEARNING OBJECTIVES

This chapter provides information that addresses the following objectives of NFPA 1035, *Standard for Professional Qualifications for Public Fire and Life Safety Educator* (1993 edition):

Fire and Life Safety Educator I

3-4.1 Select instructional materials, given a subject, program objective, the intended audience, and related resources, so that the materials are appropriate to the audience and program objectives.

3-4.1.1 *Prerequisite Knowledge:* Basic learning characteristics of preschool children, elementary school-age children, secondary school-age children, adults, and senior adults.

Fire and Life Safety Educator II

4-4.1 Develop informational materials, given an identified issue, so that information provided is accurate, relevant to the issue, and comprehensible to the audience.

4-4.2 Develop instructional materials, given course objectives, lesson plans, and a specified audience, so that the materials support the program objectives and lesson plans and are appropriate to the audience.

4-4.2.1 *Prerequisite Knowledge:* Learning theory for all age, social, and developmental audiences; needs assessment; development of written and visual educational materials; development of learning objectives, course development based on specified learning objectives and audiences, lesson plan development, and selection and use of evaluation instruments.

4-4.4 Adapt a lesson plan, given a specific audience, so that a modified lesson plan is responsive to the specific characteristics of the intended audience.

4-4.5 Design a public fire and life safety education program, given an identified need and audience(s), so that the public fire and life safety education program includes the behavioral objectives, lesson plan, informational materials, and evaluation instruments.

Fire and Life Safety Educator III

5-3.2 Evaluate current and future trends, given trend data, so that current and anticipated fire and life safety issues are identified.

5-3.2.1 *Prerequisite Knowledge:* Demographics, cultural and value shifts, governmental regulations environmental issues, and technological changes.

5-3.2.2 *Prerequisite Skills:* Trend analysis.

Questions and Notes

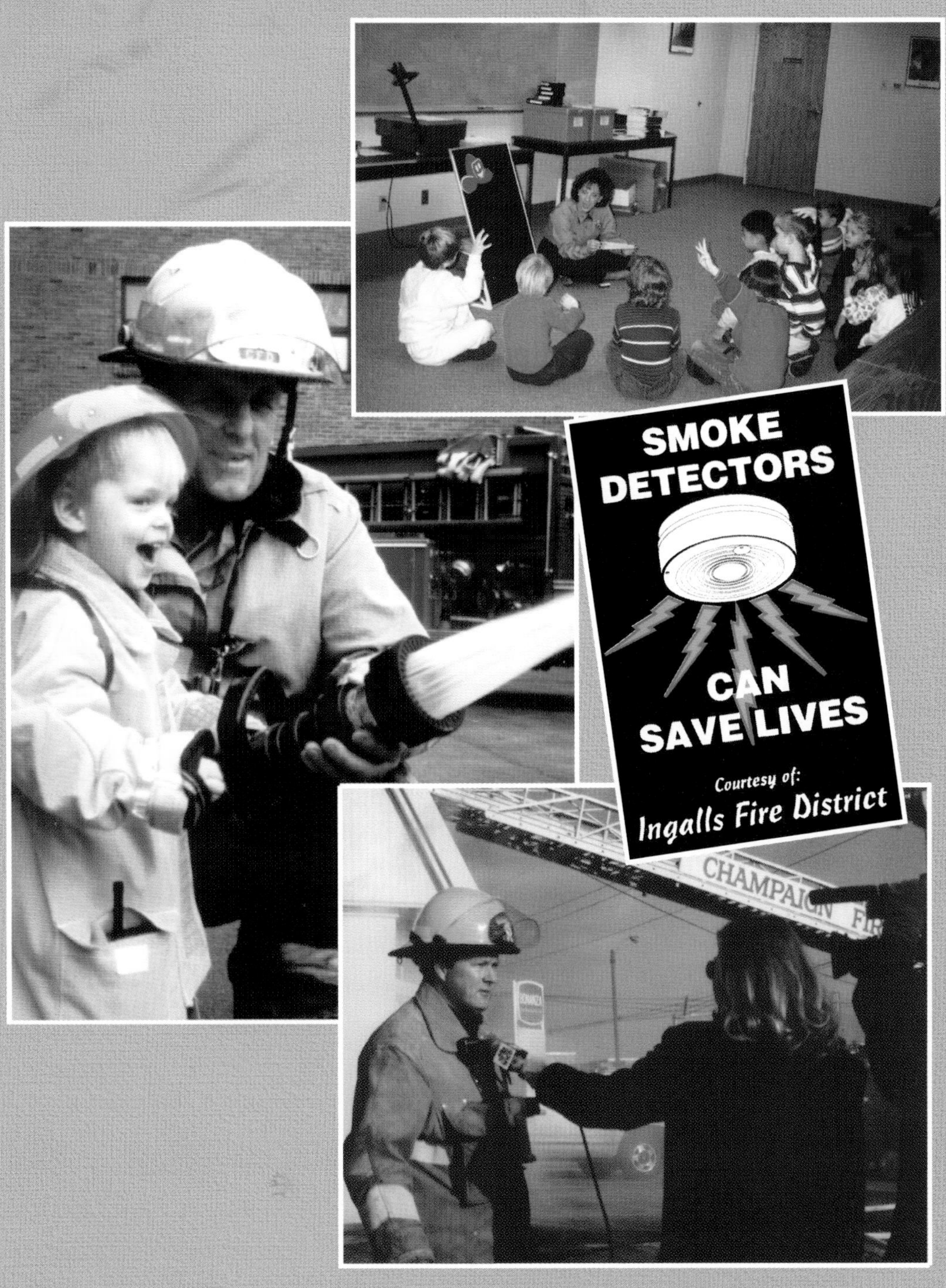
SMOKE
DETECTORS
CAN
SAVE LIVES
Courtesy of:
Ingalls Fire District
CHAMPAIGN

10 Developing the Program Curriculum

LEARNING OBJECTIVES

This chapter provides information that addresses the following objectives of NFPA 1035, *Standard for Professional Qualifications for Public Fire and Life Safety Educator* (1993 edition):

Public Fire and Life Safety Educator I

3-2.2.1 *Prerequisite Knowledge:* Types of educational programs, classifications for programs, types of documentation methods and authority having jurisdiction preferred methods, the purpose of the forms or formats, and implications of not appropriately documenting programs.

3-4.1 Select instructional materials, given a subject, program objective, the intended audience, and related resources, so that the materials are appropriate to the audience and program objectives.

3-4.1.2 *Prerequisite Skills:* Communication skills, use of prepared lesson plans with identified learning objectives, methods for active participation/involvement, methods of developing and maintaining a positive learning environment for the student including physical environment and student/instructor relationships, and proper use and care of audiovisual equipment and materials.

3-4.2 Present a prepared program, given lesson content, time allotments, and identified audience, so that program objectives are met.

Public Fire and Life Safety Educator II

4-4.2 Develop instructional materials, given course objectives, lesson plans, and a specified audience, so that the materials support the program objectives and lesson plans and are appropriate to the audience.

4-4.2.1 *Prerequisite Knowledge:* Learning theory for all age, social, and developmental audiences; needs assessment; development of written and visual educational materials; development of learning objectives, course development based on specified learning objectives and audiences, lesson plan development, and selection and use of evaluation instruments.

4-4.3 Develop a lesson plan, given a specific behavior, learning objectives, and a specified audience, so that the lesson plan reflects the learning characteristics and abilities of the intended audience.

4-4.4 Adapt a lesson plan, given a specific audience, so that a modified lesson plan is responsive to the specific characteristics of the intended audience.

4-4.5 Design a public fire and life safety education program, given an identified need and audience(s), so that the public fire and life safety education program includes the behavioral objectives, lesson plan, informational materials, and evaluation instruments.

4-4.5.1 *Prerequisite Knowledge:* Educational methodology.

Chapter 10
Developing the Program Curriculum

INTRODUCTION

Effective fire and life safety education programs do not just happen. Instead, they are the result of deciding carefully what to teach and how to teach it. This decision-making process is called *curriculum development* or *instructional design*.

Curriculum development has three basic components: *analysis*, *design*, and *evaluation* (deciding how to measure the learning that took place). This chapter covers the analysis and design components of curriculum development and also discusses how to develop a lesson plan (Figure 10.1). Evaluation is covered in Chapter 11, "Evaluating Presentations and Programs." A much more detailed discussion of the three major components of curriculum development is provided in Chapter 5, "Planning Instruction," of IFSTA **Fire Service Instructor**.[1]

The following four terms and definitions are used in this chapter:

- *Curriculum* — A sequence of presentations on fire and life safety education
- *Lesson plan* — A guide for making a presentation
- *Program* — A comprehensive strategy that addresses fire and life safety issues via educational means
- *Presentation* — A single delivery of fire and life safety information; also called a *lesson*

ANALYSIS

Three basic steps make up the analysis component of curriculum development. These steps are (1) assess the educational needs of the audience, (2) determine the characteristics of the learner, and (3) establish desired levels of learning or performance (Figure 10.2). For a complete discussion of the levels of learning and how they apply to analysis, see IFSTA **Fire Service Instructor**, 5th edition.

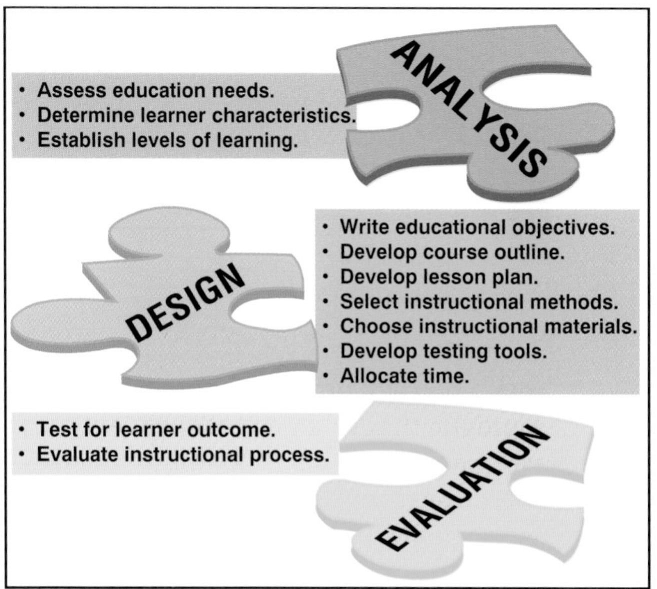

ANALYSIS
• Assess education needs.
• Determine learner characteristics.
• Establish levels of learning.
DESIGN
• Write educational objectives.
• Develop course outline.
• Develop lesson plan.
• Select instructional methods.
• Choose instructional materials.
• Develop testing tools.
• Allocate time.
EVALUATION
• Test for learner outcome.
• Evaluate instructional process.

Figure 10.1 *Instructional design* is the analysis of training needs, the systematic design of teaching/learning activities, and the assessment of the teaching/learning process.

Assessing Audience Needs

An entire art and science of needs assessment has been developed over the last few decades. In general, an educational needs assessment uses one or more of these approaches[2]:

- Observation
- Consultation/interview
- Questionnaires/surveys

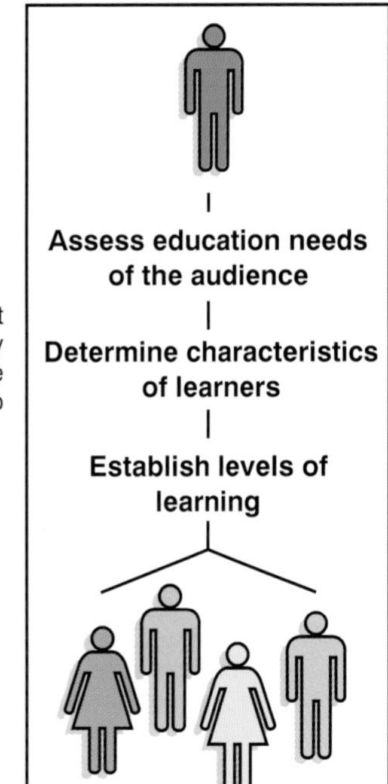
Assess education needs of the audience
Determine characteristics of learners
Establish levels of learning

Figure 10.2 The analysis component of curriculum development is simply identifying the gap between what the audience knows and what it needs to learn.

- Task forces/committees
- Work samples
- Nominal group process (a decision-making technique that relies on independent ideas from each participant, round-robin feedback on each idea, discussion of each idea, and voting to rate mathematically each idea)
- Delphi technique (using a series of questionnaires in which each questionnaire is based on responses to the one before it)
- Futuristics (prediction of future needs, based on population or economic trends, for example)
- Document analysis
- Participant evaluations

The fire and life safety educator uses several of these approaches to assess education needs. For example, an educator who is considering a program to teach kindergarten children to "stop, drop, and roll" could observe kindergartners who are asked what to do when their clothes catch fire. The educator also could consult with kindergarten teachers or parents about what their students/children do when asked to pretend that their clothes are on fire or could interview children. More elaborate approaches, such as the nominal group process or the Delphi technique, may be needed for developing more complex curricula such as high-rise fire safety.

Information gained from existing programs, including participant evaluations or pretest/posttest scores, can also be valuable in assessing educational needs. Regardless of the approach used, an assessment uncovers situations shown in Table 10.1.

TABLE 10.1
Education Needs And Learning Domains

Audience Situation	Audience Needs	Target Domain
Does not know something	Information/ knowledge	Cognitive
Cannot do something	Skills	Psychomotor
Does not care	Motivation	Affective

What Are the "Domains of Learning?"

The *cognitive domain* deals with facts. Textbooks teach material in the cognitive domain.

The *psychomotor domain* deals with skills. "How-to" manuals and demonstrations are ways to teach skills in the psychomotor domain.

The *affective domain* deals with attitudes, values, and habits. Testimonials, role-play, and personal examples are ways to teach the affective domain.

Determining Learner Characteristics

After assessing audience needs, the next step in curriculum development is determining the general characteristics of the expected audience. This step is not as complicated as it sounds. It can be as straightforward as thinking about the audience for a few minutes and then planning action to match the curriculum to the audience. For an employee fire safety program, for example, the educator wants to know about the employees' level of education, the kind of work they do, whether they work in shift, and whether anyone on the work team has been hurt in a fire. Table 10.2 shows common audience characteristics and sample instructional actions.

class from time to time. For this reason, complete and clear lesson plans are especially important. *In judging your lesson plans, a good rule of thumb is to ask whether someone else will be able to follow and use them.*

The lesson plan guides how the students and educator spend their class time; it is not a document that dictates what must happen during each class minute. A good lesson plan has some built-in flexibility, which is very valuable if, for example, the pretest reveals that the class lacks prerequisite knowledge.

The essence of lesson planning is to develop instructional units. In developing instructional units, the lesson plan allows for the following implementation actions:

- Emphasizing the parts of the lesson
- Effectively using training aids
- Staying within the time allotted
- Including the essential information

Lesson Plan Format

With a typical lesson plan format, an actual lesson has two main components: an *information presentation* and a *practical demonstration*.

The information presentation (sometimes called a *technical lesson*) covers theory and technical knowledge such as the facts of fire growth and spread. The information presentation gives the background (cognitive domain) that is often essential to skills development (psychomotor domain).

The practical demonstration (sometimes called a *manipulative lesson*) teaches psychomotor skills such as installing a smoke detector or using a portable fire extinguisher safely.

What about the affective domain? The critical area of attitudes, values, and opinions can be covered in a session that comes before the information presentation and practical demonstration. Other educators prefer to weave the affective domain throughout the entire presentation. The important thing is to make sure that the affective domain is covered somewhere in the lesson plan.

This sections covers the information presentation. To learn about demonstrations and other instructional methods, see Chapter 14, "Applying Fire and Life Safety Educational Theory."

Information Presentation Format

In its simplest form, an information presentation is formatted by identifying all learning objectives to be achieved and then providing a framework for teaching to those objectives (Figure 10.6). This format organizes the lesson around what the student needs to learn, rather than around what the educator wants to teach.

Typically, the lesson plan for an information presentation includes the following components or areas:

- **Topic**. A short, descriptive title should limit the content of the lesson and should include enough information so that another fire and life safety educator would understand clearly what is to be covered.
- **Time**. This is the estimated time needed to teach the lesson. Some fire and life safety educators establish times for each objective or for each instructional unit as a way of controlling time for the overall lesson.
- **Prerequisites**. This section lists any information or skills that the student should

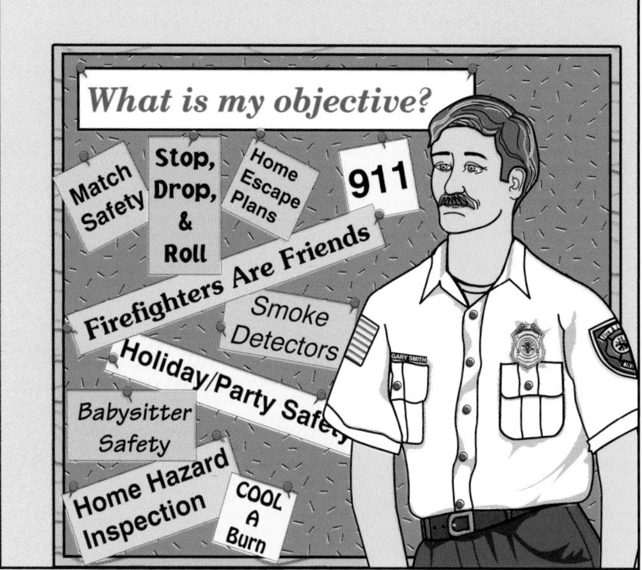

Figure 10.6 The educator must identify all learning objectives to be achieved through an information presentation.

have mastered already. As a practical matter, though, most fire and life safety educators have little or no control over the prior knowledge or skills of their audience. This is especially true of adult audiences, but it is also true of school-age audiences. Using a pretest will reveal whether or not prerequisites have been met — or whether the prerequisites will become the first topic to be covered in class.

- **Objectives**. Here, the fire and life safety educator describes the minimum acceptable behaviors (in the affective, cognitive, and psychomotor domains) that the student must be able to do after the presentation. Remember, the objectives should have been developed before writing the lesson plan. If the objectives have not been written yet, now is the time for the educator to write them.
- **Preclass preparation**. This section includes any activities that the instructor needs to complete before entering the classroom. Activities such as "collect handouts" or "preview videotape" are included.
- **References**. Specific references (including page numbers) that the fire and life safety educator must study are cited. In some cases, the materials used to develop the lesson plan may also be listed.
- **Preparation**. In the preparation step, the educator prepares the student to learn. In this part of the lesson plan, the fire and life safety educator shows why the material to be covered matters (especially to the student), thus beginning the process of motivation to learn.
- **Presentation**. The lesson plan lists, in teaching order, the information to be covered, how it will be covered, and what methods the fire and life safety educator must use to teach the lesson.
- **Application**. This part of the lesson plan includes activities, exercises, and tasks for the student to do to apply the information from the lesson. These application activities do not necessarily need to be listed under application, but they may be integrated into the presentation information. Blending application with the technical presentation has the advantage of allowing the students to be more involved in their own learning.

  In short, it is more important to be sure that application activities are included than to list them separately.
- **Lesson summary**. Here, the fire and life safety educator restates and reemphasizes important concepts, facts, and skills. The purpose of the summary is to clear up uncertainties, prevent misconceptions, and increase retention.
- **Evaluation**. The fire and life safety educator tests students to assess just how much learning took place and whether or not the objectives were met. Although the students are the ones taking the test, it is really the fire and life safety presentation and curriculum that are being judged during evaluation. (**NOTE**: For more information, see Chapter 11, "Evaluating Presentations and Programs.")

Using Lesson Plans

After developing lesson plans, fire and life safety educators should remember six keys to their effective use (Figure 10.7)[5]:

- **Review the lesson plan**. With your own lesson, visual aids, and handouts, it is very easy to be trapped into a false sense of security.

  Even the best lesson plan needs to be reviewed before class. During this review, fire and life safety educators refresh themselves on the content and skills to be taught. At the same time, educators ask themselves questions such as "How is this group different from the last one?" "What worked especially well during the last presentation?" "What didn't work well the last time?" "What will be on people's minds today?" "Has the information or proce-

Chapter 10 Review

Directions

The following activities are designed to help you comprehend and apply the information in Chapter 10 of **Fire and Life Safety Educator**, second edition. To receive the maximum learning experience from these activities, it is recommended that you use the following procedure:

1. Read the chapter, underlining or highlighting important terms, topics, and subject matter. Read the sidebar material, study the photographs and illustrations, and read the captions with each.
2. Review the list of vocabulary words to ensure that you know the chapter-related meaning of each. If you are unsure of the meaning of a vocabulary word, look up the word in the glossary or a dictionary, and then study its context in the chapter.
3. On a separate sheet of paper, complete all assigned or selected application and review activities before checking your answers.
4. After you have finished, check your answers against those on the pages referenced in parentheses.
5. Correct any incorrect answers, and review material that was answered incorrectly.

Vocabulary

Be sure that you know the chapter-related meanings of the following words:

- affective *(172)*
- analysis *(171)*
- cognitive *(172)*
- criterion/criteria *(174)*
- curriculum *(171)*
- domain *(172)*
- educational objective *(173, 174)*
- lesson plan *(171)*
- motivation *(175)*
- preparation *(175)*
- presentation *(171)*
- program *(171)*
- psychomotor *(172)*
- standard *(174)*

Application of Knowledge

1. Assume that you must teach the information and skills covered in this chapter to a group of fire and life safety educators. Write two cognitive and two psychomotor educational objectives for your lesson. Make sure that your objectives include minimum standards and are measurable.
2. Create the lesson plan you will need to teach this chapter to a group of fire and life safety educators. Base your lesson plan on the objectives you developed in Activity 1 if you desire.
3. When you have completed the two previous activities, swap your lesson plan with that of one of your classmates. Pretend that you must use your classmate's lesson plan to make a presentation to the fire and life safety educators in another city. Critique and discuss each other's lesson plans.

Review Activities

1. Name a synonym for curriculum development. *(171)*
2. List the three basic components of curriculum development. *(171)*
3. Explain the three steps in the analysis component of curriculum development. *(171)*
4. Explain methods by which the educator can conduct a needs assessment. *(172, 173)*
5. Describe how you might teach each of the following types of objectives: *(172)*
   - affective objective
   - cognitive objective
   - psychomotor objective
6. List learner characteristics of common audiences faced by fire and life safety educators. *(172, 173)*
7. Provide examples of instructional actions the educator might use to teach each of the audiences with characteristics listed in Activity 6. *(173)*
8. List the seven steps in the design component of curriculum development. *(173)*

9. Name three synonyms for educational objective. *(173)*
10. Describe the two keys to writing effective educational objectives. *(173, 174)*
11. List the advantages of educational objectives. *(174)*
12. Explain Robert F. Mager's format for writing educational objectives. *(174)*
13. State and briefly explain the four steps to effective lesson design and teaching; list the optional step that can precede these four steps. *(175)*
14. Explain some of the uses of pretests. *(175)*
15. Describe the major disadvantage of written and oral pretests. *(175)*
16. Explain the meaning of the word *preparation* as it applies to the four-part teaching process. *(175)*
17. List some advantages of a lesson plan. *(177)*
18. Explain the information presentation and the practical demonstration components of lesson plan format. *(177)*
19. Outline the format of a typical information presentation. *(177, 178)*
20. List and briefly explain the six keys to using lesson plans effectively. *(178)*
21. Briefly explain the steps in the Hunter lesson plan model. *(179, 180)*
    - anticipatory set
    - objective/purpose
    - input
    - modeling
    - checking for understanding
    - guided practice
    - independent practice
    - closure

Questions and Notes

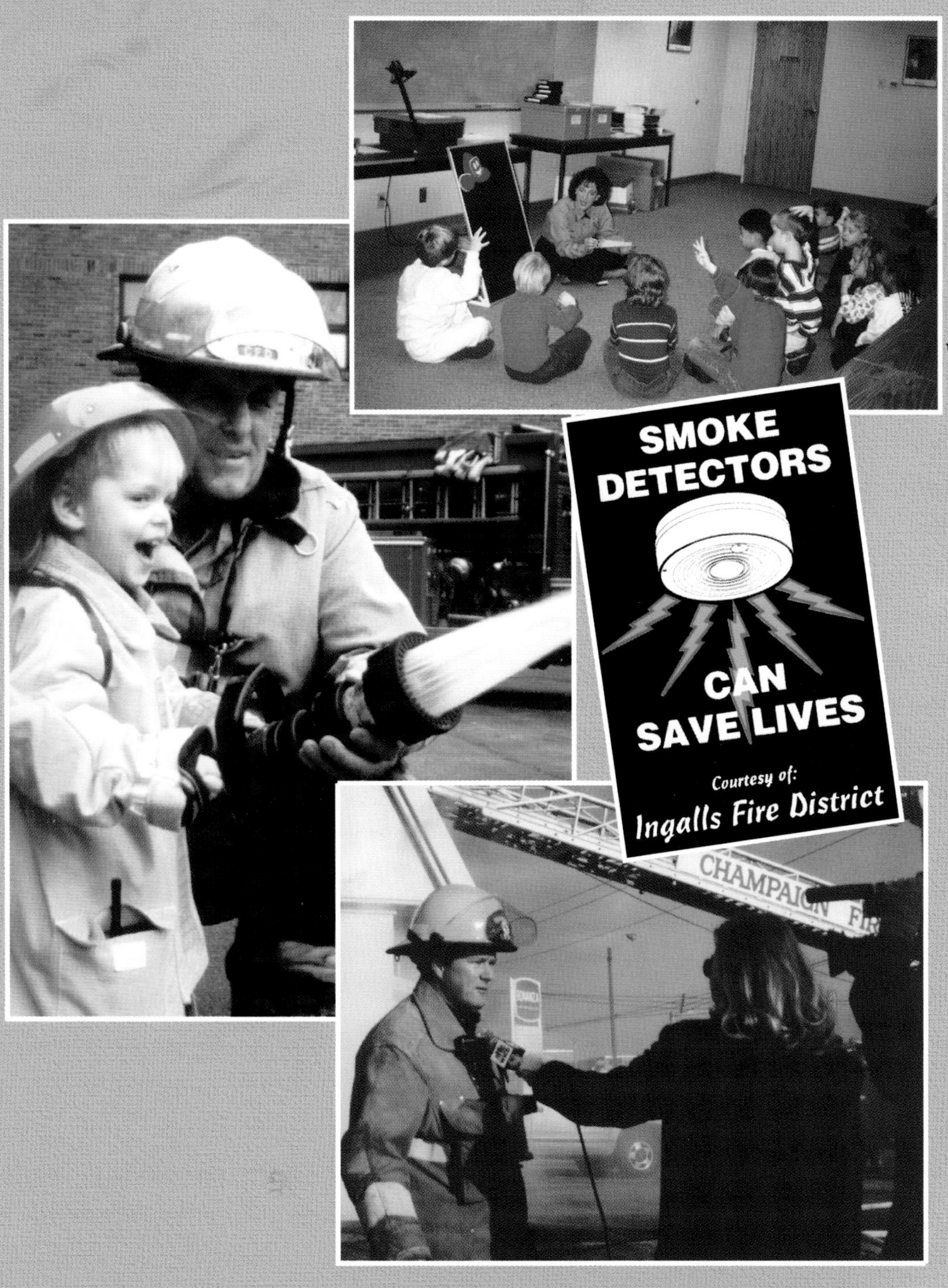
SMOKE
DETECTORS
CAN
SAVE LIVES
Courtesy of:
Ingalls Fire District
CHAMPAIGN

11 Evaluating Presentations and Programs

LEARNING OBJECTIVES

This chapter provides information that addresses the following objectives of NFPA 1035, *Standard for Professional Qualifications for Public Fire and Life Safety Educator* (1993 edition):

Public Fire and Life Safety Educator II

4-3.2 Implement an evaluation process, given an evaluation method and overall program goals and objectives, so that program effectiveness is measured.

4-3.2.1 *Prerequisite Knowledge:* Basic evaluation methods.

Public Fire and Life Safety Educator III

5-4.6 Design an evaluation instrument, given an educational or informational objective, so that the evaluation instrument measures the educational outcome.

5-4.6.1 *Prerequisite Knowledge:* Basic statistical methods and resources.

Chapter 11
Evaluating Presentations and Programs

INTRODUCTION

One of the most important components of any successful public fire and life safety education program is effective evaluation (Figure 11.1). Yet, it is one component that is most often missing from programs. In fact, many public educators fear evaluation, viewing it as something that is complicated, detailed, and time-consuming. In reality, it is a task that can be successfully accomplished by most public educators using local resources. It is a critical tool for every fire and life safety educator.

Every day fire and life safety educators conduct a myriad of different types of educational presentations to a variety of diverse audiences in their communities. Often, these educators depend upon their own experiences and "gut instincts" to determine the effectiveness of their efforts. In some cases, their conclusions may be accurate; in others, their conclusions may be inaccurate and off the mark. This is because there is no way to quantify an instinct or feeling.

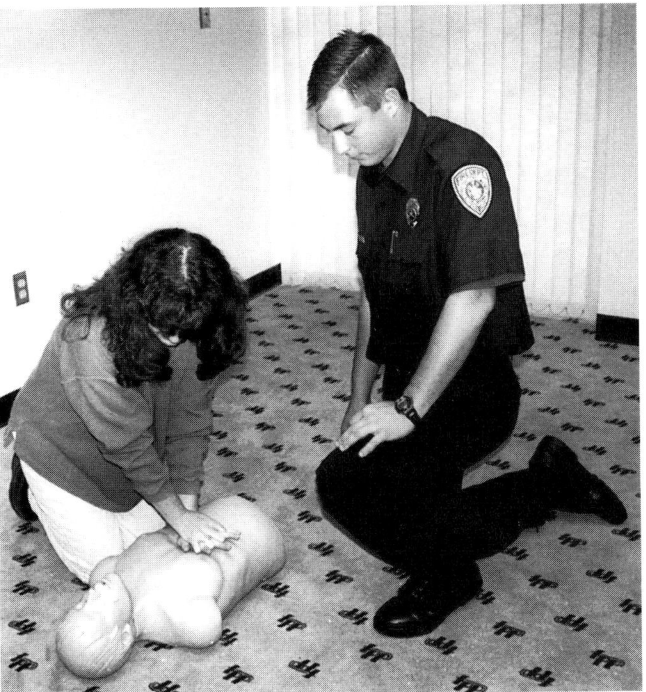

Figure 11.1 The effectiveness of a life safety presentation becomes apparent as a participant demonstrates skills learned during the presentation.

It is critical, however, that today's fire and life safety educators know that the audience understands and, more important, can apply the behaviors taught during the presentation. For example, a fire and life safety educator makes a presentation on prevention of slips and falls to a group of senior citizens. At the end of the presentation the educator receives a standing ovation and lots of hugs. The educator is proud of a job well done and is obviously well liked by the participants. But, are the hugs a sign of success? How many of the seniors will go home and apply the new information? Without formal evaluation, the educator will never know whether the objectives were really achieved.

Another example is cardiopulmonary resuscitation (CPR) training. It goes without saying that evaluation during a CPR class is essential. Every participant must be able to demonstrate the ability to properly perform CPR on a mannequin to complete the course. Obviously, CPR is a valuable life-saving skill that does not allow any margin for error or misunderstanding. But are not many of the behaviors taught by public educators also valuable life-saving skills that do not allow any margin for error? Yet, little effort is put forth to evaluate learning following public fire and life safety education presentations.

It is also important to note the difference between evaluation of results and the evaluation of the educator. When evaluating the educator, feedback is sought on his or her performance. While this information may be useful, this chapter addresses evaluation of results — in other words, evaluation of changes (in areas such as loss) due to the presentations and programs. Information on evaluation of the educator is available through local schools and through other educators.

Finally, it is important to distinguish between evaluation of a single presentation and evaluation of a program. A presentation is but one part of a program. The evaluation of an individual presentation or part of an overall program is called *formative evaluation*. The evaluation of the overall program following completion is known as *summative evaluation* (Figure 11.2).

In most programs, there are many additional methods used to reach the target audience, including public service announcements, written materials, and news stories. Because of the variety of components of a program, program evaluation is a complex process. Yet, the same basic rules and methods used for presentation evaluation can be used to evaluate an overall program. Evaluation of overall programs is addressed later in the chapter.

ELEMENTS OF A SUCCESSFUL PROGRAM

Each successful fire and life safety education program progresses through several distinct elements. When developing an evaluation plan for a specific type of presentation, it is necessary to identify which step will be achieved by the presentation or program and which of the steps will be evaluated. There are five steps a program goes through that result in reduction in fires and injuries. These steps include the following (Figure 11.3):

- Outreach activity
- Knowledge change
- Behavior change
- Environmental change
- End impact

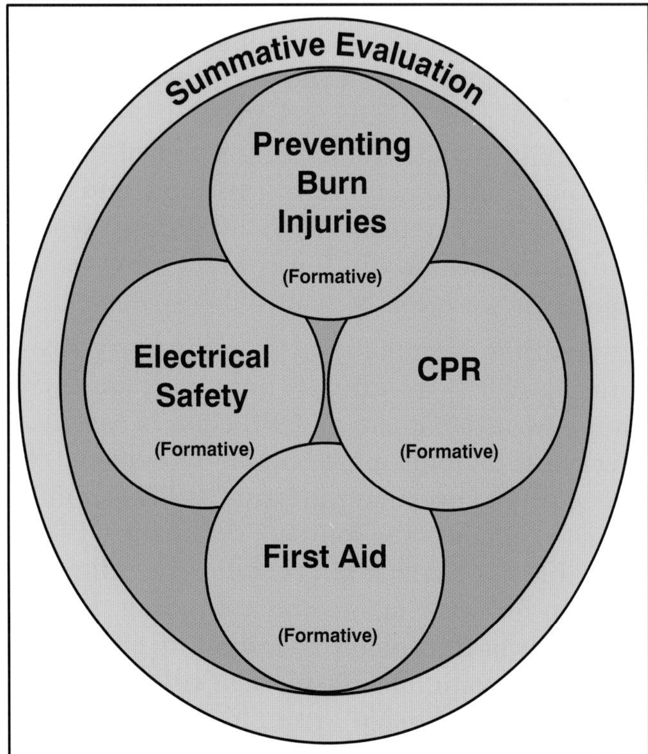

Figure 11.2 Formative evaluation is the evaluation of part of a program while summative evaluation encompasses the overall program.

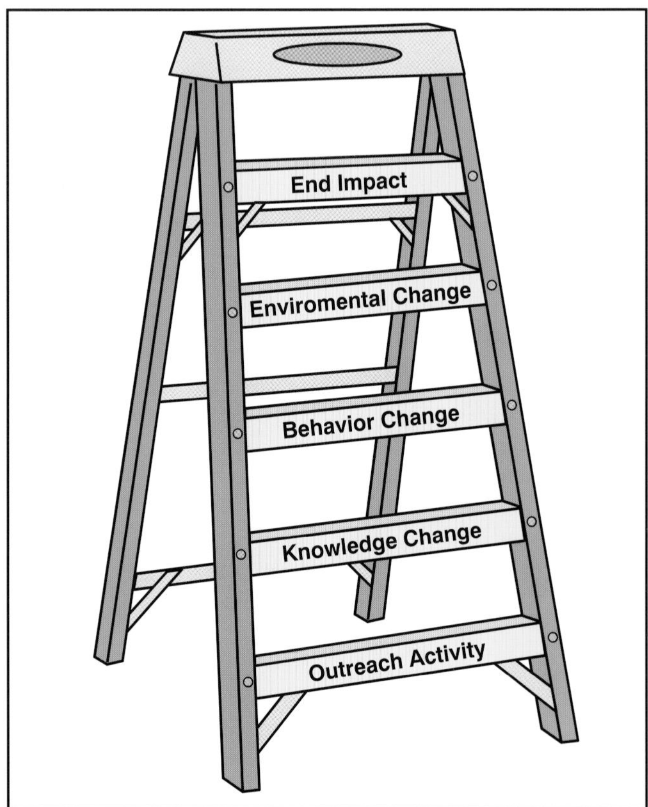

Figure 11.3 The five steps of a successful fire and life safety education program.

The *outreach activity* can be considered as the actual public education presentation. Before it is possible to change any behaviors or attitudes, it is necessary to have contact with the target audience. This contact could be a public service announcement, a brochure, or some other method or material. In most cases, the most effective outreach activity is a direct presentation to the target audience delivered by a public fire and life safety educator.

The step that occurs after the outreach activity is a knowledge change. The *knowledge change* is an increase in the understanding of fire and life safety practices. A presentation provides the target audience with the knowledge that creates an increase in awareness. The knowledge can be new information, or it may be old information presented again. Remember, before any change in behavior or attitude can occur, the target audience must be provided with the knowledge necessary to make those changes.

A behavior change follows a change in knowledge. The *behavior change* is a change in a person's actions. This behavior change was brought about because of an increase in knowledge. For example, a member of the target audience quits smoking in bed after attending a fire and life safety education presentation on careless smoking. There was a knowledge change due to the information in the presentation. This knowledge change brought about a change in personal behavior. Even though the outcome objective was a change in behavior, it would not have been accomplished without the knowledge change.

An environmental change can also occur after a knowledge change. An *environmental change* is a change in the home or workplace following a presentation. The environmental change involves making a change in the surroundings or in the fire and life safety equipment in the home or workplace. For example, mounting a smoke detector would be changing the environment in the home. Also, installing handicap rails in a bathtub would be a change in the environment. By adding the smoke detector and the rails, the safety of the environment is increased.

Generally, a change in the environment must be accompanied by a change in behavior. Consider the installation of the smoke detector. The change in the environment will be effective only if the person is willing to test and maintain the smoke detector. This requires a change in behavior. Often, changes in the environment are brought about by legislation and codes, but no thought is given to changing behaviors through public education. Remember, environmental changes are most effective when accompanied by behavior changes.

The final step in this process is end impact. The end impact is the decrease in fires and injuries due to other elements including knowledge change, behavior change, and environmental change. Most of the time the end impact occurs after months and in many cases, years. Because of this, end impact is not a good measure for evaluation of individual presentations. However, *end impact is the element most often considered when evaluating an overall program. Keep in mind though, end impact is a result of the cumulative effects of many individual presentations.*

When developing an evaluation plan, consider which of the elements are to be evaluated. The outcome objectives — or the type of presentation — may identify the element to evaluate. For evaluation of individual presentations, it is necessary to consider only knowledge change, behavior change, and environmental change. The outreach activity occurs every time a fire and life safety educator delivers a presentation. The end impact will be evaluated after many presentations are given.

For example, consider a presentation to a high-school class on cooking fire safety. The presentation provides the target audience with information. This means that the objective is a knowledge change resulting in a behavior change. However, it is not possible to evaluate a behavior change in the classroom. It is possible to measure the *knowledge change* through a written pretest and posttest.

An example of a presentation targeting a change in behavior would be a presentation to children on "stop, drop, and roll." The objective of the presentation would be to develop the behavior: stop, drop, and roll. Even though a knowledge change must precede the behavior change, the final goal is for all the children to be able to do the behavior. Another example of a presentation targeting a behavior change would be a presentation on testing a smoke detector properly. The testing of the detector is a specific behavior that incorporates knowledge and behavior.

An example of a presentation targeting environmental change would be a presentation on the installation of hot-water tempering valves. The information in the presentation would motivate the target audience to install a tempering valve, resulting in a change in the environment.

BENEFITS OF EVALUATION

It is obvious that evaluation is a vital part of the duties of a fire and life safety educator. Evaluation provides the educator with the information necessary to determine whether the objectives of a program or presentation have been achieved. Evaluation also provides feedback on the educator's presentation skills.

Evaluation is also part of the overall educational process known as the *five-step process.* This process includes identifying the local fire and injury problem, selecting achievable program objectives, designing the program, implementing the program, and evaluating the program (Figure 11.4). Keep in mind that fire and life safety education is a dynamic, ongoing process in which evaluation provides information that is used to revise and modify the program or presentation.

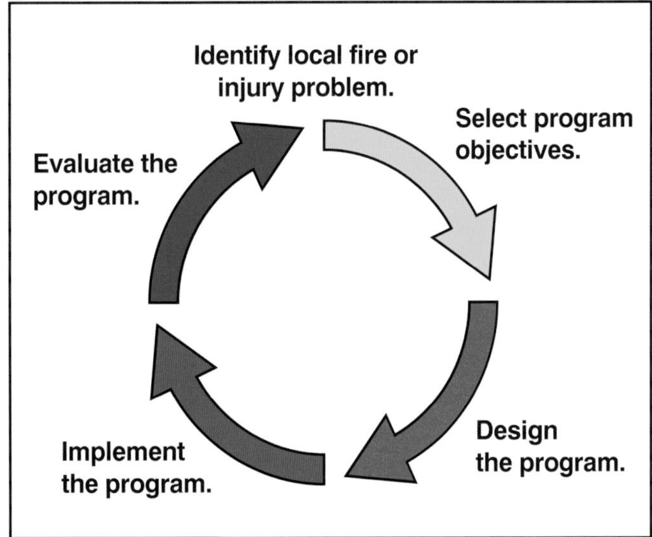

Figure 11.4 In the continual cycle of the education process, evaluation provides important feedback for improving programs.

Evaluation is a planned process with a distinct series of steps. It requires careful consideration during the planning process, as well as careful implementation. Effective evaluation can show the fire and life safety educator the following information:

- The level of knowledge or skills of the target audience before the presentation or program
- Whether the target audience learned the desired information from the presentation or program
- Whether the target audience can perform the behavior(s) presented
- Whether members of the target audience have applied the information in their homes or workplaces
- The strengths and weaknesses of the instructional methods used by the educator

Specifically, evaluation is a process that examines the results of a presentation or program to determine whether the participants have learned the information or behaviors. Sometimes, this evaluation is immediate. For example, a written test is given to a grade-school class following a presentation on burn prevention. In other situations, the evaluation is completed at a later date. A good example of this is with a presentation on proper placement and testing of carbon monoxide detectors. The evaluation is a survey sent to each participant to find out whether or not they mounted a carbon monoxide detector following the presentation. In both cases evaluation is used to determine whether the outcome objectives were achieved.

A major benefit of evaluating education programs is to justify — and quantify — their worth in the department's overall fire and injury prevention efforts. In today's organizations it is necessary to justify the worth of each program in a cost-benefit evaluation. Without the information provided by evaluation, it is difficult for decision makers to determine whether a program is worth continuing. *The days of doing something just because it seems to be the right thing to do are over; the fire and life safety educator must be able to prove that a program is effective in changing behaviors and reducing loss* (Figure 11.5).

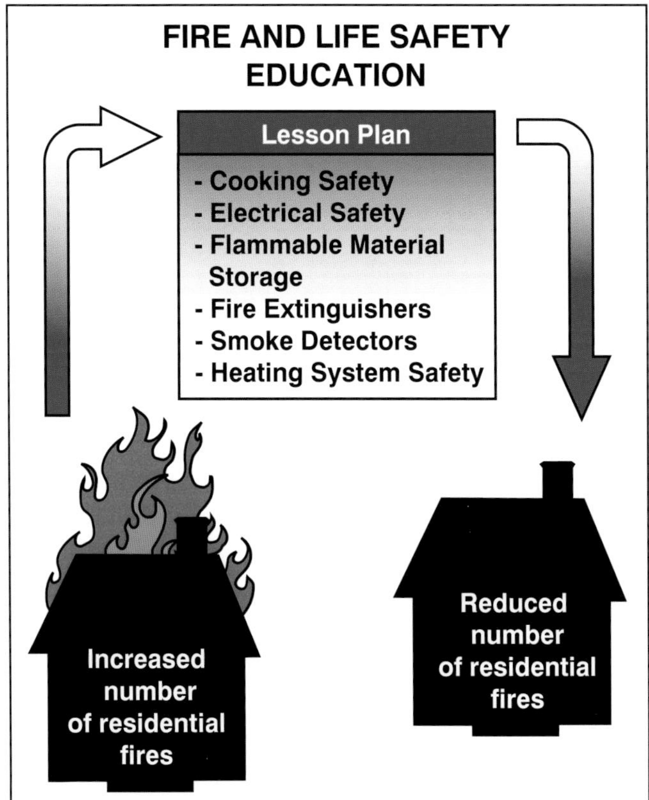

Figure 11.5 A reduction in the number of residential fires is a benefit that may be used to justify the cost of fire and injury prevention programs.

Another benefit of evaluation is that it identifies the strengths and weaknesses of individual presentations. The best planned presentation may have problems. For example, an educator may use a presentation on swimming pool safety that was borrowed from a different department. The educator takes time to prepare for the presentation but discovers through evaluation of the presentation that the information does not apply to the educator's area. In this case, a change in the presentation content is required. Evaluation points out those problems so that they can be corrected as soon as possible. If the necessary changes are made after the first few presentations, there is much less chance of participants confusing the information or behaviors. Also, identifying the presentation's strengths helps when developing and conducting future presentations. Effective educators capitalize on the strengths of a presentation while always working to improve the weak areas. Keep in mind that the long-term success of any program is due to the success of its many individual presentations. In short, it is critical that each and every presentation be as effective as possible.

Often, evaluation will provide a motivational boost to the educator. For example, most educators take great pride in a job well done, especially when that affirmation comes from the participants. When the evaluation shows that the objectives were achieved and that the target audience was pleased with the presentation, it is a positive boost to the educator. However, not every evaluation will be positive. Educators should not take negative evaluations personally or be demoralized by them. Evaluations should be used as a guide to improve presentation skills or the content of the presentation.

In some cases, the evaluation will also motivate the target audience. This is especially true with an audience of children. Children work hard to please fire and life safety educators. Evaluation provides the children with valuable feedback, reinforcing their efforts and developing positive attitudes toward fire and life safety. Also, this recognition of efforts will motivate them to be attentive and receptive to future presentations. For example, an educator from the Red Cross goes to an elementary school to do a presentation of the American Red Cross course, Basic Aid Training (BAT). The children are evaluated after the first session and are all able to perform the skills. This success creates a positive perception toward the program and helps to motivate the children for the subsequent sessions.

Also, evaluation can provide feedback on the effectiveness of any needs analysis, part of identifying the local fire and injury problem. This is conducted prior to the development of the program or presentation. Post-presentation evaluation can identify whether the information was what the target audience expected and can use.

The information gathered by the evaluation can be used to change the data on the target audience or to modify the content of the presentation. In either case, the evaluation helps to ensure that future presentations will more effectively meet the particular needs of the target audience. A good example is the pilot testing of new presentations. Through the pilot process, participants provide feedback on the presentation. This feedback is then used to make changes, resulting in a more effective presentation.

LIMITATIONS OF EVALUATION

Evaluation has its limitations, just as does any other tool used in fire and life safety education. There are several limitations to evaluation:

- Requires thoughtful preparation
- May require assistance to design, administer, and interpret
- May not provide the information desired
- May be affected by the bias of the target audience

As mentioned earlier, evaluation is more than an audience survey or a multiple-choice test used with children; it is a *process* that considers outcome objectives, the characteristics of the target audience, and the nature of the information and behaviors being presented (Figure 11.6). This information is used to develop an evaluation strategy. The *evaluation strategy* is the plan for conducting the evaluation, including the type of evaluation instrument to be used, the information or behaviors to be evaluated, and the methods to be used to interpret the information provided through evaluation. This process requires that careful thought and planning be given to the purpose of the evaluation and the best method of achieving that purpose.

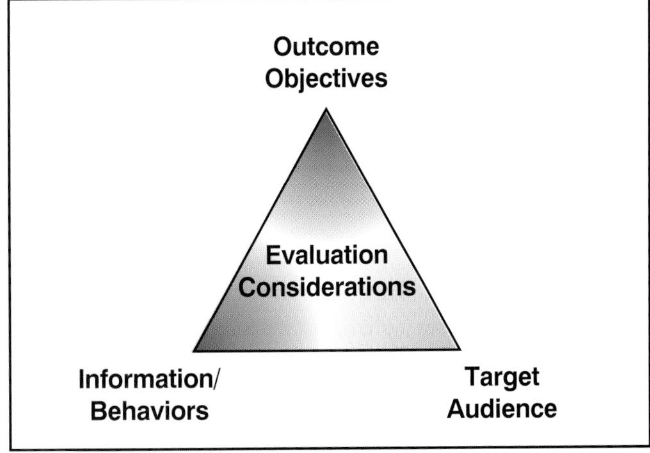

Figure 11.6 When planning for evaluation, the fire and life safety educator must consider each part of the process.

Often, it is necessary to gain the assistance of other educators or educational professionals to help design, administer, or interpret the information provided by an evaluation. Evaluation is a new tool to many fire and life safety educators, and it may be beneficial for them to seek help in the beginning of the planning process. This ensures that the evaluation method used meets the objectives identified in the evaluation strategy.

Another limitation of evaluation is that it may not provide the information needed or desired. Even though careful planning will help make sure that the evaluation is effective, there are things that are beyond the control of the educator. For example, surveys sent to participants after a presentation can provide valuable information. Unfortunately, many people do not return surveys. If the surveys are not returned, the evaluation cannot be completed.

Finally, the biases of the target audience may result in inaccurate information. Often, participants will provide the "right" information even though it does not reflect the truth. For example, someone may mark "yes" to a question about conducting home fire escape drills because they know that "yes" is the desired answer. However, in reality they do not have a home escape plan. Also, some target audiences may resent the authority of the educator. In these situations, the evaluation may not provide any information.

EVALUATION METHODS

There are many different methods of evaluation. However, there are six methods that are straightforward and can be easily used by fire and life safety educators to effectively evaluate individual presentations (Figure 11.7):

- Pretest/posttest
- Skills test
- Survey
- Inspection

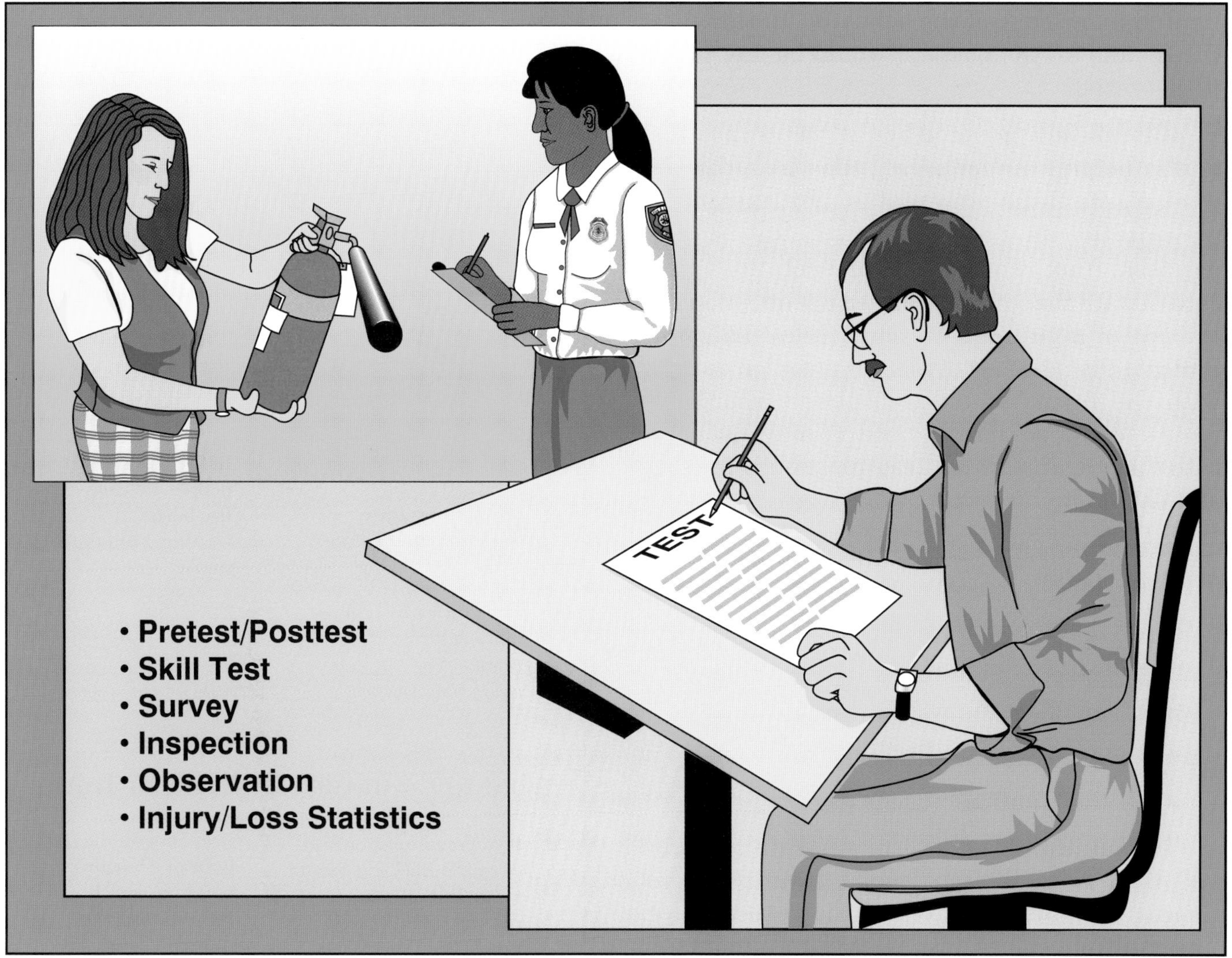
TEST
• Pretest/Posttest
• Skill Test
• Survey
• Inspection
• Observation
• Injury/Loss Statistics

Figure 11.7 Evaluation methods available to the fire and life safety educator.

- Observation
- Injury/loss statistics

These six methods lend themselves to evaluation of fire and life safety because they have the following characteristics:

- Have a simple design
- Provide accurate, usable information
- Are easily administered
- Are well-accepted by participants

Pretest/Posttest

The pretest/posttest is used to compare knowledge or skills before and after a presentation. The advantage of comparing the knowledge of the target audience before and after is that it indicates the amount of knowledge gained (educational gain) from the presentation. This type of evaluation can be used for evaluating behavior as well, but doing so is time-consuming and may not be practical for most public education programs. Here, however, it is used to refer to the use of written tests that evaluate knowledge.

In some cases, the target audience will already have knowledge of the information or specific behavior(s). In these instances, the presentation may not provide any new information. For example, young school children may receive many different presentations of the behavior "stop, drop, and roll." A pretest will show that the behavior has already been mastered and further presentations on the behavior are not necessary.

The opposite situation may also be true when the pretest shows that the target audience had a limited knowledge of the behavior. In this case, the results on the posttest would be due to the presentation.

Information provided by the pretest/posttest is also helpful in identifying the strengths and weaknesses of the presentation. For example, a presentation is given on bicycle safety. The posttests from two different presentations indicate that all the children missed the questions on the proper fitting of a bicycle helmet. This may indicate that the part of the presentation dealing with the fitting of bicycle helmets should be reviewed and possibly revised. It may also indicate that the individual test question is unclear and should be revised.

Five of the most common formats of pretests/posttests follow:

- Multiple-choice
- Fill-in-the-blank
- True/false
- Picture-identification
- A combination of the above

The multiple-choice format asks a question and then gives the participant several answer choices. The participant selects the correct choice. The multiple-choice test is easy to administer and to score. However, the person taking the test must be able to read and understand the questions. A multiple-choice test used in the *Learn Not to Burn® Curriculum* is shown in Figure 11.8.

A fill-in-the-blank test gives the participant a statement with a key word or phrase missing. The participant then fills in the correct word or phrase. The fill-in-the-blank test is very basic and does not provide in-depth information to the level of understanding. Here is one example of a fill-in-the-blank test question:

1. Each home escape plan should identify at least __________ way(s) out of every room.

A true/false test gives the participant a statement regarding the information. The participant must identify whether the statement is true or false. As with a fill-in-the-blank test, this type of test is very basic and lends itself to guessing.

Knowledge Test: Level 2

Please mark your answers.

The Nature of Fire

1. The three elements necessary for fire to occur are
   a. heat + fuel + oxygen.
   b. oxygen + nitrogen + hydrogen.

2. Smoke from fires
   a. stays close to the floor.
   b. rises to the ceiling.

3. The fabric which burns more easily is
   a. wool.
   b. nylon polyester.

4. The liquid which burns more quickly is
   a. gasoline.
   b. kerosene.

5. In fire tragedies, more people die from
   a. fire burns.
   b. breathing too much smoke.

What to do in Case of a Fire or Burn

6. If you see smoke or fire in your home, you should
   a. try to find out what is causing the smoke or fire.
   b. shout "Fire!" and alert everyone to get out.

7. When you see smoke coming from under a closed door, you should first
   a. open the door to see if there is a fire.
   b. feel the closed door to see if it is hot.

8. If you are in a smoke-filled house, you should
   a. hold your breath and run through the smoke.
   b. crawl low out of the smoke.

9. If you are on the sixth floor of a burning building, you should get out using the
   a. stairs.
   b. elevator.

10. If your clothes are on fire, you should
    a. drop to the ground and roll over and over to smother the flames.
    b. run to put out the flames.

Figure 11.8 A multiple-choice test used in the *Learn Not to Burn® Curriculum. Reprinted with permission from* Learn Not to Burn®, The Pre-School Program/Resource Book, *National Fire Protection Association, Quincy, MA 02269. This reprinted material is not the complete and official position of the National Fire Protection Association, on the referenced subject which is represented only by the Curriculum in its entirety.*

Here is an example of a true/false question:

2. T F Rugs used on a well-polished wood floor should be skid-resistant.

A picture-identification test is used primarily with younger children. Although younger children cannot read, they have the ability to identify pictures that show proper behaviors. However, this type of test requires providing detailed information to the participants so that they understand the situation being depicted by the pictures in addition to the directions for completing the test. An example of a picture-identification test from the *Learn Not to Burn® Curriculum* is shown in Figure 11.9.

Finally, a pretest/posttest can be a combination of these four types of test items. This type of test can evaluate several different levels of understanding, from basic understanding to application of the new information.

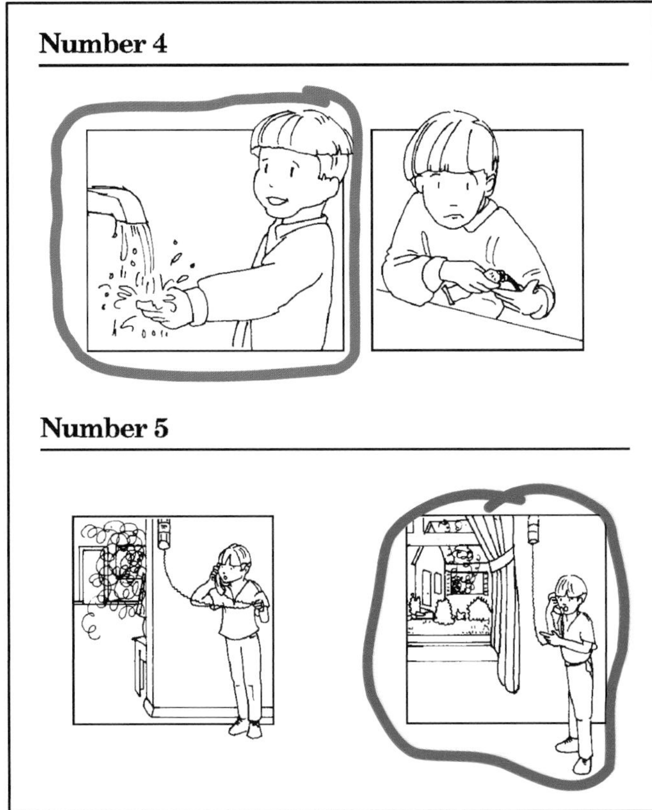

Figure 11.9 A picture-identification test from the *Learn Not to Burn® Curriculum. Reprinted with permission from* Learn Not to Burn®, The Pre-School Program/Resource Book, *National Fire Protection Association, Quincy, MA 02269. This reprinted material is not the complete and official position of the National Fire Protection Association, on the referenced subject which is represented only by the Curriculum in its entirety.*

In general, pretests/posttests are most effective when used in classroom settings. In these settings, the target audience can be managed during the evaluation process. Also, in most cases, the audience will be familiar with these types of tests. A pretest/posttest is not as effective with informal audiences such as adults and seniors. In these situations, surveys are best used to evaluate knowledge or behavior before and after the presentation.

Skills Test

Skills tests (performance tests) are used to evaluate the student's ability to perform a specific physical behavior such as testing a smoke detector or crawling low under smoke. Fire and life safety educators often assume that because someone can verbally explain the behavior they can also properly perform the behavior. This is not always the case. In fact, the only way to be *certain* that a person can perform a behavior is to conduct a skills-based evaluation (Figure 11.10).

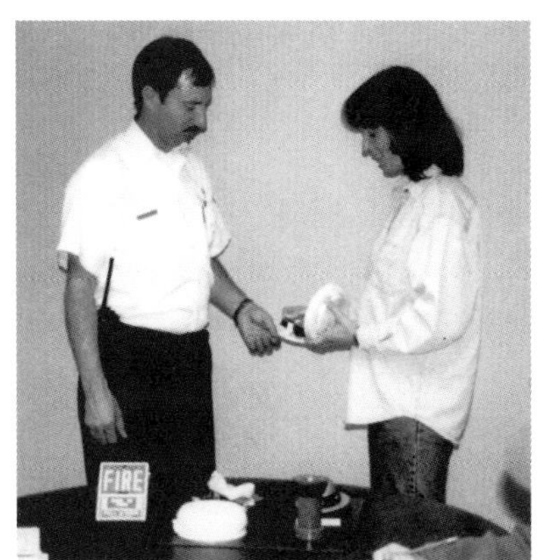

Figure 11.10 An educator watches a student demonstrate the ability to change a smoke detector battery.

Consider the earlier example of CPR. Immediately following the lecture about CPR the participant can probably explain the proper procedure for chest compressions and ventilations. However, he or she probably could not properly perform the behavior on a mannequin at that point in the course. Remember, a primary objective of fire and life safety education is the development of behaviors that can be successfully applied during an emergency. Skills test evaluations are the only ways of determining whether these objectives have been achieved.

A skills test uses an evaluation sheet that identifies the proper steps in the behavior. (Figure 11.11). This sheet is used as a guide to ensure that each specific step of the behavior has been

OPERATE A MULTIPURPOSE BASE DRY CHEMICAL FIRE EXTINGUISHER

Name ________________________ **Date** ____________

Evaluator ________________ **Overall Competency Rating** ____________

Equipment
- Multipurpose base, hand-carried, dry chemical fire extinguisher
- Simulated or small, live Class A or B fire

Job Steps	Key Points	Attempt No. 1	2	3
1. Size up fire.	1. Safe to fight with an extinguisher			
2. Carry extinguisher to within stream reach of fire.	2. a. 5 to 20 feet (1.5 m to 6 m) of fire			
	b. Upright position			
	c. By handle			
	d. Upwind of fire			
	e. Back to an escape route			
	f. Quickly but without running			
3. Pull pin at top of extinguisher.	3. Inspection band broken			
4. Release and aim discharge hose.	4. Toward base of fire			
5. Discharge extinguishing agent.	5. a. Squeezing handle			
	b. Slow side-to-side sweep to cover burning surface			
6. Make sure that fire is out.	6. a. Entire surface coated			
	b. Intermittently discharging to glowing areas after flames are extinguished			
7. Tag extinguisher for recharge and inspection.	7. a. Red tag			
	b. Initialed and dated			
	Time (Total)			

Evaluator's Comments ________________________________

____

____

Figure 11.11 An evaluation sheet helps the educator check that the required steps are completed.

successfully completed. This also ensures consistent evaluation of different audiences. When administering a skills test, the educator should give the participant a scenario appropriate for the desired behavior and then provide an opportunity for the participant to perform the behavior.

A skills test requires more time to administer than a written test. Also, space is needed to allow the participant to perform the behavior safely and out of the view of others. When giving a skills test, it is very important that the educator not provide any feedback during the evaluation that would assist the participant. Coaching or prompting the participant eliminates the objectivity of the evaluation. If the participant is unable to do the behavior, then the educator should provide more instruction until the participant can properly perform the behavior.

A final thought about skills testing. It is imperative that young children be evaluated on every skill they are taught. An evaluation ensures that each child clearly understands the correct behavior for the situation and that the child can correctly perform the behavior.

In many cases, the best method to use to evaluate performance with young children is to create a game which incorporates the behavior (Figure 11.12). For example, a blanket can be used to simulate smoke in a room. The children are asked to demonstrate the proper behavior if there is smoke in the room. The game is nonthreatening and allows the teacher to evaluate the child's understanding and performance. However, when a game is used, the same rules that apply to formalized evaluation should be followed, such as avoiding prompting and ensuring that the game is out of view of the other children while the evaluation is being conducted.

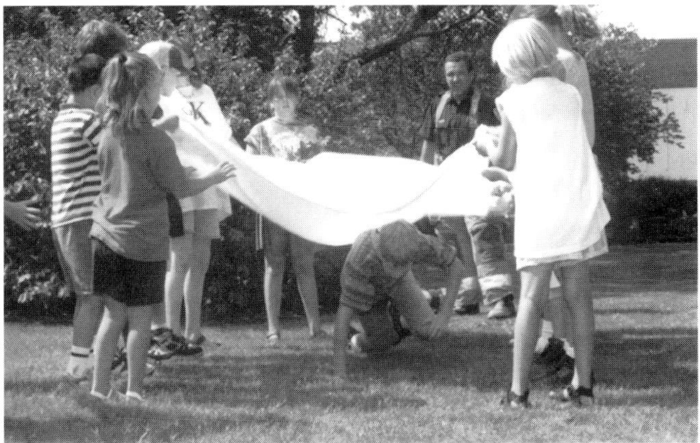

Figure 11.12 By playing the "blanket game" with the children, the educator teaches a desired behavior — crawl low under smoke.

Survey

A *survey* is an instrument used to identify the behavior and/or attitude of the target audience, both before and after the presentation. Generally, it is a series of questions about a specific safety issue and is an ideal method of determining whether the presentation resulted in the target audience acting on the information. It is best used with adults.

A survey must be carefully designed to be effective. It must ask for information that applies directly to the presentation. It must be easy to understand and not require a lot of time to complete. Remember, if a survey is very time-consuming or hard to complete, the participant will not complete it.

Also, the questions used in the survey should be written so that the question does not create the desired response. None of the questions should be leading questions. For example, you may want to determine the participants' understanding of testing a smoke detector. An appropriate question is:

1. A smoke detector should be tested every _________.

Conversely, the following question suggests the answer to the participant.

2. You do not need to test your smoke detector everyday, do you?

It is also important to keep in mind that information gained by a survey can be inaccurate. Participants may respond with information that they think the survey-taker wants to hear, even if it is not the truth. The best way to prevent this is to inform the participants about the purpose of the survey and how the information obtained will be used.

It may seem like a giant task to survey all the participants of any given presentation or program. However, it is only necessary to survey a sample of the participants. Generally, surveying 5 to 10 percent of the participants for any given program is adequate. Statistically, the results gained should represent the changes for all the participants. It is best to discuss the evaluation plan with a local resource, such as an educator at a local college, to determine the appropriate sample size to ensure a valid evaluation.

Inspection and Observation

The next two evaluation methods are more accurate than others because the evaluation is actually completed by the educator. The first of these two, inspection, has been used for years to ensure compliance with fire codes. However, inspections can also be used to determine the extent to which fire and life safety behaviors are being implemented in the community. For example, a voluntary home inspection program will provide information such as the number of smoke detectors installed in homes, the number of functioning detectors, and so on.

Heed these three important considerations for conducting inspections: It is essential that participants of the inspections be informed of the purpose of the inspections, that the inspection is an educational tool — not an enforcement tool — and that those personnel conducting the inspections be properly trained in inspection practices (Figure 11.13).

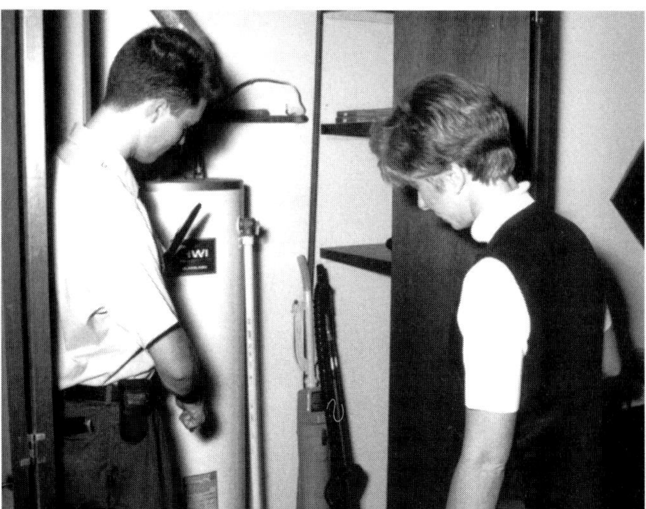

Figure 11.13 For the fire and life safety educator, inspection is an educational tool for preventing fires and accidents that could take the lives of occupants and destroy the home.

The other of these two evaluation methods is observation. Observation is useful in cases where it is possible for the educator to observe behaviors in a natural setting. Direct observation provides very reliable information on the effects of programs. For example, observation would be an ideal method of evaluating the effectiveness of a presentation to students at a specific school on the use of bicycle helmets. The educator can determine how many students wore helmets prior to the presentation by observing the children who ride their bikes to and from school. Then, following the presentation, observation will identify the increase or decrease in the use of helmets (Figure 11.14).

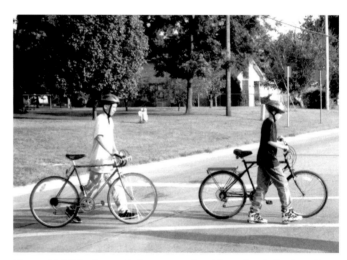

Figure 11.14 By demonstrating appropriate bike safety behaviors, these cyclists provide the educator with direct feedback concerning the effectiveness of the educational program.

Techniques for Observation

- Identify the group that you wish to evaluate. The group should be the target audience of the presentation. Also, determine the appropriate sample for the evaluation.
- Determine the best time and location to conduct the observation.
- When observing the group, be discrete. It is important for the group to be unaware that it is being evaluated.
- Clearly define the behavior or changes which you wish to observe.
- Have an evaluation form for recording your observations. This is helpful and adds consistency and accuracy to the evaluation over a period of time. It is essential that the observations be recorded accurately.

However, the information gained through observation, if the evaluation is not carefully designed, may not reflect the actual impact of educational programs or presentations. For instance, in the previous example the information gained through observation might reflect the effects of a television public service announcement, a discount for helmets in the local paper, or another influencing factor.

Injury/Loss Statistics

The final evaluation method is the use of injury/loss statistics such as dollar loss, incidents, causes of fire and injury, mortality/morbidity figures, etc. This information is available from many sources which are discussed in Chapter 7, "Using Data to Plan Programs." The other methods previously discussed provide information soon after the presentation. Injury/loss statistics reflect the effects of change, and it may take years before a realistic evaluation is possible. However, the information provided by evaluating injury/loss statistics is the most reliable indicator of the success of the program. In fact, this method of evaluation is best suited for long-term evaluation of overall programs (Figure 11.15).

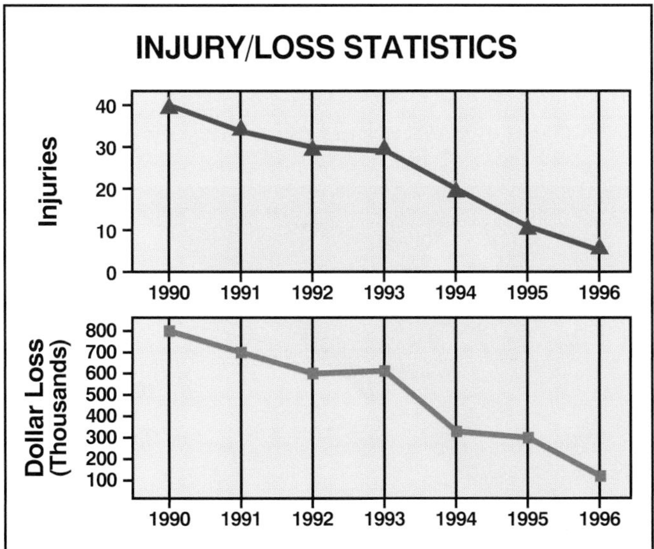

Figure 11.15 Injury/loss statistics represent information gathered over a period of time and provide the most reliable feedback on program effectiveness.

INTERPRETING THE DATA

One of the most difficult yet most important parts of the evaluation process is the interpretation of the gathered information. The methods described earlier provide only data and information that must be interpreted. The purpose of interpreting the evaluation results is to determine whether there has been an educational gain. An *educational gain* is a gain in knowledge, a positive change in behavior, or a positive change in the environment following a presentation. In other words, the educational gain is the amount of change that has occurred in the target audience because of the presentation or program.

Educational gain is determined by comparing knowledge or behaviors before the presentation with knowledge or behavior after the presentation. For example, an evaluation of a presentation to a third-grade class showed that the average posttest score was 30 points higher than the pretest. This indicates that there was an educational gain because of the presentation.

However, it is important to realize that educational gain is often a subjective interpretation on the part of the educator or evaluator. There may not be any guidelines that say, "These results clearly show an educational gain!" This is why it is so important for fire and life safety educators to seek the assistance of others when they are unsure of proper interpretation methods; the interpretation of the results must be correct. For example, an educator receives the posttest results from five classrooms using the *Learn Not to Burn® Curriculum*. The scores do not seem to show any conclusive educational gain. The educator should meet with the teachers to discuss the results from the individual classrooms. This will help to ensure accurate interpretation of the results.

There are generally two different types of calculations used to interpret the data:

- Mean of scores
- Percentages

Mean

The *mean* of a set of scores is simply the average score. To calculate the mean, add all the scores of the test, and divide by the number of scores. Use the following formula:

$$\text{Mean} = \frac{\text{Sum of the Participants' Test Scores}}{\text{Number of Participants}}$$

This may look like a complicated math problem, but it is really an easy calculation. Consider the test results from a presentation on cooking safety to a middle-school class. There were 20 children who participated in the presentation. The scores of the students are listed below.

95	90	85	85	60
90	95	65	90	85
65	50	95	75	45
85	90	90	100	80

To calculate the mean, you must first total the scores. The total, or sum, of the 20 scores is 1,615. In the next step, divide the sum by the number of participants, which in this example is 20.

$$\text{Mean} = \frac{1{,}615}{20} = 81$$

So, in this example, the mean (rounded to the nearest whole number) is 81. This shows that the average posttest score of the children is 81.

Percentage

Determining percentages is the other calculation commonly performed during the evaluation process. A *percentage* is a part of a whole expressed in hundredths. An example is the best way to demonstrate calculating percentages.

Recently, a presentation on home escape plans was presented to a civic group. There were 40 in the audience. A week after the presentation, a survey was sent to each participant to determine whether or not they had completed a home escape plan because of the presentation. Thirty of the participants returned the survey. Of those, 20 had completed a home escape plan because of the presentation.

In this example it is necessary to calculate two percentages:

- Percentage of participants who returned the survey
- Percentage of participants who did a home escape plan because of the presentation

To calculate the percentage of participants who returned the survey, divide the *number of participants who returned the survey by the total number of participants who received the survey:*

$$\text{Percentage (\%)} = \frac{30}{40} = 75\%$$

Based on this calculation, 75 percent of the participants completed the survey. This is a good response to the survey.

The next calculation is the percentage of participants who did a home escape plan because of the presentation (Figure 11.16). To calculate the percentage, divide the *number of participants who completed a home escape plan by the number of participants who returned the survey:*

$$\text{Percentage (\%)} = \frac{20}{30} = 66\%$$

Based on this calculation, 66 percent of the participants who returned the survey developed a home escape plan because of the presentation. This may not represent the actual number of participants who did the home escape plan because all the surveys were not returned.

Another use of percentages is in the evaluation of skills test. For example, assume it is necessary to evaluate a presentation given to 25 new fathers on proper placement of children in safety seats. The evaluation requires calculating the percentage of fathers who successfully com-

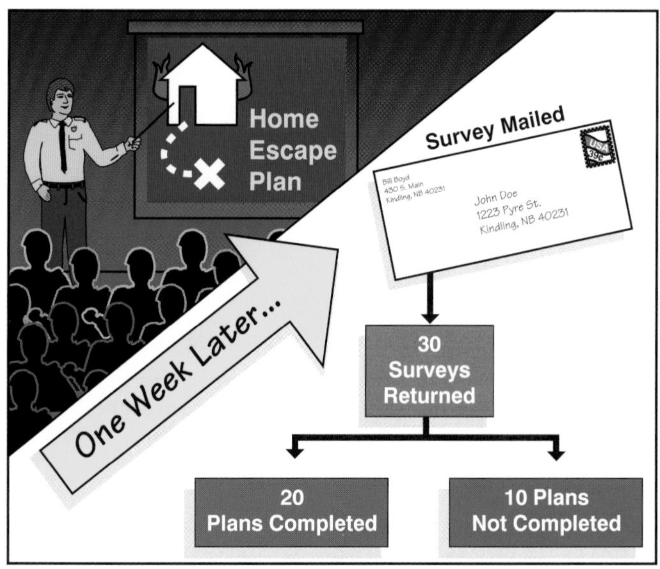

Figure 11.16 One area of data interpretation involves determining the percentage of those respondents who demonstrated the appropriate behavior as a result of a presentation.

pleted the skills test. There were 19 fathers who successfully placed the child in the safety seat during the skills test.

To calculate this percentage, divide the *number of fathers who successfully completed the skills test by the number of fathers taking the skills test:*

$$\text{Percentage } (\%) = \frac{19}{25} = 76\%$$

Based on this calculation, 76 percent of the fathers were successful in the skills test.

Remember, the calculation of the mean and of percentages help only to clarify the data obtained in evaluation. The experience and judgment of the educator are required to interpret the data and to determine the educational gain.

Interpretation

The final step in the evaluation process is to develop a conclusion about the effectiveness of the presentation. This conclusion is always based on an *objective* interpretation of the results. After the calculations have been completed, it is necessary to consider one or all of the following to develop a conclusion:

- The difference between the average pretest and posttest scores
- Any patterns in the scores such as specific questions that are missed, lack of improvement in any one area, confusion about specific behaviors, etc.
- The differences in scores from one presentation to another or from one target audience to another
- The outcome objectives for the presentation

For example, consider the third-grade class discussed in one of the previous examples. The difference in the average of pretest and posttest scores was 30 percentage points. If the average pretest score was 65 percent, then this would mean that the average posttest score was 95 percent. This is an excellent score and shows an important and acceptable educational gain. However, if the average pretest score was only 35 percent, the average posttest score would be 65 percent. This is a low score and is probably not acceptable. In both cases the difference was 30 percentage points. When determining whether the educational gain is acceptable, the educator compares the educational gain with the desired outcome identified in the learning objectives. This determines whether the gain is acceptable or whether further education is necessary with the audience. If there is any confusion, the educator should seek help from a qualified educator. (**NOTE:** See the "Local Resources" section at the end of this chapter.)

Another example is the home escape plan survey discussed earlier. In that example, 80 percent of those attending the presentation completed and returned the survey. Depending on the outcome objectives, this may be an acceptable level of participation. However, if the outcome objective calls for more than 80 percent participation, it will be important to find out *why* the other 20 percent did not return the surveys. In this type of situation, it is critical to contact participants who did not return the survey and determine the reason(s) for the lack of participation. It is also important to contact those who did return the survey and find out why they returned the survey. In short, consider all the information; do not base conclusions on just one piece of information or data.

Each type of fire and life safety education presentation or program presents different evaluation needs and criteria. Regardless of the type of presentation, take the time to carefully review all the information and the meaning of the information. Use the following tips to guide the interpretation of the results of the evaluation:

- Make sure the evaluation method is appropriate for the presentation.
- Spend the necessary time to develop a good evaluation plan before the presentation.
- If you need assistance in developing an evaluation tool, get it during the planning stage.
- Explain the purpose of the evaluation to the target audience, especially if they are adults. This will help to ensure that information obtained from the audience is accurate.

- Consider each piece of information gained from the evaluation. Look for any patterns, differences in scores, desired outcome objectives, etc. Consider also the evaluation results of other similar presentations.
- If the evaluation indicates the outcome objectives were not achieved, ask "Why?" Think about how the presentation affected the outcome and especially about any changes that could be made to improve the presentation.
- If the results are unclear or if it is difficult to develop a conclusion, ask for help from an educational resource. The results of the evaluation could have a significant impact on the presentation; do not make presentation changes based on bad conclusions.

SELECTING EVALUATION INSTRUMENTS

It is important to note that in every presentation it is possible to evaluate a change in knowledge. However, if the objective of the presentation is for the target audience to act on the information — for example to install a smoke detector — evaluating the knowledge change is not enough. It is important to go further and to evaluate the behavior change or environmental change.

Different types of evaluation instruments (methods) are best suited for each of the steps and for specific types of audiences. These are presented in Table 11.1.

The best method of evaluating knowledge change is through written tests such as multiple-choice and picture-identification tests. For younger children, oral questions can be used effectively. *Remember that this type of evaluation must be specifically designed for the characteristics of the target audience.* This is one of the reasons that effective audience analysis is so critical.

The best methods for evaluating behavior change include skills tests and surveys. Skills tests are a method of immediate evaluation. They can be used when teaching physical behaviors such as crawling low under smoke. For behaviors that are performed in the home or workplace, such as testing a smoke detector, a survey must be used after the presentation.

TABLE 11.1
Methods For Evaluating Change

Type Of Change	Evaluation Methods
Knowledge	Multiple-choice written test
	True/false written test
	Oral or written picture-identification test
	Oral questions
Behavior	Skills test
	Survey
	Observation
Environmental	Survey
	Inspection

The best methods for evaluating environmental change are surveys and inspections. A survey can be sent to the target audience after the presentation to find out whether participants acted on the information. It is important to give them time to act. Another method is to perform a home or workplace inspection to check for the desired environmental changes. This is a labor-intensive method. An additional drawback is that many people will not allow you to inspect their homes.

In all cases, the evaluation process provides the best results when there is information on the knowledge, behaviors, or environment — both before and after the presentation. This information can be gathered through written pretests and posttests. Or, in the case of surveys, the questions can all be asked in one survey given after the presentation. Regardless of how the educator obtains it, she or he always should try to get the information so that a comparison is possible. This comparison will provide the best conclusions about the effectiveness of the presentation.

ADMINISTERING EVALUATION INSTRUMENTS

A reliable evaluation process is totally dependent on the proper administration of evaluation instruments. It is the responsibility of the educator to ensure that evaluation instruments, such as tests and surveys, are presented appropriately. Often, the acceptance of the evaluation by the target audience hinges on the way it is presented. The directions for the evaluation instruments probably will have already been developed; it is only necessary to provide the directions.

Consider three things when administering an evaluation instrument:

- The environment where the evaluation instrument is being used
- The evaluator's attitude toward the target audience and the evaluation process
- The instructions for the target audience

Environment

The *environment* is the physical area in which the evaluation is done. For example, in a grade school the environment will be the classroom. In some cases, such as a survey, there is little control over the environment. The following recommendations help to ensure a proper environment for the evaluation:

- Keep the environment free from all distractions. The target audience must be able to concentrate on the questions.
- Create a relaxed setting for the target audience. They should understand the importance of the evaluation but should not feel as though they are taking a college-entrance exam.
- Be sure the environment is well-lit.
- Check to see that the environment is free of hazards. This is especially important when evaluating physical behaviors.
- Always be prepared with the proper material and equipment to do the evaluation. For example, always be ready with the proper evaluation forms, pencils, instructions, props, etc.

Evaluator's Attitude

The evaluator's attitude will have a dramatic impact on the process. The target audience must believe that the evaluator values their feedback and that their feedback will be used to improve the presentation in the future. If they are given the impression that the evaluation is not a valuable process, they will not take it seriously. Consequently, the information provided will not be accurate. The following recommendations help to demonstrate the proper attitude:

- Always be positive about the presentation and the evaluation process. Express the importance of evaluation and that the information provided will be used to improve the presentation.
- Avoid influencing the participants. The evaluation instrument should elicit objective information. If a participant does not know the answer or cannot perform the behavior, avoid providing the needed information.
- Follow the instructions for administration provided with the evaluation instrument. For example, most prepared evaluation instruments are provided with instructions on how to administer the evaluation. Follow these instructions explicitly to ensure the reliability and credibility of the evaluation.
- Provide clear instructions to the target audience before the evaluation. If you are using a survey, make sure the written instructions are clear. (**NOTE:** The survey may be done through the mail — without the educator being present to clarify the instructions.)
- Provide feedback to the target audience after the completion of the evaluation. Tell them that their participation is appreciated.
- Always maintain and respect the anonymity of those taking the evaluation. It is seldom necessary to share the results of a certain participant's evaluation with others. However, it may be helpful in certain instances such as with school children to have the child's name on the evaluation so that it can be returned after it is scored. (**NOTE:** The evaluator probably wants to share the information gained with other evaluators — but not with other participants.)

Audience Instructions

Finally, the instructions to the target audience must be very clear. The instructions should include not only how to complete the evaluation instrument but also the purpose of the evaluation. With a survey, it is critical that the survey instructions are easy to understand because it is not possible for the educator to answer questions. The following recommendations help the fire and life safety educator provide good instructions to the target audience:

- Ensure that participants are able to understand the instructions. For written tests and skills tests, explain the instructions before giving the evaluation.
- Be sure that instructions are easy to read. Also, see that the instructions are written at the education and reading level of the target audience.
- Make sure instructions are concise.
- Explain the purpose of the evaluation to the target audience. This is very important, especially with adults.

EVALUATING THE OVERALL PROGRAM

Up to this point, the focus has been on the evaluation methods for individual presentations. However, there may be a need to evaluate an overall program. This section discusses this type of evaluation.

(**NOTE:** As mentioned at the beginning of the chapter, the evaluation of an individual presentation or part of an overall program is called *formative evaluation.* The evaluation of the overall program following completion is known as *summative evaluation.*)

A *program,* as defined in Chapter 10, "Developing the Program Curriculum," is a comprehensive strategy that addresses fire and life safety issues via educational means. A program consists of more than one component. For example, a program on heating safety may include public service announcements, presentations to civic groups, and advertisements in the local paper.

In this example, it is possible to evaluate each of the individual components. It is also possible to evaluate the overall program by using a survey or through loss statistics. In either case, the scope of the evaluation must be identified in the planning process, and an appropriate evaluation strategy must be developed.

It may be helpful to evaluate both the components and the effectiveness of the overall program. By evaluating the individual components, the successful components are identified as well as those that need improvement. By also evaluating the overall program, the total effect of the components is identified.

When evaluating the overall program, the same guidelines and methods previously discussed apply. It is best to get assistance with program evaluation to ensure a valid and reliable process.

One other change that can occur due to an effective program is institutional change. *Institutional change* is a change in the values or attitudes of the organization. For example, following a series of fire safety presentations, a company decides to provide residential smoke detectors to their employees at no charge. This commitment to the residential fire safety of the employees represents a change in the values of the company toward fire safety. This is an institutional change.

Local Resources

Many fire and life safety educators use predeveloped curricula such as NFPA's Learn Not to Burn® material. Most of these types of programs come with evaluation instruments as well as an evaluation strategy. It is best to use these prepared evaluation instruments because they have already been validated and are designed to specifically evaluate the information presented in the program.

When a curriculum that does not have an evaluation instrument is purchased or when a curriculum is developed locally, it is necessary to develop an evaluation instrument.

Assistance may be needed to develop the new evaluation instrument as well as to interpret the information or to help conduct the evaluation. Also, it is sometimes necessary to review questions in prepared evaluation instruments to ensure that they are appropriate. Using outside resources can add credibility to the evaluation process, reduce bias, and improve the quality of information gained through interpretation. For all these needs, assistance is generally available locally.

The best local resources for help with evaluation are other professional educators. Teachers, college professors, principals, and injury prevention specialists routinely develop and implement evaluation instruments. These resources are generally qualified and willing to provide help with fire and life safety programs (Figure 11.17).

Several other local and state individuals/groups are potential resources for help with evaluation:

- County health departments
- State extension offices

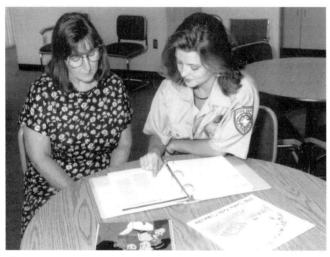

Figure 11.17 A teacher and a fire and life safety educator discuss an evaluation instrument for an education program presentation.

- County and state fire marshals
- State fire training agencies
- Marketing firms
- Other fire and life safety educators
- Local governmental analysts
- Community colleges

CONCLUSION

Evaluation is a planned process that is used to measure the success of a presentation. It requires careful planning by the fire and life safety educator. In some cases, evaluation will require assistance of other educators. In all cases, evaluation is a valuable tool that should be an integral part of every program.

The evaluation process provides the fire and life safety educator with feedback in the following areas:

- Effectiveness of the presentation
- Educational gain of the target audience
- Appropriateness of the instructional methods used in the presentation

The information provided by evaluation must be acted on to be of any value. The information should be used to refine and improve the presentation. Evaluation must be an ongoing process used with every presentation.

Finally, evaluation must be given the same importance as any tool or process used by the fire and life safety educator. Effective evaluation is the only way to know whether presentation and program outcome objectives are being achieved.

Chapter 11 Notes

(**NOTE:** A bibliography of references is provided for this chapter.)

American Red Cross, *Community Disaster Education Guide*, American Red Cross, Washington, DC, 1992.

Fire Service Programs Across America, U.S. Fire Administration, 1990.

Herman, Joan, *A Practical Guide to Alternative Assessment,* 1st ed., Association for Supervision and Curriculum Development, 1992.

Lofquist, William, *Discovering the Meaning of Prevention,* 1st ed., AYD Publications, 1983.

National Academy of Sciences, *Injury in America,* National Academy Press, Washington, DC, 1985.

The National Committee for Injury Prevention and Control, *Injury Prevention: Meeting the Challenge,* Oxford Press, New York, 1989.

Presenting Effective Public Education Presentations, U.S. Fire Administration, 1994.

Proving Public Fire Education Works, U.S. Fire Administration, 1990.

Public Fire Education Resource Directory, U.S. Fire Administration, 1988.

Stanford Center for Research in Disease Prevention, *How-To Guides on Community Health Promotion,* 2nd ed., Health Promotion Research Center, 1991.

Chapter 12
Networking, Forming Coalitions, and Working Cooperatively

INTRODUCTION

Fire and life safety is not solely a fire department responsibility but rather a responsibility that requires community-wide action. In recent years, fire departments across North America have enlisted the help of community-based organizations and of active citizens for education programs. In other cases — especially in communities participating in USFA's National Community Volunteer Fire Prevention Program (NCVFPP) — community organizations took the lead in education programs, and the fire department was one of many community partners. The trend is clear: Fire departments and other organizations are working cooperatively as equal partners for fire and life safety.

This chapter introduces skills and techniques for community action. The chapter begins with information about networking and discusses the "how tos" of coalition building. Tips for working with steering committees and task forces are also presented, as well as techniques for facilitating group action.

This chapter also includes a section about volunteers. This section covers the role of volunteer educators, ideas for expanding volunteer resources, and suggestions for working with volunteers from other community agencies and organizations.

NETWORKING

In the last several years of the twentieth century there has been a major organizational shift from hierarchies to networks, according to social observer John Naisbitt. In other words, loosely knit networks of equals are replacing pyramid-shaped hierarchies in the workplace and in other organizations (Figure 12.1).

Just what are networks? "Simply stated, networks are people talking to each other, sharing ideas, information, and resources. The point is often made that networking is a verb, not a noun. The important part is not the network, the finished product, but the process of getting there — the communication that creates the linkages between people and clusters of people."[1]

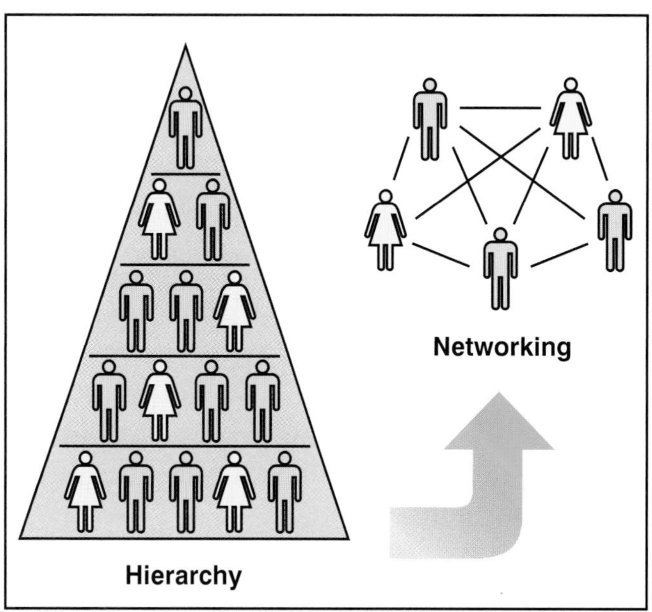

Figure 12.1 A growing number of organizations are changing from hierarchies to networks.

Like other network users, fire and life safety educators use networks to do the following:

- Network through conferences, newsletters (including Oklahoma State University's *Public Fire Education Digest* and NFPA's *Education Section Newslet-*

ter), state and national public education organizations, other organizations (such as the American Burn Association or SAFE KIDS® Coalitions) with similar interests, telephone calls, faxes and letters, photocopied materials, shared materials, and specialized organizations (such as statewide public fire education associations).

- Use networks as an easy and fast way to get information they trust.
- Provide a cross-disciplinary approach to problems through networking.
- Gain access to influential people through networking.
- Know that effective networks spread outward, like ripples in a pond.

Because fire and life safety educators often do not have peers — "someone to talk to" — at work, networking is especially important. Fire and life safety educators can take several specific steps to expand their network of contacts and information:

- Join a statewide fire education association. If there is no group in your state, join an association in a neighboring state, or start one in your state. For contact names, addresses, and program descriptions, see the *Directory of National Community Volunteer Fire Prevention Programs, Community Based Fire Prevention Education Initiatives* published by the United States Fire Administration.
- Make it a personal and professional goal to attend a fire and life safety education conference or similar meeting within the next year.
- Keep the attendance list from any conference that you attend. Note which people you met and what topics you discussed. These notes are helpful for reestablishing contact later.
- Keep a business-card collection. Note where you met each person and what you talked about (Figure 12.2).
- Always carry business cards. (**NOTE**: An order of 500 two-color cards will probably cost less than $50.)

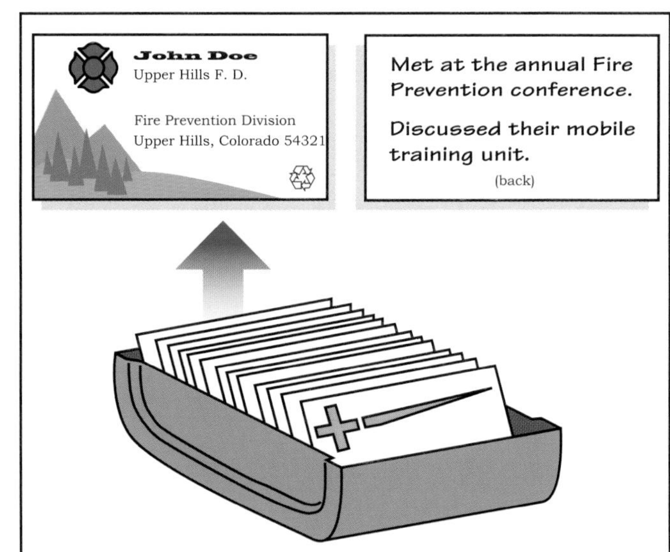
John Doe
Upper Hills F. D.
Fire Prevention Division
Upper Hills, Colorado 54321
Met at the annual Fire Prevention conference.
Discussed their mobile training unit.
(back)

Figure 12.2 By obtaining business cards from peers and making notes for reference, educators can acquire a significant number of network contacts.

- Expand your network to include nonfire resource people. Include public and private school teachers, other school professionals such as counselors and librarians, health care professionals, and community leaders in the list of people you know — and can contact for help with your programs.

Fire Education Network

One example of successful networking has taken place in the state of North Carolina. In order to share information about fire and life safety education, a handful of local and state fire educators coordinated efforts to establish the North Carolina Fire Education Regional Network. The state was divided into four geographic regions: southeast, northeast, central, and western. Individuals involved in fire and life safety education in these regions meet quarterly to share experiences and ideas, identify problems, and work cooperatively to address issues in their region.

In addition, five representatives from each of the fire education regional committees (networks) serve on an advisory council, the North Carolina State Fire Education Committee. This advisory council coordinates an annual conference, disseminates information on safety education issues to fire and injury prevention personnel, promotes fire and life safety educator certification, and serves as a focal point for safety education within the state.

The North Carolina Fire Education Regional Network has been successful: It is used by the majority of fire and life safety educators in North Carolina, and information is exchanged and used.

COALITION BUILDING

Networks are usually informal groups of persons with a common interest (Figure 12.3). Coalitions, on the other hand, are more formal relationships between or among *organizations* (Figure 12.4). Coalitions often start from an existing network. Coalitions have a specific goal, but networks do not.

Both networking and coalition building are familiar to fire and life safety educators and to the fire service. As USFA said in *Leadership for Public Fire Safety Education*, "In some departments, fire safety education programs are being redefined in broader terms as injury prevention education programs. Because of the pressure of such responsibilities in a time of shrinking budgets, fire departments must increasingly work through coalitions to solve problems. Overall, fire departments are showing a marked increase of interest in networking — a positive trend that can help them cope with their diverse responsibilities."[2]

Coalitions have some of the following advantages[3]:

- Grass-roots coalitions have more credibility than individuals or single organizations and agencies.
- Participants in coalitions are actively involved in a common cause, giving them ownership in the project.
- Because organizations have ownership in the coalition, they are generally more willing to provide resources for coalition projects.
- Coalitions have fewer organizational restrictions than government agencies. This may allow them to react more quickly to community needs and operate more efficiently than other agencies and organizations.
- Grass-roots coalitions may more easily gain the support of local media because they deal with specific issues.
- Because many organizations are working together on a single issue, community resources are used more efficiently and effectively.

Coalitions

Coalitions are like mutual aid agreements. Two or more organizations agree to help each other in specific ways. There is often a written agreement that spells out what kind of help each will provide to the other.

Coalitions, like mutual aid agreements, are *mutual*. Because coalitions are not one-sided, fire and life safety educators must be as ready to help with nonfire programs as they are to ask nonfire organizations for help.

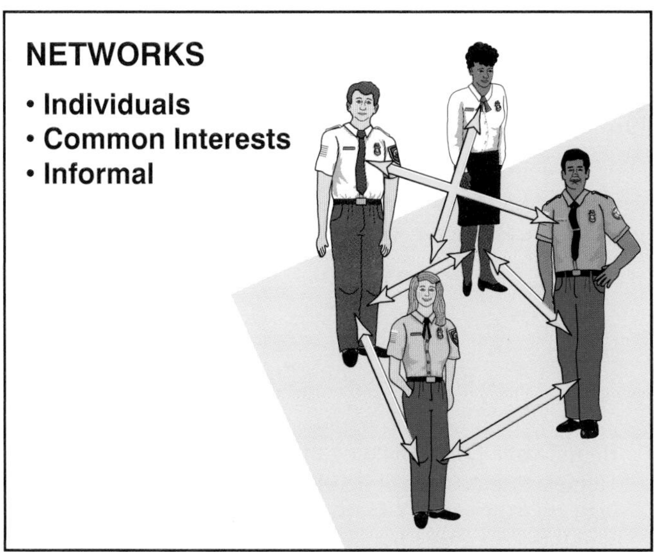

Figure 12.3 Characteristics of networks.

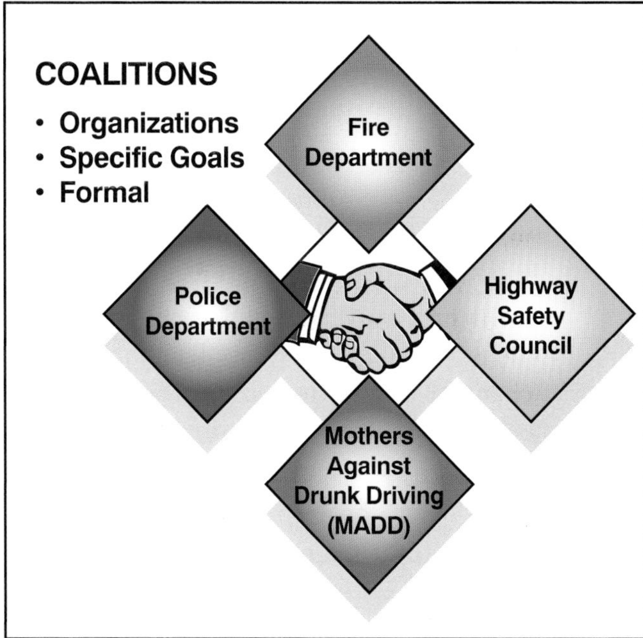

Figure 12.4 Characteristics of coalitions.

Networking Leads to Coalition

An example of a coalition-building effort began in 1988 in Minnesota when two public educators (from Minneapolis and the State Fire Marshal Division) began networking regarding the need to develop a statewide focus on fire safety issues based on MFIRS data. The lack of smoke detectors or nonworking smoke detectors coupled with home-escape planning was determined as the priority issue.

A list of organizations and individuals interested in fire and life safety issues were identified, and subsequently their undertaking became known as the Minnesota Fire Safety Project. By 1990, the results of their efforts created a statewide fire drill program called "Gopher It Minnesota," using the University of Minnesota team mascot, Goldy Gopher.

The program included six messages (visual/print) relating to home fire drills:

- "Gopher" the smoke detector every month to make sure it works.
- "Gopher" the floor and crawl under smoke.
- "Gopher" the bedroom door and close it when going to bed.
- "Gopher" the family meeting place once out of a burning home.
- "Gopher" the neighbor's phone and call 9-1-1 in case of fire.
- "Gopher" the window if fire blocks the door.

So should you.

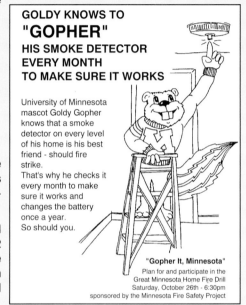

GOLDY KNOWS TO

Saturday, October 26th - 6:30pm

The statewide fire drill was held on the last Saturday in October to coincide with the "Change your clock, change your battery" program. Program materials were mailed to fire departments explaining the program and the steps departments could take to be a part of the statewide fire drill.

Following the event, the Minnesota State Fire Marshal Division conducted a survey to evaluate the program's effectiveness. The survey was sent to 802 fire departments in Minnesota, and 345 surveys (43 percent of those sent) were returned. These fire departments protect 51 percent of Minnesota's 4.5 million population. Nearly 75 percent of the fire departments returning surveys stated they participated in the program.

A member of the coalition from the Minnesota news network identified 450 media markets for the program's media kit. A clipping service identified media coverage by gathering 93 articles from 75 newspapers — and an additional 25 articles related to the "Change your clock, change your battery" program. Additional media coverage included 250 radio PSAs, which reached a potential listening audience of half a million people.

The program continues on an annual basis, and the coalition has moved on to address the fire problems associated with senior citizens. Over the past five years, this Minnesota coalition has helped reduce the state's fire deaths from 90 in 1989, to 46 in 1995.

Conversely, there are challenges associated with coalitions:

- Generally, coalitions do not have any legal authority to carry out interventions that involve enforcement or legal action.
- Coalitions may not have dedicated staff whose primary role is carrying out the activities and mission of the coalition, making tasks such as planning, implementation, and evaluation hard to accomplish.
- Because of the diversity of the organizations in a coalition, different agendas may be advocated on a single issue, making consensus difficult.

Of course, the fire department and the groups that participate in the community's education programs both need to feel that the coalition benefits *them*. USFA's *Partnerships Against Fire Action Pak*[4] identifies incentives to the fire department for working with community groups — and incentives to community groups for working with the fire department.

A Way to Reach the Community

Coalition-building extends to the community's residents, too. For example, the Colorado Springs Fire Department hosts neighborhood meetings — complete with refreshments — for residents to meet the fire chief and the firefighters that serve the neighborhood.

Fire departments can receive three types of benefits from working with community groups: management incentives, political incentives, and financial/productivity incentives.

The following management incentives benefit the fire department:

- Finding a community-supported solution to the community-wide needs of fire and life safety
- Donated resources of time, manpower, and money
- The potential for creating networks
- Reduced fire losses through public education
- Fire department visibility and recognition
- Demonstrated community support

Political incentives have some similarities to management incentives:

- Enhanced visibility
- Identifying the fire department as a "partner in life safety"
- Goodwill of influential individuals and organizations
- Enhanced fire department image among elected officials
- Demonstrated fire department involvement in comprehensive activities that extend beyond fire suppression and vehicle maintenance

And, finally, there are financial/productivity incentives for working with community groups:

- A demonstration of fire department effort to maximize the impact of the taxpayers' dollars
- A way to augment fire department funding
- A way to strengthen the fire marshal's office and other fire prevention agencies
- A way to reduce the number and severity of fires

Likewise, community groups and individuals receive benefits from working with the fire department. Their benefits include the following incentives:

- Increased and positive media coverage
- Contributing to community well-being
- A way to create positive opportunities for community organizations
- The excitement of association with a fire department
- The chance of meeting their own organization's objectives through fire education
- Increased membership

Building a Successful Coalition

The National Fire Academy's Developing Fire and Life Safety Strategies course recommends eight guidelines to follow when setting up a coalition[5]:

- Use people who are credible in their fields.

Click It or Ticket

North Carolina's statewide "Click It or Ticket" program to encourage the use of seat belts and child safety seats relies heavily on coalition-building. The Department of Transportation and its Governor's Highway Safety Program, various law enforcement agencies, and the Department of Insurance are among the public agencies participating in the Click It or Ticket coalition. The North Carolina Medical Society, the state chapter of the American Academy of Pediatrics, and the Carolina Association of Professional Insurance Agents are among the community groups that have shown their support for the program.

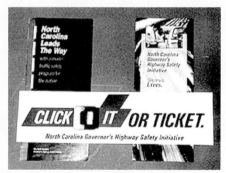

The program is successful on several levels. Nearly nine out of ten residents were familiar with the program and supported enforcement efforts for the use of seat belts and child safety seats. U.S. Secretary of Transportation Federico Pena reported that six other states will use the North Carolina model as a blueprint for their own programs. After the program began, seat-belt use rose to about eight out of ten drivers — one of the highest rates in the nation.

- Select people whose primary role is compatible with injury prevention.
- Select people with the ability to carry out prevention activities.
- Be sure that representatives have the authority to commit their agency.
- Select a chair and members with ability and time for leadership roles.
- Insist on a program plan with clear goals, objectives, and responsibilities; provide technical assistance in developing the plan.
- Donate personnel — or volunteer — to staff the meetings, keep minutes, and follow up on assignments.
- Inform the community about the coalition, using the existing public recognition of the participating organizations.

Sample Coalitions

Coalitions come in many shapes and sizes. For example, the National SAFE KIDS Campaign® is a nationwide effort with the goal of reducing preventable injuries, the number one killer of children age 14 and under. The campaign is a program of the Children's National Medical Center in Washington, D.C. Fire and burn prevention are part of the SAFE KIDS® focus, along with traffic safety, water safety, poisoning prevention, choking prevention, and playground safety. This high-profile and well-funded program (Vice President and Mrs. Al Gore are Honorary Chairs, and Johnson & Johnson is the founding sponsor) includes an annual National SAFE KIDS® Week. Highlights of 1993 activities included a special episode of the CBS program *Rescue 911* on preventable childhood injuries, several public service announcements by well-known television personalities, participation by thousands of retailers who gave away free injury-prevention materials, and a newspaper advertising supplement (funded by Johnson & Johnson) that reached 55 million homes and offered free First Alert® smoke detectors.

The National SAFE KIDS Campaign® has very active local and state components. The cam-

A Successful Coalition

Another example of a successful coalition is the Colorado Springs, Colorado, SAFE KIDS® Coalition. The Coalition was established in 1993 as a joint effort of the Colorado Springs Fire Department and the Colorado Springs Junior League. Both organizations had an interest in prevention of childhood injuries and understood the benefits of a community-based approach to the problem.

After establishing the Coalition, several other community organizations and agencies were asked to become involved. By the spring of 1994 over 20 individual organizations were actively participating in the Coalition, including law enforcement, school districts, local media, and child welfare agencies. The Coalition has implemented several injury prevention education campaigns as summarized below:

- **A bicycle safety campaign that provided information to parents on the need for wearing bicycle helmets**. Parents and children were provided with discount coupons for bicycle helmets at local stores. Helmets were provided at no cost to those children who could not afford them.
- **A smoke detector campaign that provided free smoke detectors and batteries at local fire stations and child-care providers**. The detectors were purchased through a grant from BRK (First Alert®); Everready® provided the batteries. Local media members of the Coalition produced and broadcast public service announcements on the program.
- **A child safety seat campaign that educated young parents about the use of child safety seats**. The SAFE KIDS® Coalition worked with another local coalition, Drive Smart Colorado Springs, on the development and implementation of the campaign. The SAFE KIDS® Coalition used their other programs to reach young parents with the information on the safety seats.
- **A child fire play awareness campaign**. At the time of the campaign, child fire play was the leading cause of fire in Colorado Springs. The goal of the campaign was early detection and intervention of fire play behaviors. The Coalition gained the support and participation of law enforcement, the District Attorney's Office, and the Department of Social Services. Through the Coalition, an informational campaign was implemented with expansion of the program planned in the immediate future.

13. List the seven fundamental steps to coalition building outlined in the National SAFE KIDS Campaign® *Leader's Guide*. *(218)*

14. Name the groups that may be included in the Sesame Street® Fire Safety Program coalition. *(219)*

15. Describe techniques that help fire and life safety educators become effective facilitators. *(220)*

16. Identify and briefly contrast the three basic forms of brainstorming. *(221)*

17. Describe guidelines for facilitating a brainstorming session. *(221, 222)*

18. Describe techniques for bringing a group to consensus. *(222)*

19. Explain why people volunteer to work with fire and life safety educators. *(223, 224)*

20. Identify the following names, abbreviations, and acronyms:
    - USFA *(213)*
    - NCVFPP *(213)*
    - John Naisbitt *(213)*
    - SAFE KIDS® *(214)*
    - Sesame Street® Fire Safety Program *(219)*
    - *Partnerships Against Fire Action Pak (220)*
    - Alex Osborn *(221)*
    - Peter Drucker *(223)*
    - CDF VIP *(223)*

Questions and Notes

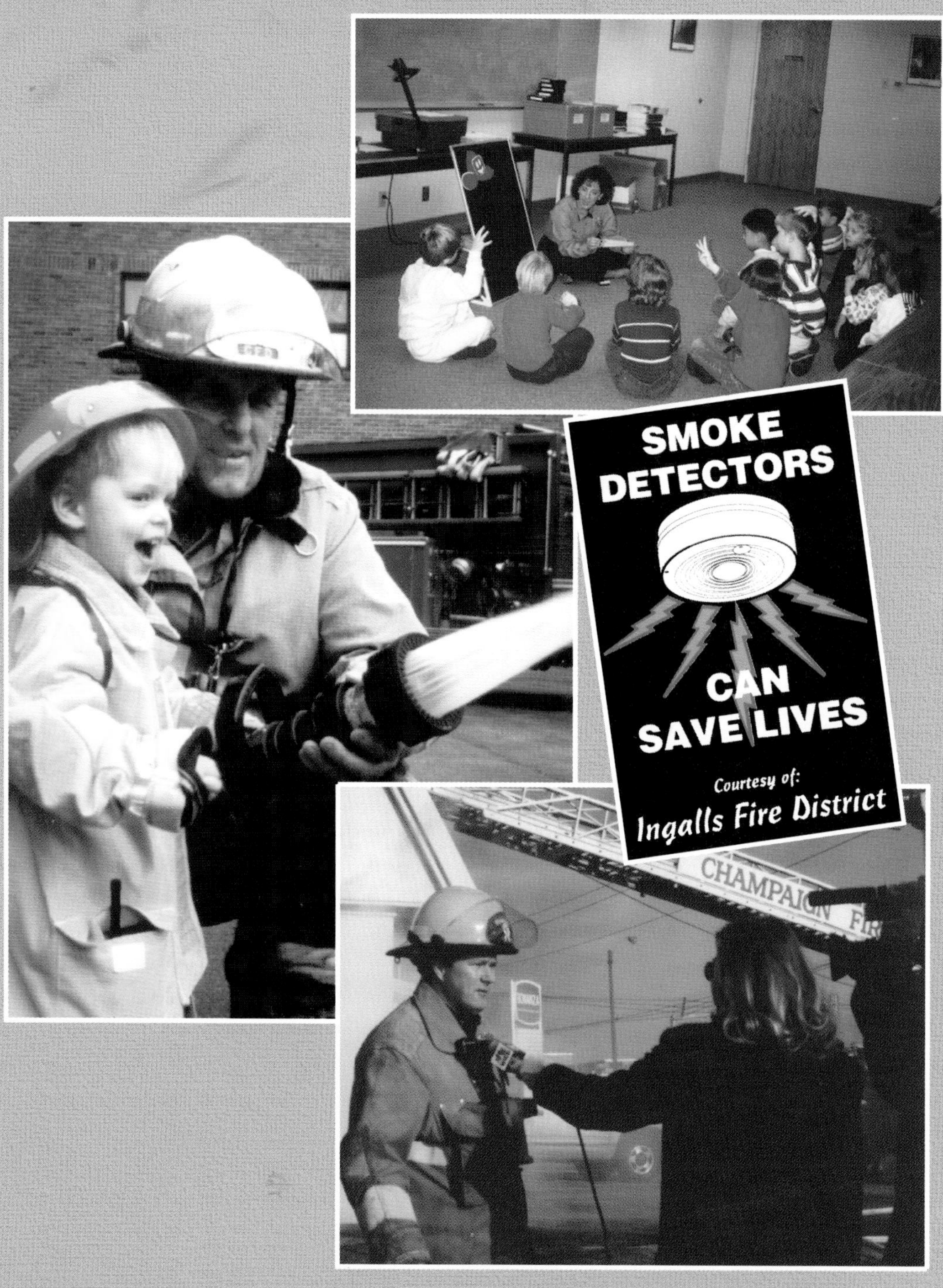
SMOKE
DETECTORS
CAN
SAVE LIVES
Courtesy of:
Ingalls Fire District
CHAMPAIGN

13 Learning Fire and Life Safety Educational Theory

LEARNING OBJECTIVES

This chapter provides information that addresses the following objectives of NFPA 1035, *Standard for Professional Qualifications for Public Fire and Life Safety Educator* (1993 edition):

Public Fire and Life Safety Educator I

3-4.1.1 *Prerequisite Knowledge:* Basic learning characteristics of preschool children, elementary school-age children, secondary school-age children, adults, and senior adults.

Public Fire and Life Safety Educator II

4-4.1 Develop informational materials, given an identified issue, so that information provided is accurate, relevant to the issue, and comprehensible to the audience.

4-4.2.1 *Prerequisite Knowledge:* Learning theory for all age, social, and developmental audiences; needs assessment; development of written and visual educational materials; development of learning objectives, course development based on specified learning objectives and audiences, lesson plan development, and selection and use of evaluation instruments.

4-4.3 Develop a lesson plan, given a specific behavior, learning objectives, and a specified audience, so that the lesson plan reflects the learning characteristics and abilities of the intended audience.

4-4.5.1 *Prerequisite Knowledge:* Educational methodology.

Chapter 13
Learning Fire and Life Safety Educational Theory

INTRODUCTION

Fire and life safety educators work in fire departments, in other fire service organizations, in hospitals, and in corporations. Wherever they work or whatever other duties they have, fire and life safety educators are educators — so they need to have a working knowledge of how people learn.

This chapter covers the differences among learning, education, and information. The chapter also addresses the basics of what motivates people to learn and how people learn differently at different stages of life. Finally, the chapter discusses how to evaluate whether or not learning has taken place.

It is important to be able to distinguish among the definitions of four key terms used in this chapter (Figure 13.1):

- *Curriculum* — A sequence of presentations on fire and life safety education
- *Lesson plan* — A guide for making a presentation
- *Program* — A comprehensive strategy that addresses fire and life safety issues via educational means
- *Presentation* — A single delivery of fire and life safety information; also called a lesson

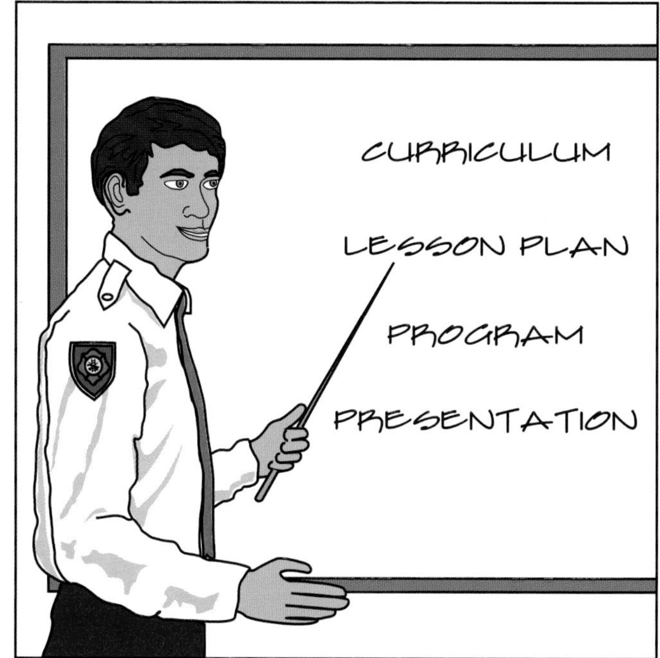

Figure 13.1 Key terms in fire and life safety educational theory.

WHAT IS LEARNING?

The terms *learning, education,* and *information* are related, but there are important differences among these three concepts.

Learning is knowledge gained through observation and study, resulting in a change of attitude or behavior.[1] Stated another way, *learning cannot take place without change.* Learning is what students do.

Education is the process of teaching, instructing, or training students in new skills. Teaching, instruction, and training all deal with preparing students for some kind of action or activity. Teaching or instruction shows students how to master a new skill, such as swimming or playing the piano. Training prepares the individual for a test of some kind (such as a driver's test, an athletic contest, or an effort to better one's time to run five miles) of the skill. Education is what teachers do to bring about learning in their students.

Information is facts, knowledge, data, or publicity. Information is the raw material upon which the learner bases the new skills of education and the change of learning. However, information transfer can happen without learning or education.

Some so-called education programs provide more entertainment than learning. For example, a program for school children that features a Dalmation trained to bark when a smoke detector sounds may get children's attention, but it does not teach the children what actions to take when the smoke detector sounds. The diversion or amusement of entertainment can be a helpful attention-grabber. If, on the other hand, the Dalmation crawls low, the children can model that behavior (Figure 13.2).

Remember though, by itself, entertainment is not information, education, or learning. The line between entertainment and information, education, or learning can seem very fine. Ask the following questions to distinguish between entertainment and the other activities:

- What will the audience most remember about the presentation? If the answer is attention-getting devices, the presentation was probably entertainment.
- What specific change has taken place as a result of the presentation? Remember, without change, there is no learning.
- What specific new information (facts, knowledge, or data) does the audience have about fire and life safety? Without new information about fire and life safety, the presentation was probably entertainment.

CHARACTERISTICS OF LEARNING

Entire books have been written about learning. Much of learning theory can be summarized in a few points[2]:

- **Learning is a lifelong activity**, beginning at birth and ending at death. Learning does not stop when school ends.
- **Learning can be very uncomfortable and stressful** because it necessitates a change in attitude or behavior. For example, it is stressful to change a fire safety attitude from "It can't happen to me" to "I need to be more careful about smoking." In fact, the higher the level of stress, the less likely the learner is to learn the material.

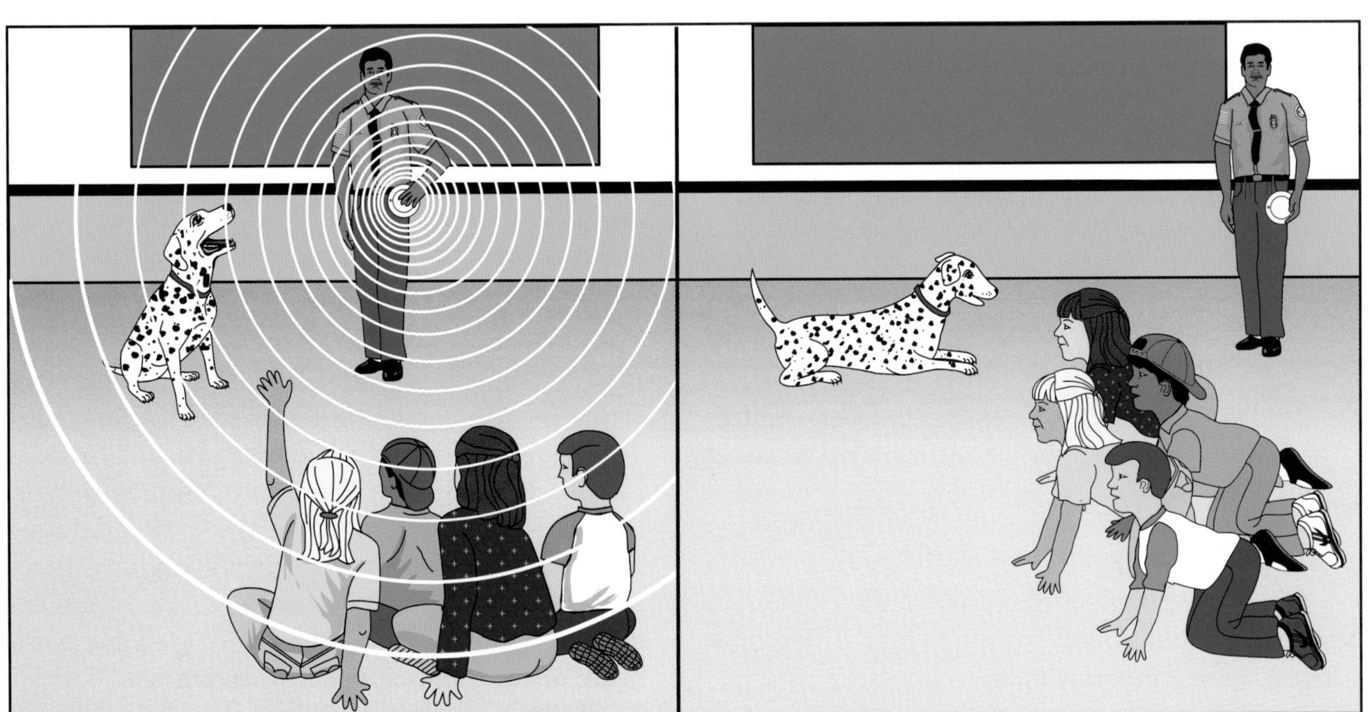

Figure 13.2 The educator must determine whether the activities presented are entertainment (attention-grabbers) or are designed to teach a specific behavior.

Public Education or Public Information?

Public education and public information (or public relations) are sometimes confused — and no wonder! Public education and public information involve similar skills. Often one person is responsible for both important functions.

A presentation for the Kiwanis on how to develop an occupant emergency plan for the workplace is a public education activity. It teaches a skill (how to develop an occupant emergency plan). Later, when the participants actually develop their plans, a change has happened. The change means that learning has taken place.

A presentation to the same Kiwanis group about how the fire department is organized or how the community's Insurance Services Office (ISO) rating is set is a public information activity. Interesting facts have been shared. However, while information has been exchanged, the participants have not demonstrated any new skills; they do not know how to manage the fire department or use an ISO grading schedule.

Sometimes, a single presentation will have elements of both public education and public information. Public education *and* public information are each valuable activities. But the differences between them are real.

- **People learn at different rates**. Learning quickly or slowly is not related to intelligence.
- **People learn in a variety of ways**. Some people learn more, for example, from what they see than from what they hear. For this reason, fire and life safety educators need to vary their teaching methods.
- **To be effective, learning must be reinforced**. Learning cannot sustain itself in a vacuum. Learning must be practiced and applied. Practice must be repeated to be effective. This characteristic of learning argues against once-a-year fire and life safety education programs, but it is a strong argument for ongoing activity.
- **Effective learning requires support from the people who influence or control the students**. For example, supervisors should support an employee's interest in moving stored cardboard boxes that block workplace exits. Parents need to support a child's pressure to test the smoke detectors.
- **Learning is enhanced when the senses are stimulated**. The chances of learning are greater when students not only *hear* words but also *see* illustrations. Providing props (such as burned items from a house fire) that relate to the instructional message lets students *touch* and even smell the effects of fire. Practicing an exit drill under simulated emergency conditions would also involve multiple senses. This characteristic of learning applies to adults as well as children.
- **Learning is most effective when it is focused** on a specific behavior. In focused learning, the fire and life safety educator begins with an overview ("This morning, we will learn what to do in case your clothes catch fire") and then explains the components (the "stop, drop, and roll" technique, how to cool a burn, when to get medical attention). When an audience knows the big picture, absorbing the individual pieces of information is easier.
- **Learning is incremental**. Even an apparently simple message such as "crawl low under smoke" is impossibly complex to a preschool child who may not know what smoke is. For this reason, the fire and life safety educator may have to teach about smoke before teaching how to crawl low.

A Change of Values

In recent years, public educators have begun to understand that fire and life safety is more than just behaviors and information. In fact, fire and life safety involves an individual's values, and such values guide personal behavior. For example, if someone does not value the safety provided by a seat belt, that person probably is not going to use one.

Because of this, a goal of fire and life safety education becomes developing or changing personal values. The task of developing safety behaviors can be achieved in young children because they have not yet developed any contrary values. However, adults have developed values which may not support safety. In these cases, the fire and life safety educator must change an adult's existing value and then develop a new safety value. This is a challenging task and requires the educator to use the best possible programs that incorporate adult learning theory and appropriate instructional methods.

- **Learners must identify with the importance or personal significance of the message**. In many ways, this means that the learners must change what they value. (See the accompanying sidebar, "A Change of Values.")

MOTIVATION AND LEARNING[3]

Fire and life safety educators often describe the need to motivate their audiences. Since 1954, motivation has often been described according to a hierarchy of needs identified by researcher Abraham H. Maslow.

According to Maslow, people have five basic needs that motivate all actions. The needs can be drawn as a pyramid, with the more urgent needs at the bottom (Figure 13.3). People must first satisfy the needs at the bottom of the triangle before they can move on to the needs higher up. However, *once a need is satisfied, it no longer motivates action.*

Physiological needs are immediate and include items such as food, water, and shelter that are essential to sustain life. Physiological needs also include escaping from situations, such as a fire, that are immediately life-threatening.

Safety and security needs are similar to physiological needs, but they deal more with the long term or with dangers that are not immediately threatening. Fire prevention activities fall into this category.

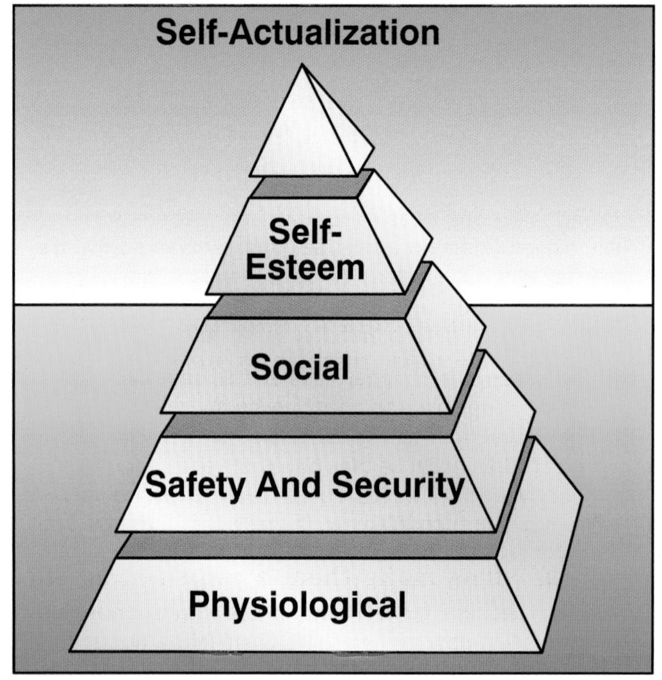

Figure 13.3 Maslow's Hierarchy of Needs

The *need for a sense of belonging and social activity* falls in the middle of the hierarchy. Identifying with a group and doing things with a group are actions that fulfill this need. For children, completing a home hazard inspection — along with the rest of their classmates — would satisfy the need for a sense of belonging or social activity. For adults, team jackets or decals that announce membership in an organization are very common ways of expressing a need for belonging and social activity.

People also need *esteem and social status* within the group. When we recognize someone's worth or value, we are helping to fulfill this need for them. A sticker in a child's workbook, a scouting badge, or a certificate of achievement on the wall, for example, reflects the need for esteem and social status.

The *need for self-actualization and fulfillment* is at the very top of the pyramid. The U.S. Army recruiting slogan, "Be all you can be," is designed around the need for self-actualization.

It is possible to modify this basic pyramid. For example, a fire and life safety educator might want to add "the need for physical comfort" to the basic pyramid. This need would encompass factors such as the comfort of the chairs, how crowded the classroom is, the temperature of the room, and the time between breaks.

There has been very little research about what motivates people to practice fire safety. Existing research does, though, give clear direction to fire and life safety educators.

The landmark research of fire safety motivation is *A Study of Motivational Psychology Related to Fire Preventive Behavior in Children and Adults,* commissioned by the NFPA and completed in 1974. "That study challenged the conventionally held view of the public's apathy about firesafety by concluding that people *do* care about firesafety, even though they might not know how to prevent or respond to fires. Based on interviews with people who had and had not experi-

> **How We Think**
>
> "There is ample evidence that fear and threats of violence, unless continually maintained, have little long-term positive effect on behavior. People tend to tune out or suppress information which is disturbing or contrary to their beliefs or inclinations.
>
> Others will block out that which is creating the tension. Therefore, fire prevention information should be directed toward positive motives which already exist within the recipient of the message."
>
> Richard Strother, *A Study of Motivational Psychology Related to Fire Preventive Behavior in Children and Adults*

enced a fire, the study noted that 'awareness of a fire as a powerful and potentially tragic force is not deeply buried in most people's consciousness.' For both those who had and had not experienced a fire, 'fire prevention awareness is increased when a person is responsible for others.'[4]

A 1991 study by the American Red Cross reached similar conclusions to those brought to light in Richard Strother's study. The Red Cross study investigated whether people took more (or less) action to prepare for natural disasters after seeing slides of disasters. The following conclusions provide highlights from the American Red Cross report:

- Seeing graphic images of disasters does not encourage people to take action to get ready for a natural disaster.
- Seeing disaster images actually discourages people from taking action to prepare for a disaster. After seeing disaster images, people were more confused about what to do.
- Among those who saw the disaster images, avoiding or denying something unpleasant caused people not to take action.
- Among those who did not see the disaster images, "Just not getting around to it" caused people not to take action.[5]

The Red Cross has also concluded that recommended actions must be clear and specific. For example, the recommendation to "have one gallon of water per person" is more complete and memorable than "have enough water on hand" (Figure 13.4).[6]

LIFELONG LEARNING

People learn from cradle to grave. But *how* people learn changes throughout life. The twin factors of psychological development stage and age determine how people learn throughout their lives.

Life Stages

Generally, people pass through the six development stages outlined in Table 13.1.[7] Unlike aging (which happens automatically), psychological development or passing through life stages does not happen automatically. Psychological development happens only when the person is ready and when the environment is right. Environmental factors such as family, friends, school, and work may restrict or encourage psychological growth.

People may remain in a particular developmental stage even though they continue to age. People may also regress to an earlier developmental stage.

Age and Learning

The second factor that influences learning is age. Preschoolers, elementary school children, adolescents, adults, and seniors all learn in very different ways — simply because of their age. In learning, age combines the influences of psychological/social/personal development with the effects of motor ability and communication skills. Being aware of how people learn at different ages is the first step in making sure that fire and life safety education programs and materials are age appropriate for their intended audiences.

PRESCHOOL CHILDREN

Preschoolers present a double challenge for fire and life safety educators: Their high risk of fire and burns make them a priority audience, yet they are a very difficult audience to reach.

Children aged three to five grow and change more rapidly than any other fire safety audience.

TORNADO • FLASH FLOOD • EARTHQUAKE • WINTER STORM • HURRICANE • FIRE • HAZARDOUS MATERIALS SPILL

EmergencyPreparedness Checklist

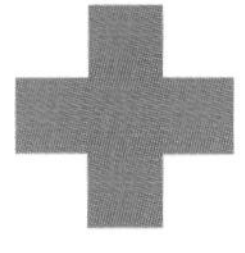

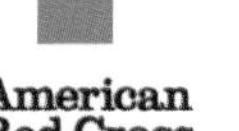

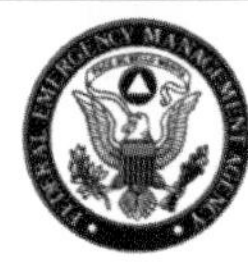

Federal Emergency Management Agency

The next time disaster strikes, you may not have much time to act. Prepare now for a sudden emergency.

Learn how to protect yourself and cope with disaster by planning ahead. This checklist will help you get started. Discuss these ideas with your family, then prepare an emergency plan. Post the plan where everyone will see it—on the refrigerator or bulletin board.

For additional information about how to prepare for hazards in your community, contact your local emergency management or civil defense office and American Red Cross chapter.

Emergency Checklist

Call Your Emergency Management Office or American Red Cross Chapter

- ❏ Find out which disasters could occur in your area.
- ❏ Ask how to prepare for each disaster.
- ❏ Ask how you would be warned of an emergency.
- ❏ Learn your community's evacuation routes.
- ❏ Ask about special assistance for elderly or disabled persons.

Also . . .

- ❏ Ask your workplace about emergency plans.
- ❏ Learn about emergency plans for your children's school or day care center.

Create an Emergency Plan

- ❏ Meet with household members. Discuss with children the dangers of fire, severe weather, earthquakes and other emergencies.
- ❏ Discuss how to respond to each disaster that could occur.
- ❏ Discuss what to do about power outages and personal injuries.
- ❏ Draw a floor plan of your home. Mark two escape routes from each room.
- ❏ Learn how to turn off the water, gas and electricity at main switches.
- ❏ Post emergency telephone numbers near telephones.
- ❏ Teach children how and when to call 911, police and fire.
- ❏ Instruct household members to turn on the radio for emergency information.
- ❏ Pick one out-of-state and one local friend or relative for family members to call if separated by disaster (it is often easier to call out-of-state than within the affected area).
- ❏ Teach children how to make long distance telephone calls.
- ❏ Pick two meeting places.

  1) A place near your home in case of a fire.

  2) A place outside your neighborhood in case you cannot return home after a disaster.
- ❏ Take a basic first aid and CPR class.
- ❏ Keep family records in a water and fire-proof container.

Prepare a Disaster Supplies Kit

Assemble supplies you might need in an evacuation. Store them in an easy-to-carry container such as a backpack or duffle bag.

Include:

- ❏ A supply of water (one gallon per person per day). Store water in sealed, unbreakable containers. Identify the storage date and replace every six months.
- ❏ A supply of non-perishable packaged or canned food and a non-electric can opener.
- ❏ A change of clothing, rain gear, and sturdy shoes.
- ❏ Blankets or sleeping bags.
- ❏ A first aid kit and prescription medications.
- ❏ An extra pair of glasses.
- ❏ A battery-powered radio, flashlight and plenty of extra batteries.
- ❏ Credit cards and cash.
- ❏ An extra set of car keys.
- ❏ A list of family physicians.
- ❏ A list of important family information; the style and serial number of medical devices such as pacemakers.
- ❏ Special items for infants, elderly or disabled family members.

Figure 13.4 Recommended actions when preparing for emergencies must be clear and specific.

Chapter 13 Notes

1. Clark Lambert, *Secrets of a Successful Trainer: A Simplified Guide for Survival*, copyright ©1986 John Wiley & Sons, p. 36.

2. Ibid., pp. 36-37. Reprinted by permission of John Wiley & Sons, Inc.

3. This discussion is largely based on R. Custer and P. Powell, "Teaching Firesafety in the Workplace" in *Firesafety at NYNEX: Your Piece of the Action*, 1991.

4. Reprinted with permission from "Learn Not to Burn®: A Decade of Progress," *Fire Journal* (Mar./Apr., Vol. 79, No. 2), p. 8. Copyright ©1985, National Fire Protection Association, Quincy, MA 02269.

5. Rocky Lopes, "Public Perception of Disaster Preparedness Presentation Using Disaster Damage Images," *NFPA Education Section Newsletter*, Fall/Winter 1992. Reprinted with permission from *NFPA Education Section Newsletter*, Fall/Winter, Copyright ©1992, National Fire Protection Association, Quincy, MA 02269.

6. Copies of the *Emergency Preparedness Checklist* shown in Figure 13.4 and other personal and family disaster preparedness materials are available at cost through your local Red Cross chapter or by calling FEMA Publications at 1-800-480-2520.

7. The National Fire Academy's course *Developing Fire and Life Safety Strategies* covers the concept of life stages in some detail.

8. For more information on teaching methods for preschool children, see Theresa Smalley, "Preschool Children," *Firesafety Educator's Handbook*, National Fire Protection Association, Quincy, MA, 1983, pp. 43-51.

9. See *Fire Safety on Television for Preschoolers*, prepared by the Children's Television Workshop™ under a grant from the U.S. Fire Administration/Federal Emergency Management Agency, FA-2A, July 1980, and *Sesame Street® Fire Safety Resource Book*, prepared by the Children's Television Workshop™ under a grant from the U.S. Fire Administration/Federal Emergency Management Agency, 1982.

10. Available from USFA or Children's Education Services, Children's Television Workshop™, One Lincoln Plaza, Department FS, New York, NY 10023; telephone 212-595-3456.

11. Much of this material is based on Carol Gross, "Elementary School Children," *Firesafety Educator's Handbook*. Reprinted with permission from *Firesafety Educator's Handbook*, Copyright ©1983, National Fire Protection Association, Quincy, MA 02269.

12. Dean Pedrotti, Phoenix Fire Department, Community Services Division, Phoenix, AZ 85003. ©1991 City of Phoenix.

13. Much of this section is based on Jacqui Sowers, "Adolescents," *Firedafety Educator's Handbook*. Reprinted with permission from *Firesafety Educator's Handbook*, Copyright ©1983, National Fire Protection Association, Quincy, MA 02269.

14. This discussion is largely based on R. Custer and P. Powell, "Teaching Firesafety in the Workplace" in *Firesafety at NYNEX: Your Piece of the Action*, 1991.

15. For more information, see Robert Lightman, "Elderly," *Firesafety Educator's Handbook*, National Fire Protection Association, Quincy, MA, 1983.

Chapter 13 Review

Directions

The following activities are designed to help you comprehend and apply the information in Chapter 13 of **Fire and Life Safety Educator**, second edition. To receive the maximum learning experience from these activities, it is recommended that you use the following procedure:

1. Read the chapter, underlining or highlighting important terms, topics, and subject matter. Read the sidebar material, study the photographs and illustrations, and read the captions with each.
2. Review the list of vocabulary words to ensure that you know the chapter-related meaning of each. If you are unsure of the meaning of a vocabulary word, look up the word in the glossary or a dictionary, and then study its context in the chapter.
3. On a separate sheet of paper, complete all assigned or selected application and review activities before checking your answers.
4. After you have finished, check your answers against those on the pages referenced in parentheses.
5. Correct any incorrect answers, and review material that was answered incorrectly.

Vocabulary

Be sure that you know the chapter-related meanings of the following words:

- curriculum *(231)*
- program *(231)*
- comprehensive education *(244)*
- lesson plan *(231)*
- presentation *(231)*
- service learning *(245)*

Application of Knowledge

Explain how you would apply each of the following basics of learning theory in a fire and life safety context:

- Learning is a lifelong activity.
- Learning can be very uncomfortable and stressful.
- People learn at different rates.
- People learn in a variety of ways.
- To be effective, learning must be reinforced.
- Effective learning requires support from people who influence or control the students.
- Learning is enhanced when the senses are stimulated.
- Learning is most effective when it is focused on a specific behavior.
- Learning is incremental.
- Learners must identify with the importance or personal significance of the message.

Review Activities

1. Distinguish among learning, education, and information. *(231)*
2. Draw a pyramid or stair-step representation of Maslow's Hierarchy of Needs. *(234)*
3. Explain how Maslow's Hierarchy of Needs relates to fire and life safety education. *(234)*
4. List the six psychological developmental stages through which all people pass. *(237)*
5. List the five physiological developmental stages (age brackets) into which people are often categorized. *(235, 241, 245, 247, 248)*
6. Explain how one's life stage (psychological development) differs from one's physiological level (age/physical development). *(235)*
7. Describe facts that affect the way in which preschool children learn. *(237, 238)*
8. Summarize the Children's Television Workshop™ study of preschoolers that resulted in the *Sesame Street® Fire Safety Resource Book. (238)*
9. Explain the nine major groups of developmental learning tasks faced by elementary children. *(241 and 244)*
   - physical skills
   - social skills
   - academic skills
   - values
   - social attitudes
   - self-attitude
   - social roles
   - living concepts
   - independence

10. Describe the Phoenix Fire Department's comprehensive Urban Survival Program. *(245)*
11. Explain the seven developmental tasks faced by adolescents. *(245)*
12. Outline the key points in the adolescent's learning style. *(245, 246)*
13. List characteristics of adult learners. *(247, 248)*
14. Provide four examples of external motivators and four examples of internal motivators. *(248)*
15. Describe guidelines that the fire and life safety educator should follow when planning programs for older adults. *(249, 250)*
16. Identify the following:
    - Abraham H. Maslow *(234)*
    - Maslow's Hierarchy of Needs *(234)*
    - Children's Television Workshop *(238)*
    - *Learn Not to Burn®: The Pre-School Program (238)*
    - *Sesame Street® Fire Safety Book (238)*
    - Robert Havighurst *(241)*
    - Urban Survival Program *(245)*
    - H.D. Thornburg *(245)*

Questions and Notes

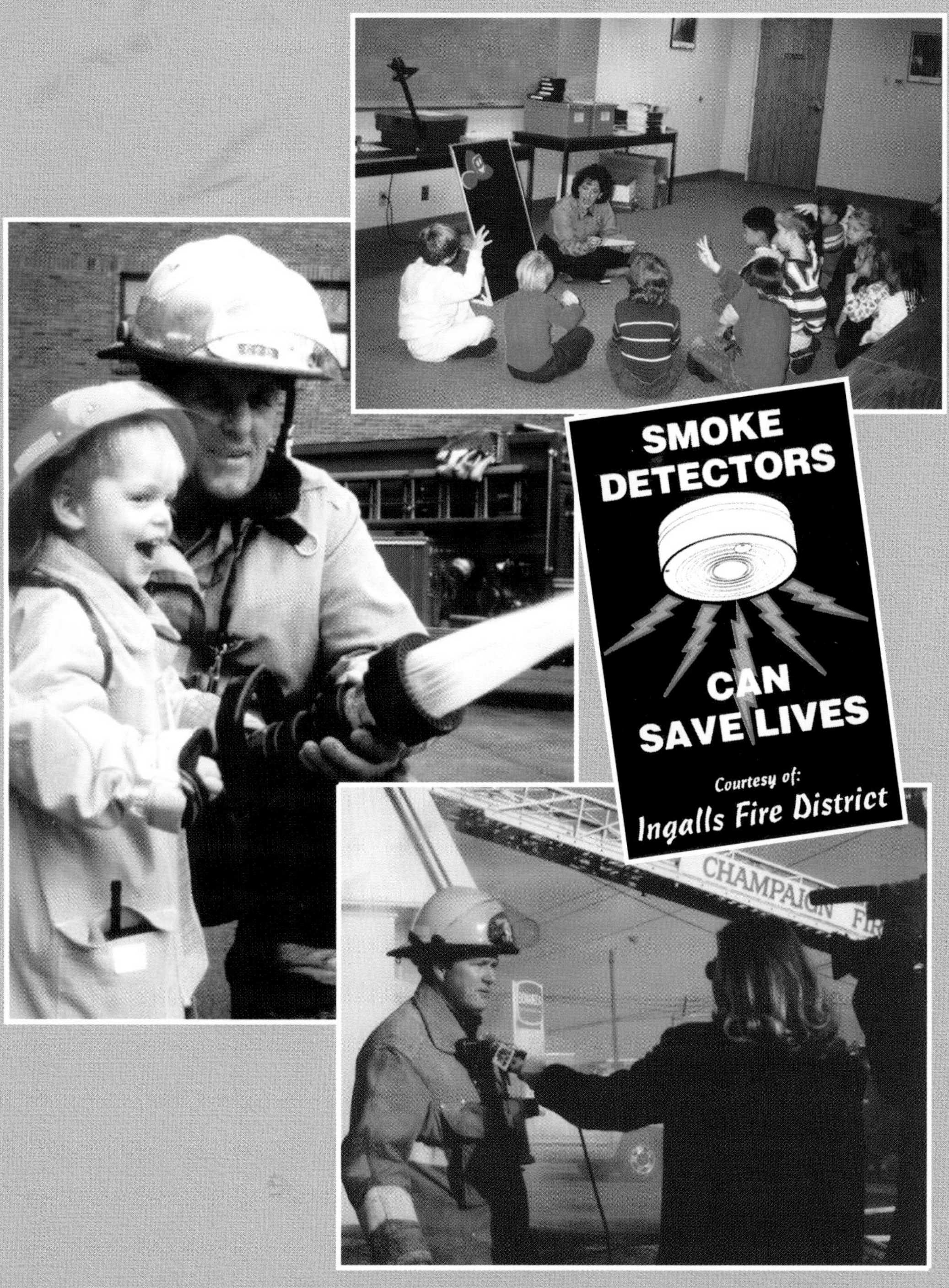
SMOKE
DETECTORS
CAN
SAVE LIVES
Courtesy of:
Ingalls Fire District
CHAMPAIGN

14 Applying Fire and Life Safety Educational Theory

LEARNING OBJECTIVES

This chapter provides information that addresses the following objectives of NFPA 1035, *Standard for Professional Qualifications for Public Fire and Life Safety Educator* (1993 edition):

Public Fire and Life Safety Educator I

3-4.1.2 *Prerequisite Skills:* Communication skills, use of prepared lesson plans with identified learning objectives, methods for active participation/involvement, methods of developing and maintaining a positive learning environment for the student including physical environment and student/instructor relationships, and proper use and care of audiovisual equipment and materials.

3-4.2 Present a prepared program, given lesson content, time allotments, and identified audience, so that program objectives are met.

3-4.3 Use multiple presentation methods when presenting prepared programs, given program objectives, time allotments, and a specified audience, so that the chosen presentation methods are used.

Public Fire and Life Safety Educator II

4-4.2.1 *Prerequisite Knowledge:* Learning theory for all age, social, and developmental audiences; needs assessment; development of written and visual educational materials; development of learning objectives, course development based on specified learning objectives and audiences, lesson plan development, and selection and use of evaluation instruments.

4-4.3 Develop a lesson plan, given a specific behavior, learning objectives, and a specified audience, so that the lesson plan reflects the learning characteristics and abilities of the intended audience.

4-4.5.1 *Prerequisite Knowledge:* Educational methodology.

4-4.5.2 *Prerequisite Skills:* Instructional techniques.

Chapter 14
Applying Fire and Life Safety Educational Theory

INTRODUCTION

Outstanding fire and life safety education programs often share two common characteristics. First, these programs are firmly based in educational theory (covered in Chapter 13, "Learning Fire and Life Safety Educational Theory"). Second, these outstanding programs use very practical techniques based on that educational theory. Those techniques are what this chapter is all about.

This chapter covers communication techniques used in fire and life safety education programs. Chapter highlights include fire and life safety instructional methods and the process of matching those instructional methods to educational objectives. Questioning techniques are also introduced. Finally, the chapter covers the physical learning environment, including preparing the classroom and providing for safety during education programs.

COMMUNICATION TECHNIQUES

Effective fire and life safety educators are effective communicators. Like other skills, good communication depends on knowing how the process works and on practicing techniques.[1]

"Communication" is more than the ability to speak before a group or to write clearly. Communication has been described as both a process that explains how people interact with each other and as a cycle of interchanged information. In this chapter, *communication* is defined as *the ongoing process that educators and their audiences use to complete the exchange of information and attitudes about fire and life safety.*

Communication appears to be a fairly straightforward process. The process usually begins when the educator (who might be called the *sender* or the *source*) decides to transmit information or attitude/opinion (the *message*) to the audience (the *receiver*). Putting the message into words is called *encoding* the message. The educator picks a medium, method, or vehicle for sending the encoded message.

The audience (receiver) listens to the message — decoding, translating, and evaluating it almost simultaneously. Through feedback, the audience and the educator determine whether or not the exchange of information or attitude was completed (Figure 14.1).

Communication is actually much more complicated than it appears in Figure 14.1. In fact, each step is complex, and each arrow represents

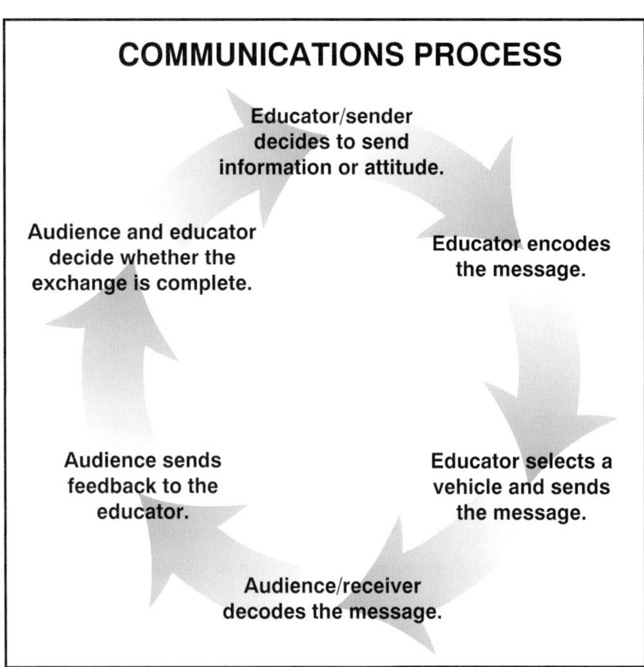

Figure 14.1 Communication is accomplished when the receiver confirms the intended message has been received.

a potential breakdown in the communication process. Knowing how to avoid those breakdowns makes the fire and life safety educator more effective. Communication techniques are tools to prevent breakdowns.

Encoding the Message

Whenever a fire and life safety educator puts a message (information or attitude) into words, she or he is encoding and interpreting. Several factors influence how educators encode their messages:

- The educator's subject knowledge, experience, and commitment, as well as overall health and well-being
- The educator's attitude toward the audience
- The educator's overall mood at the moment
- The good or bad experiences that the educator had earlier in the day or week (sometimes called the *frame of reference*)
- The physical environment

As a professional, the educator is responsible for making sure that whatever happened at home or at work *before* a presentation does not interfere with delivering an effective presentation (Figure 14.2). For example, consider two educators who are teaching a group of caregivers at a local child-care center about fire and burn safety for preschoolers.

The first educator, who is a rookie, has a headache and bad memories of a frustrating class at another child-care center. He is running late and skipped lunch. Just before he left the office, the first educator was assigned responsibility for the science fair, which will be held on his son's birthday. The day-care center is hot and noisy.

The second educator worked out at the gym on the way to work. She was a preschool teacher before joining the fire department and so always looks forward to presentations at the day-care center. In fact, the supervisor has just assigned her the job of overhauling the preschool fire safety program. The children are napping when she arrives at the center.

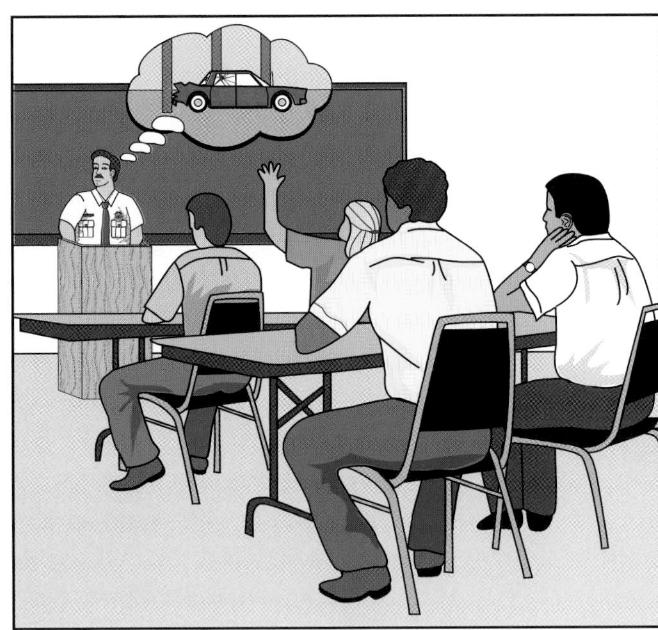

Figure 14.2 Outside events in the educator's personal life should not interfere with the delivery of an effective presentation.

Both educators sincerely want to send information and instill an attitude in the audience that will keep preschool children safe from fire and burns. Both educators are equally responsible for doing a good job — regardless of what kind of day they have had.

Note that several factors that affect the interpretation of the encoded message are somewhat beyond the educator's control. As a result, educators need to be especially careful to attend to the factors that they *can* control. The educator does have some control over health and well-being (through rest, nutrition, and exercise), attitude, and environment (planning to arrive at the day-care center during nap time rather than at the end of the day, for example) (Figure 14.3).

Sending the Message

A message can be sent through the spoken word (orally), through the written word, or through nonverbal communication. Nonverbal communication includes facial expression, gestures, and other body language. It even includes the kind of illustrations, the style of typeface, and the color of ink used in handout or audiovisual materials!

The form that a message takes is sometimes called its *medium* or *communication vehicle.* Lectures, role-playing, and question-and-answer

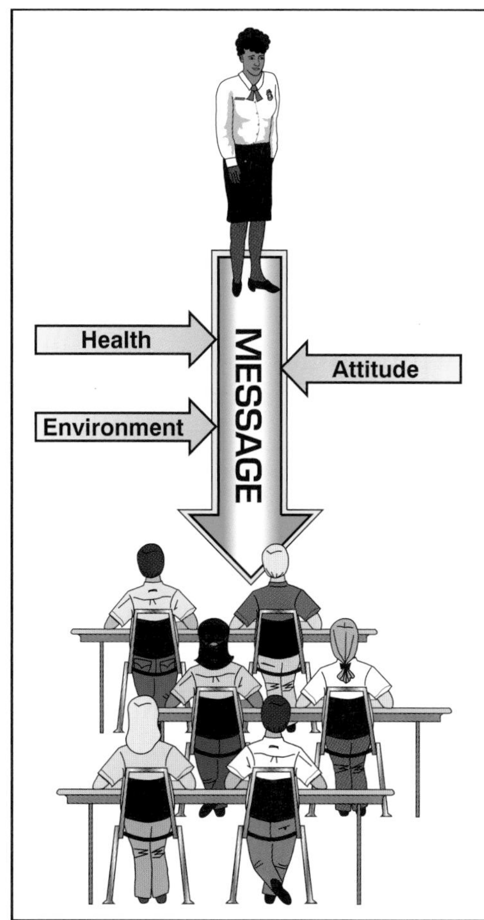

Figure 14.3 Educators should look closely at the factors affecting messages that are *not* beyond their control.

series are among the many oral communication vehicles. Slide shows, films, and videotapes can also be considered as forms of oral communication. Written communication vehicles in education include brochures, flyers, posters, and so forth. Nonverbal communication can have an impact on both oral and written communication vehicles.

Fire and life safety educators carefully match their message with the most appropriate communications vehicle. The "Instructional Methods" section of this chapter and Chapter 15, "Selecting Educational Materials," covers techniques for selecting the most effective communication vehicle.

Receiving and Decoding the Message

Members of the audience begin to interpret the fire and life safety educator's message as soon as they see and hear it. Several factors affect their interpretation:

- The audience's overall health and well-being
- The audience's attitude toward the educator
- The audience's overall mood
- The audience's recent good or bad experiences (that is, the frame of reference)
- The physical environment (including noise, uncomfortable temperature or other distractions).
- The audience's general understanding of the subject of the message

Receiving a message is more than simply "hearing" a message. Decoding and listening are what people do to find the meaning in what they hear and in what they observe (Figure 14.4). *Commonly, there are things that get in the way of communication; these are generally called barriers. Poor listening habits or environments are examples of communication barriers.*

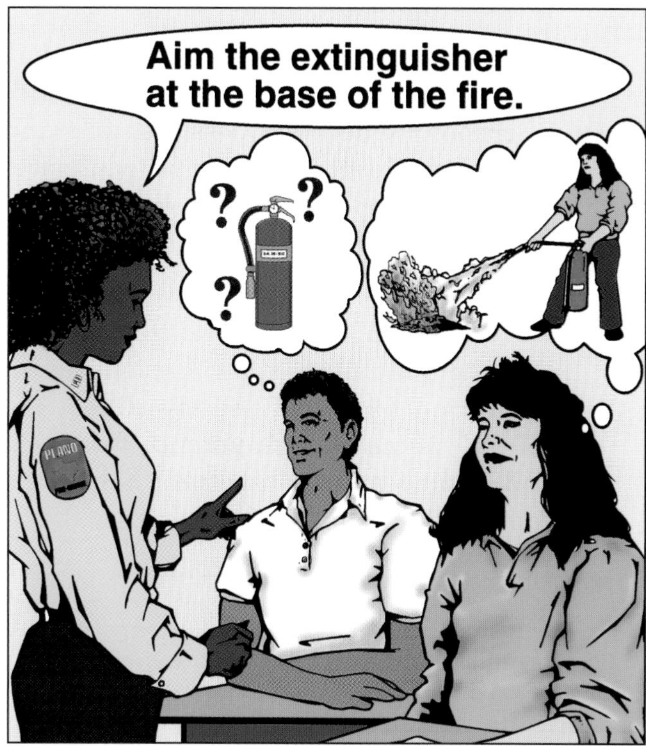

Figure 14.4 The receiver must apply meaning to the message rather than just hear the words.

There are very few born listeners. In fact, the average person remembers only 25 to 30 percent of the average conversation![2] The following barriers make listening, and thus communication, difficult (Figure 14.5):

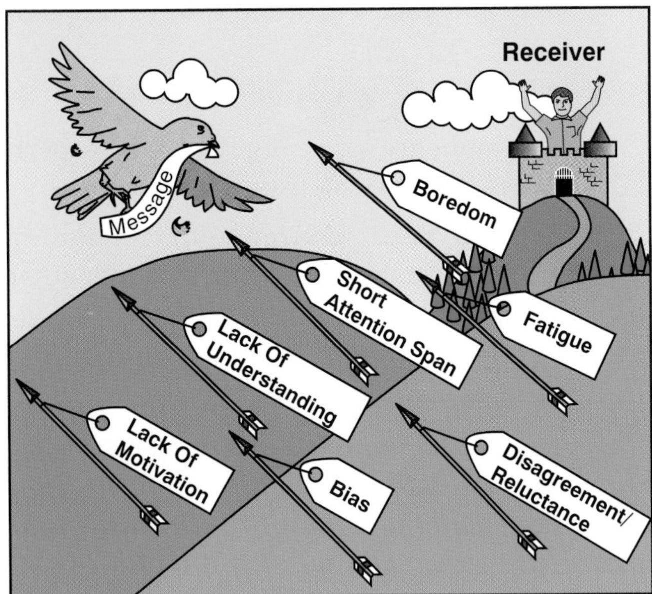

Figure 14.5 Barriers to communication.

- **Short attention span**. A short attention span is one that lasts from a few seconds to a few minutes.
- **Fatigue**. No matter how well-rested they are in the morning, people tire by mid-afternoon. Whenever possible, fire and life safety educators should schedule presentations for late morning and early afternoon — times when most people are more alert.
- **Boredom**. This is a natural consequence of a short attention span. Presenting information in small, easily digestible "bites," watching for audience feedback, and adding attention-getters help overcome audience boredom.

A Quick Tip

For every 30 minutes of instruction, schedule an audience-participation activity to lessen fatigue and boredom.

- **Lack of motivation**. Listeners may have a sense that the message being sent does not matter to them.
- **Bias**. Listeners simply may not care for the educator because of mannerisms or differences in race, gender, age, weight, accent, or even style of hair or dress.
- **Disagreement or reluctance**. The audience may disagree with what is being said or may be reluctant to take the actions being proposed.
- **Lack of understanding.** When people do not understand what is being said to them, they may tune out — in other words, listen less.

Decoding really depends on what are commonly know as *listening skills* or *active listening*. Listening skills include maintaining eye contact with the message sender, imagining the sender's upcoming points, taking notes or mentally summarizing key points, and paraphrasing especially important points. Nodding the head and thinking or saying something like "I understand" are other listening skills.

The fire and life safety educator is not responsible for teaching listening skills to the audience. However, the educator *is* responsible for making sure that the audience is listening. Observing the audience — whether they are sitting through a presentation, watching a demonstration, or seeing a videotape — is vital. For example, the educator can see whether or not people in the audience are maintaining eye contact with the speaker (or the screen), taking notes, and nodding their heads.

Other ways to check for understanding include sampling, signaled responses, group choral response, and individual private response.[3]

Through sampling, the fire and life safety educator asks the entire group a question, giving them time to think about the answer, before calling on one person to answer. "Why is it important to test your smoke detector? I'll give you a minute to think" is an example of a sampling question.

Signaled responses are particularly popular with elementary-age children. The educator makes a statement and then asks the class to signal silently whether they agree with the statement. "Nod your head if you agree, and shake it if you don't." In another form of the signaled response, the educator could, for example, ask the audience to point to an object ("Show me where the exit sign is").

In a group choral response, everyone theoretically answers a question together. Group choral responses are useful when there is a clear, simple answer, but they are less useful when searching for more complex answers. Group choral responses give information about the group's understanding but do not provide information about how much individuals understand.

Finally, the individual private response can be used to check understanding. Short notes or even whispered responses to a question are forms of individual private responses. Individual private responses give solid information on an individual's understanding. They may be used with children, but they are not particularly appropriate for adult audiences.

QUESTIONS AND FEEDBACK

What the fire and life safety educator *asks* the audience may be as important as what the educator *tells* the audience. What the audience asks the educator is also critically important. This is especially true in the feedback stage of the communication process — the point at which the audience and the educator decide whether or not the exchange of information/attitude has been completed.

Questions can also be an effective way for the audience to learn. Why? Questions encourage thinking, the exchange of ideas, and the molding of opinion, attitude, and values (Figure 14.6). Effective questions exhibit the following qualities:

- **They are open-ended, requiring more than a "yes" or a "no" to answer**. The response to the question "Why do you need to test your smoke detector?" gives more information than the response to "Do you need to test your smoke detector?"
- **They do not suggest the answer**. For example, "You do not need to test your smoke detector everyday, do you?" will not result in as much of a response as "How often do you need to test your smoke detector."
- **They seek information but do not make the audience feel uninformed**.

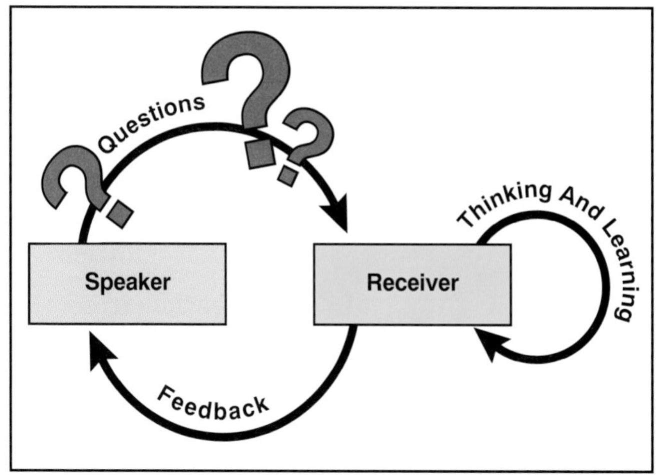

Figure 14.6 Students learn by thinking through and answering the educator's questions.

Educators should avoid using questions (during a verbal pretest, for example) as a way of "showing off" how much they know or how little the audience knows. After all, the audience is there to learn!

TYPES OF QUESTIONS

There are four kinds of questions that fire and life safety educators use:

- **Direct questions**. Direct questions are aimed at one person in the audience. These questions can put the person "on the spot" to answer correctly. Because they can be so threatening, direct questions are not often used with adults. School children are more accustomed to direct questions in school.
- **Overhead questions**. Overhead questions are aimed at the whole group, rather than one person. Anyone is free to respond to an overhead question. These questions are particularly helpful in starting thinking or discussion or in bringing out ideas and opinions. Overhead questions are frequently part of a case study or brainstorming type of discussion.
- **Rhetorical questions**. Rhetorical questions are very similar to overhead questions. The major difference between overhead and rhetorical questions is that an answer to a rhetorical question is not expected. A rhetorical question can be an

effective "attention-getter." For example, a fire and life safety educator might open a presentation by saying, "What are the most important things that you and your family can do to protect yourselves from a home fire? By the end of this presentation, you will know how to answer that question."

- **Relay questions**. A question from the audience that the educator sends back to the audience is called a *relay question*. Using these questions is a good technique for opening up discussion, especially about affective issues. Relay questions should not be used to avoid a question that the educator cannot answer. Relay questions should not be used to force the audience into guessing about facts.

Culture and Communication

Culture plays a large role in communication and learning — a fact that is becoming more important in a society that is more and more diverse. For example, fire and life safety educators who work with Southeast Asians report that they are visual communicators and learners. Audiences of Mediterranean or Hispanic descent are often much more openly communicative than northern Europeans or Native Americans.

Effective communication takes these cultural differences into account. Fire and life safety educators can, for example, ask a member of the target audience about cultural differences as part of the normal process of planning a presentation. Acknowledging and working with cultural differences is another form of knowing the audience.

INSTRUCTIONAL METHODS

Types of Instructional Methods

Instructional methods and educational materials are the vehicles that carry the fire and life safety education message to the audience. Fire and life safety educators have many types of instructional methods available to them. The challenge is to select the most appropriate instructional method for the educational objective. The educator may choose from among several types of instructional methods:

- Lecture
- Discussion
- Illustration
- Demonstration
- Team teaching

LECTURE

In a lecture, the fire and life safety educator tells, talks, and explains (Figure 14.7). While a lecture is an efficient way to send information from the educator (source) to the audience (receiver),

When the Answer is Wrong

The audience will make mistakes simply because they do not yet know enough. An incorrect or incomplete answer (or drill) is part of learning. The audience will judge how well the fire and life safety educator deals with "wrong" answers. These following guidelines are designed to help the educator respond to incorrect or incomplete answers:

- **Dignify the audience response by pointing out the "right" parts of their answer**. "You are absolutely right about needing to test your smoke detector to keep the warranty in effect. For what other reasons is it important to test the detector?" (To make sure it is in working order, to put the family's mind at rest, etc.)
- **Assist or "prompt" the audience**. "Yes, baking soda could put out a food fire in the oven. What might be an even safer way to smother an oven fire?" (For example, close the oven door, or put a lid on the fire before closing the oven door.)
- **Hold the audience accountable**. Fire and life safety attitudes, knowledge, and skills can literally mean the difference between life and death. For that reason, the educator cannot tolerate incorrect or incomplete answers or drills. However, corrections can be done gently. For example, "Let's talk about the first aid for burns a bit more, so you'll remember when to call a doctor" or "We'll go over this at the end of the presentation, just to make sure that you have it right."
- **Never ridicule, humiliate, or laugh at a wrong answer**.

As educator Madeline Hunter says, "Our function as teachers is to help students be right, *not* to catch them being wrong!"

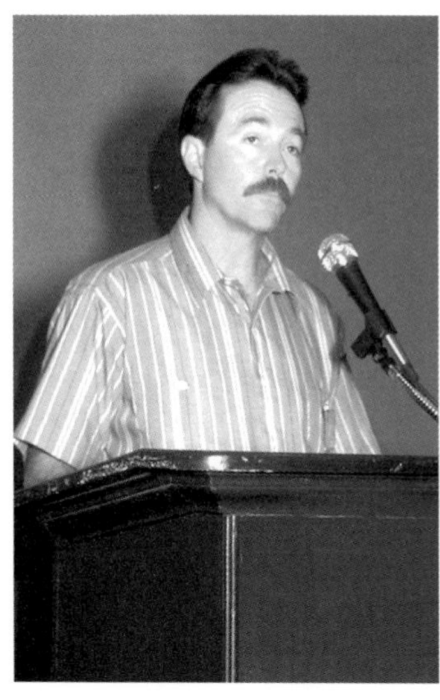
Figure 14.7 The lecture method can be used to convey information to a large audience in a short amount of time.

the information flows only one way. Seen from the standpoint of one-way information, a lecture does not fit the definition of communication (that is, the ongoing process that educators and their audiences use to complete the exchange of information and attitudes about fire and life safety).

Today's audiences are used to the fast pace — as well as the visual and audio stimulation — of television, computers, and video games. Lectures can bore the audience and may thus provide a barrier to effective communication. However this method, in moderation, is appropriate in some situations — particularly those where the educator must provide facts as a basis for learning. For example, lecture is much more appropriate for adults than for preschoolers.

Fire and life safety educators should use the lecture format sparingly — and for short periods. The use of other instructional methods and effective presentation techniques (see Chapter 17, "Using Public Speaking Techniques") is a must when the lecture format is used.

DISCUSSION

In lecture, there is little or no audience participation. When lecturing, the educator talks *to* the audience: tells what, how, and when; provides facts and examples; answers questions; and clarifies. Unlike the one-sided lecture method, however, the discussion method allows the audience and educator to interact (Figure 14.8). When discussing, the educator talks *with* the audience. This educational method allows the educator to exchange views with members of the audience to find out "why," to ask and answer questions, to provide examples based on individual experience, to arrive at joint conclusions, and to jointly reach goals. In discussion, there is much audience involvement or give-and-take (Figure 14.9). Because of this, discussion can be a very valuable instructional method — especially when the audience already has the basic knowledge.

There are several categories of discussion:

- **Guided discussion.** The group exchanges ideas directed toward reaching a common goal or conclusion.

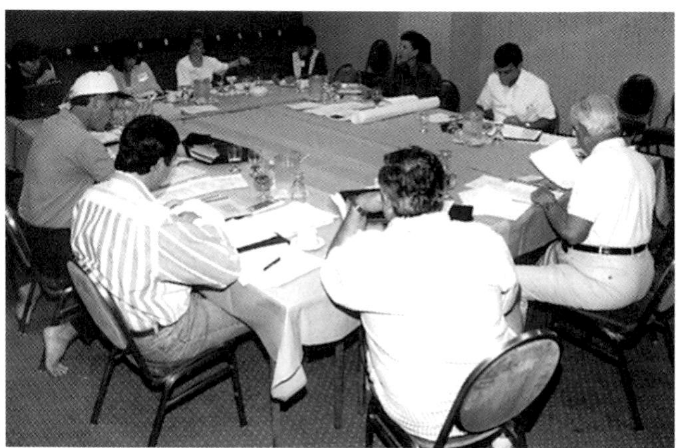
Figure 14.8 Discussion methods can arouse interest and stimulate participation.

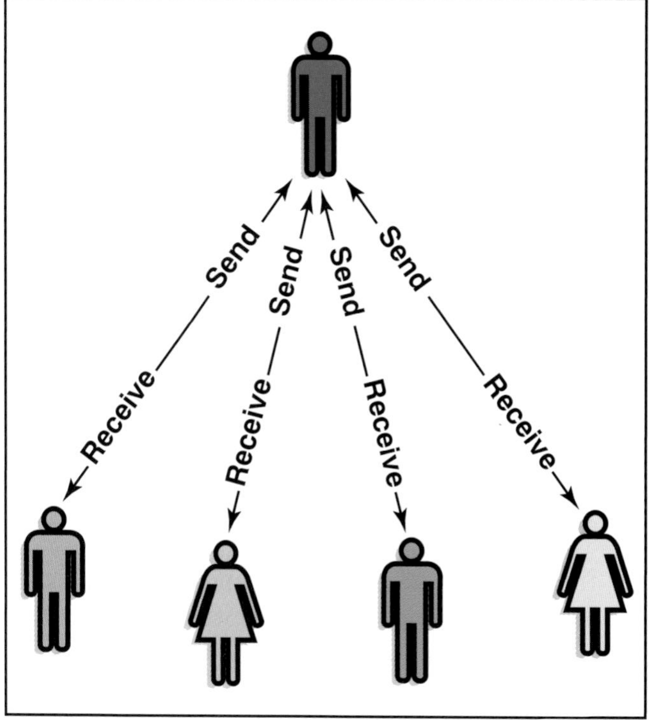

Figure 14.9 Continual interaction during a discussion often results in new ideas or methods derived from the basic knowledge of the students.

- **Conference discussion**. The group directs its thinking toward solving a common problem.
- **Case study**. The group reviews real or hypothetical events.
- **Role-playing**. The group acts out various scenarios.
- **Brainstorming**. The objective is to identify as many ideas or approaches as possible. (**NOTE**: For more information, see the Brainstorming Techniques section of Chapter 12, "Networking, Forming Coalitions, and Working Cooperatively.")

Fire and life safety educators frequently use case study and role-play discussion techniques. Asking the audience to *think* about what to do if a fire is discovered at home at night is an example of the case-study method. Inviting the audience to *show* what they would do under the same circumstances is an example of the role-play method. (**NOTE**: Demonstration and role-play are very similar.)

ILLUSTRATION

The illustration educational method is especially helpful when used in combination with either lecture or discussion format. Through illustration, the fire and life safety educator *shows* the audience something — for instance, the parts of a smoke detector or how an overloaded electrical outlet looks (Figure 14.10). However, unlike demonstration, illustration does not show the audience how to perform a task.

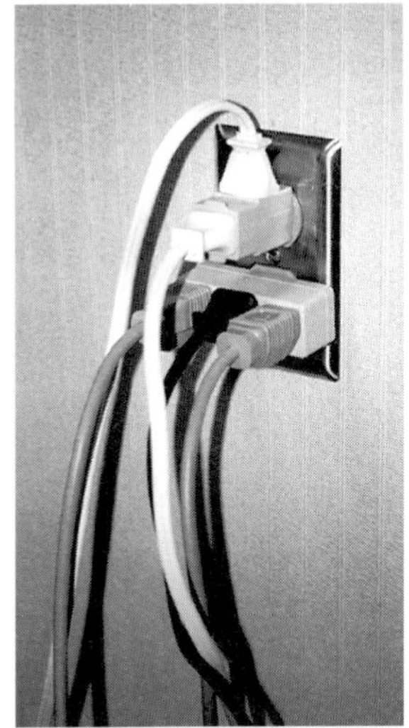

Figure 14.10 The illustration method uses visual aids to help clarify instruction.

Illustration relies heavily upon teaching aids such as drawings, posters, photos, slides, overhead transparencies, videotapes or films, models, and diagrams. (**NOTE**: Chapter 15, "Selecting Educational Materials," covers the use of educational materials.)

DEMONSTRATION

Fire and life safety educators use the demonstration method to teach their audience new skills (Figure 14.11). The educator actually performs the task, usually explaining the task step-by-step. After the educator has demonstrated the skill, the audience may then practice it through drill.

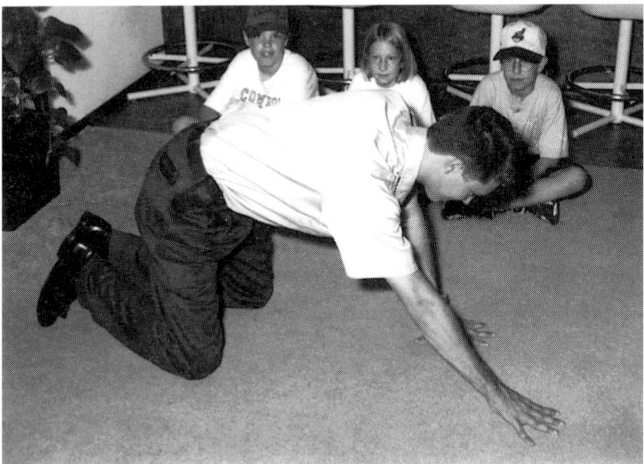

Figure 14.11 To teach the "crawl low under smoke" behavior, the educator demonstrates the appropriate action.

Five Steps to an Effective Demonstration

1. Explain what the demonstration will show the audience how to do.
2. Demonstrate the skill once at normal speed. Repeat the demonstration more slowly, step-by-step, explaining each step in turn.
3. Demonstrate the skill once again, while a member of the audience explains each step.
4. Have one member of the audience demonstrate the skill, while explaining the steps. Supervise this drill, correcting each step as needed.
5. Supervise the drill of as many people as possible. (**NOTE**: As they become skilled, members of the audience can also supervise and correct each other.)

Adapted from "Presenting the Instruction," IFSTA **Fire Service Instructor**, 5th ed., 1990, p. 144.

Safety is always a concern with demonstrations and drills. This is especially true when live fire is involved. Before using demonstrations and drills, fire and life safety educators should ask themselves the following questions:

- Will the demonstration endanger the educator? For example, could the educator get burned while demonstrating how to put a lid on a grease fire? (**NOTE**: The same question applies to the audience during a drill.)

- Will the demonstration endanger the audience? Could a shift in the wind blow flames toward the audience during a fire extinguisher demonstration? (**NOTE**: The same question applies to the audience during a drill.)
- Is a live demonstration needed, or is there another way to demonstrate a dangerous skill? For example, is live fire really needed to demonstrate how to put a lid on a grease fire? Films or videotapes can effectively — and safely — demonstrate how to use a fire extinguisher.

Whenever the safety of a live demonstration is in question, the educator should use another method or material.

TEAM TEACHING

Team teaching is a classroom method in which a group of instructors work together — combining their individual content, techniques, and materials — to meet a single educational objective.

For fire and life safety educators, team teaching not only is an effective educational tool but is also a way of cementing coalitions with other agencies and organizations. For example, a course for baby-sitters could easily involve a teaching team of people from the fire department, the police department, the Red Cross, and a local preschool, and a nurse from the maternity ward of the local hospital.

Team teaching is particularly appropriate when the material is too broad for one instructor or when more than one perspective is needed. Team teaching can also help keep the audience's attention by varying voice, pace, and style of the teachers. The team approach also gives instructors a break from long teaching sessions.

Successful team teaching requires more advance planning than solo teaching. In addition to the planning that goes into any presentation, team teaching requires the following:

- Choosing instructors whose teaching styles balance each other (matching a "high-energy" instructor, for example, with an instructor with a more relaxed teaching style)
- Agreeing (in detail!) on who will teach what
- Exchanging detailed instructor outlines
- Sticking to one format for all audiovisual and handout materials (all horizontal overhead transparencies, for example)

Team teaching can lead to stress and tension between the instructors. The most basic "survival tip" for team teaching is acknowledging — and working around — the strengths and weaknesses of each instructor. Of course, there can be only one lead teacher at a time. Each instructor must keep time commitments, as well as observe simple courtesies (never interrupting, for example) with each other.

When team teaching, an instructor may be tempted to think, "I only need to be there when I'm teaching." Actually, team partners need to attend the entire course. Having the team members in the room has a triple purpose: (1) helping the teaching member with mechanics such as handout materials and audiovisuals; (2) noting gaps, problems, and questions; and (3) providing raw material for private feedback during breaks or after the class.

Breaks

Breaks are the most frequently used method of relieving long learning sessions (Figure 14.12). The frequency of out-of-the-room breaks depends on a number of factors, including the intensity of the material, time of day, and temperature of the room. In-place stretch breaks can be very useful. Whether out of the room or in place, breaks should work with the flow of material.

One challenge is getting people back from the break. Three techniques are useful:

- Start all sessions on time — this trumpets your commitment to staying on time.
- Say exactly when the session will resume. For example, say "We'll start again at 10:30" rather than "Let's take a 10-minute break."

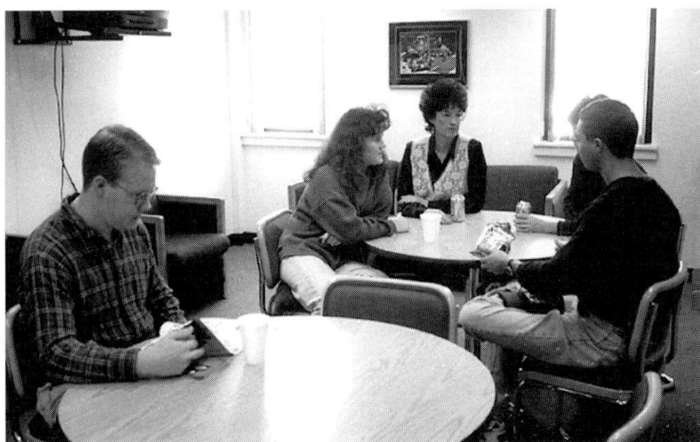

Figure 14.12 Breaks during learning sessions provide students with a change of pace and reduce fatigue.

- Designate one clock that everyone can see as the reference clock.

Matching Instructional Method and Educational Objective

Selecting the most appropriate instructional method for a specific kind of educational objective[4] is a critical skill for fire and life safety educators — it is a matter of using the right tool for the particular task. The three basic types of educational objectives — affective, cognitive, and psychomotor — are based on the way people learn, or their learning domains. The educator must select the instructional method that is most suitable for teaching to the objective's learning domain (Table 14.1). If the educator wants to teach an adult audience how to change the battery in a smoke detector (a psychomotor objective), for instance, the educator would not ask participants to write or recite the steps in changing the battery (a cognitive instructional method), but would instead demonstrate how to actually change the battery.

AFFECTIVE OBJECTIVES

Affective objectives deal with changes in the audience's values, feelings, or opinions. *At the conclusion of the presentation on residential fire safety to the Kiwanis Club, the Kiwanis participant will be able to relate two factors that illustrate the importance of testing and maintaining smoke detectors* is a sample affective objective.

Instructional methods most effective in reaching affective objectives include surveys, questionnaires, group discussion, role-play, and case studies.

COGNITIVE OBJECTIVES

Cognitive objectives deal with changes in what the audience knows or understands. For example, *At the conclusion of the presentation on residential fire safety to the Kiwanis Club, the Kiwanis participant will be able to state three reasons for testing and maintaining smoke detectors* is a cognitive objective.

Lecture, illustration, guided discussion, conference discussion, and case study are well-suited to fire and life safety education programs aimed at teaching cognitive objectives.

PSYCHOMOTOR OBJECTIVES

Changes in skill — in what the audience can do to increase their safety — are covered by psychomotor objectives. *At the conclusion of the presentation on residential fire safety to the Kiwanis Club and given a smoke detector for demonstration purposes, the Kiwanis participant will be able to change the smoke detector's battery so that the detector alarm sounds when tested* is a psychomotor objective.

TABLE 14.1
Instructional Methods For Different Types Of Objectives

Objective Type	Instructional Method
Affective	Personal survey, questionnaire, group discussion, role-play, case study
Cognitive	Lecture, illustration, guided discussion, conference discussion, and case study
Psychomotor	Illustration, demonstration, drill, and role-play

Illustration, demonstration and drill, and role-play are effective methods for teaching psychomotor objectives.

THE LEARNING ENVIRONMENT

It is a fact: the wrong learning environment can ruin even the best-planned fire and life safety education program. The term *learning environment* refers to the physical facilities where the learning takes place. Several factors make up the learning environment:

- Room size (Is it too big or too small for the audience?)
- Temperature (Is the temperature comfortable and steady?)
- Lighting level
- Ventilation
- Background noise (from neighboring rooms, the hall, the ventilation system, and outside)
- Acoustics
- Comfort of chairs and tables
- Physical arrangement of the room (floor plan, furniture and equipment arrangement)

Practiced educators inspect the classroom before arriving for the presentation. It may be possible to move the program to another room or to correct what is wrong with the room. For example, removing unneeded chairs and re-arranging chairs into a circle can make a huge room feel smaller. Videos or films can be shown in rooms with uncurtained windows — if the screen or monitor is placed so that the windows are behind the audience.

The physical arrangement of the room is one area that educators can control. Rooms can be arranged in several ways that largely depend on the size of the group and whether or not tables are used. The choice of a room arrangement lies in satisfying three criteria:

- Can everyone in the audience see and hear the educator and audiovisual materials?
- Can everyone in the audience see and hear each other?
- Does the arrangement place the maximum number of people close to the educator?

When tables are used for small groups, three common arrangements are a U-shaped setup, a hollow square, and a conference table.

The U-shape can be either flat or long (Figure 14.13). The flat U-shape allows more members of the audience to be closer to the educator and the audiovisual material. The U-shaped arrangement is very popular because it lets the participants see the educator and each other. Also, the fire and life safety educator is able to move around the open U (although this practice can be distracting and places some participants behind the educator). All participants are able to see a screen or video monitor placed behind the educator's table.

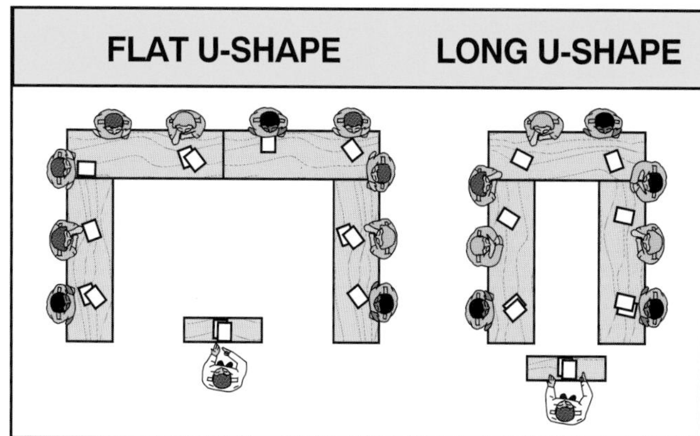

Figure 14.13 The U-shape classroom setup allows all students to see demonstrations clearly.

The hollow square is very similar to the U-shaped room setup; the only difference is that the fire and life safety educator cannot walk into the middle (Figure 14.14). Participants may feel farther away from each other, even though the distance is the same as the U-shaped arrangement.

A conference-table setup is essentially a solid U-shaped arrangement. The conference table arrangement may make the education session feel more like a meeting and less like a class (see Figure 14.14).

For larger groups that need tables, classroom styles are used. The traditional classroom-style setup is the most restrictive and provides for the least eye contact among participants. The chevron (sometimes called *herringbone*) or fan-style classroom setup places more members of the audience closer to the educator — and allows participants to see each other (Figure 14.15).

Note that these same seating arrangements can be used without tables. However, the most common way to arrange chairs without tables is the amphitheater or auditorium style. Re-arranging the chairs into a slight semicircle provides for better eye contact between the educator and the audience (and among members of the audience). The semicircle also improves the audience's line of sight to a screen or video monitor (Figure 14.16).

CONCLUSION

Communication is the heart of fire and life safety education. Through communication, educators create the change that is necessary for education.

Instructional methods are the practical tools that educators use to communicate with their audiences. Matching the instructional method and the educational objective is a key skill — and the educational objective is what drives that choice.

The learning environment supports everything that the educator does in the classroom. For this reason, managing the physical learning environment is as important as selecting the best instructional method.

FOR MORE INFORMATION

Stephen Carroll, et. al., "The Relative Effectiveness of Training Methods — Expert Opinion and Research," *Personnel Psychology*, 1972, p. 495.

John Newstrom, "Evaluating the Effectiveness of Training Methods," *Personnel Administrator*, January 1980, pp. 55-60.

David Peoples, *Presentations Plus*, John Wiley & Sons, 1988.

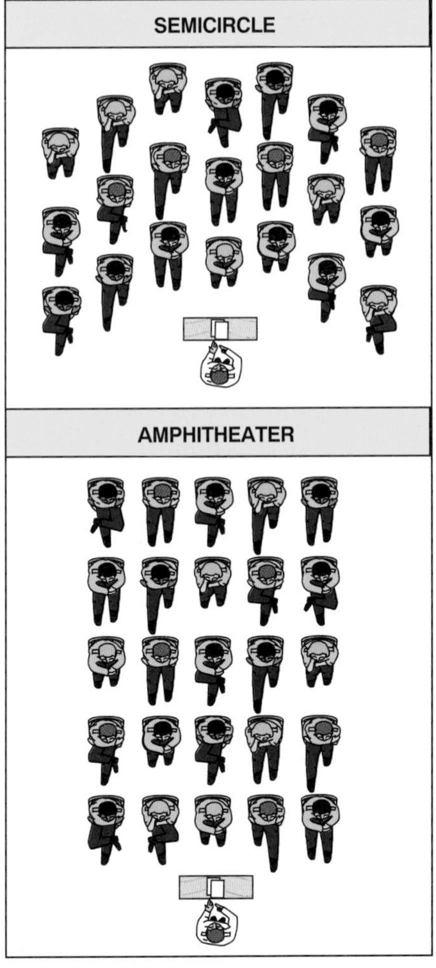

Figure 14.16 The amphitheater and semicircle have the same advantages as the classroom style; however, these setups makes it difficult for students to take notes or use training materials.

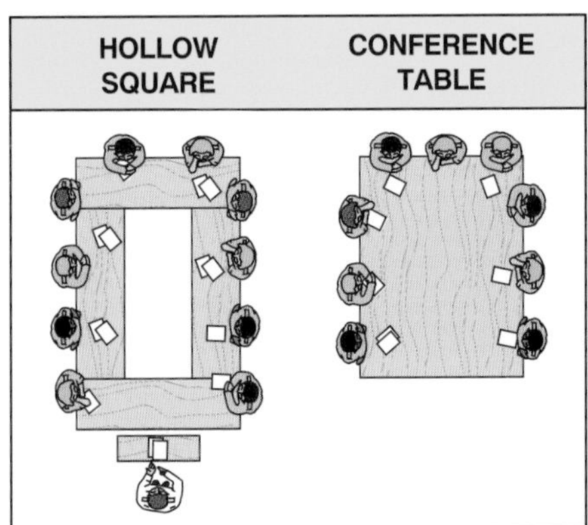

Figure 14.14 The conference and hollow squares allow all participants in a discussion group to face the center of the table or group.

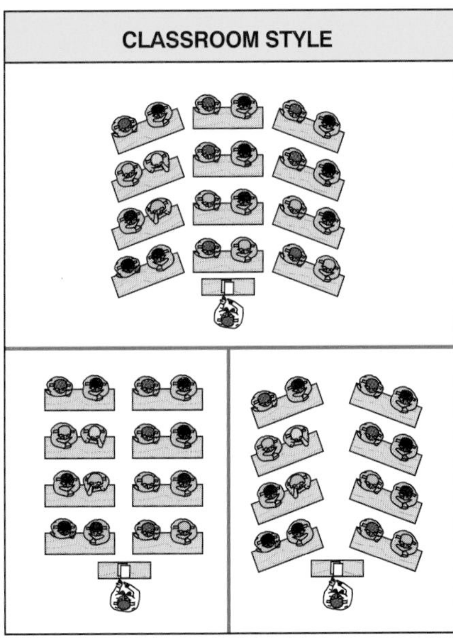

Figure 14.15 The classroom style accommodates any size group and allows individuals to move through the aisles.

Chapter 14 Notes

1. For a more detailed discussion of the communication process and communication techniques, see "Instructional Challenges of the 90s," in IFSTA **Fire Service Instructor,** 5th ed., and "Instructional Communication Skills" in Clark Lambert, *Secrets of a Successful Trainer: A Simplified Guide for Survival*, John Wiley & Sons, 1986.

2. Clark Lambert, *Secrets of a Successful Trainer*, John Wiley & Sons, 1986. p. 69.

3. See Madeline Hunter, *Mastery Teaching*, TIP Publications, El Segundo, CA, 1982, pp. 91-92.

4. To review the different kinds of educational objectives, see Chapter 10, "Developing the Program Curriculum."

Chapter 14 Review

Directions

The following activities are designed to help you comprehend and apply the information in Chapter 14 of **Fire and Life Safety Educator**, second edition. To receive the maximum learning experience from these activities, it is recommended that you use the following procedure:

1. Read the chapter, underlining or highlighting important terms, topics, and subject matter. Read the sidebar material, study the photographs and illustrations, and read the captions with each.
2. Review the list of vocabulary words to ensure that you know the chapter-related meaning of each. If you are unsure of the meaning of a vocabulary word, look up the word in the glossary or a dictionary, and then study its context in the chapter.
3. On a separate sheet of paper, complete all assigned or selected application and review activities before checking your answers.
4. After you have finished, check your answers against those on the pages referenced in parentheses.
5. Correct any incorrect answers, and review material that was answered incorrectly.

Vocabulary

Be sure that you know the chapter-related meanings of the following words:

- bias *(260)*
- communication vehicle *(258)*
- decoding *(257)*
- encoding *(257)*
- frame of reference *(259)*
- nonverbal *(258)*
- team teaching *(265)*
- verbal (oral) *(258)*

Application of Knowledge

1. Outline the specific instructional methods you would use to improve communication with each of the following audiences:
   - Third-graders with short attention spans
   - Automotive shift workers fatigued at the end of their shifts
   - Bored teens
   - Very poor, inner-city adults who appear to be uninterested in community concerns
   - Prison inmates who are biased against you
   - Belligerent male teens who are reluctant to believe what you are saying
   - Special education middle-schoolers who have difficulty understanding concepts *(xx)*
2. Draw schematics of appropriate room arrangements for each of the following situations:
   - Presentation to an audience of 75 adults who need to be able to hear and see audiovisual materials
   - Presentation to a small group of your peers who will need to take notes and prepare materials
   - Presentation to a small group of preschool children
   - Demonstration presentation to a group of 20 teens *(267, 268)*

Review Activities

1. Define *communication. (257)*
2. Expain each of the following communications terms:
   - sender
   - message
   - receiver
   - medium
   - feedback *(257)*
3. List the factors that influence how educators encode their messages. *(258)*
4. Name and explain the three primary mediums through which messages may be sent. *(258)*

5. List several examples of communication vehicles to illustrate each of the communication mediums. *(259)*

6. List factors that may affect the receiver's interpretation of the message. *(259)*

7. Provide specific examples of communication barriers. *(259, 260)*

8. List the characteristics of active listening. *(260)*

9. Explain how the fire and life safety educator uses each of the following four methods to check audience understanding. *(260, 261)*
   - sampling
   - signaled response
   - choral response
   - private response

10. Explain why asking questions is an effective educational method. *(261)*

11. Explain the following types of questions: *(261, 262)*
    - direct
    - overhead
    - rhetorical
    - relay

12. Describe guidelines for dealing with incorrect or incomplete answers to questions. *(262)*

13. Explain the role that culture plays in effective communication. Provide specific examples to illustrate your explanation. *(262)*

14. Compare and contrast each of the following instructional methods:
    - lecture *(262)*
    - discussion *(263)*
    - illustration *(264)*
    - demonstration *(264)*

15. Define each of the following categories of discussion: *(263, 264)*
    - guided
    - conference
    - case study
    - role-playing
    - brainstorming

16. List the five steps to an effective demonstration. *(264)*

17. Provide three specific examples of instances in which team teaching would be an effective teaching method. *(265)*

18. Provide four advantages of team teaching. *(265)*

19. Provide four disadvantages of team teaching. *(265)*

20. Describe methods for getting audiences back from a break. *(265, 266)*

21. Define each of the three types of educational objectives as they are tied to learning domains: *(266)*
    - affective objective
    - cognitive objective
    - psychomotor objective

22. Write one objective (other than the ones provided in the chapter) to illustrate each of the learning domains: affective, cognitive, and psychomotor. *(266)*

23. Provide at least three examples of instructional methods appropriate for each of the types of objectives: *(266)*
    - affective objective
    - cognitive objective
    - psychomotor objective

24. Define learning environment. *(267)*

25. List the eight factors that make up a learning environment. *(267)*

Questions and Notes

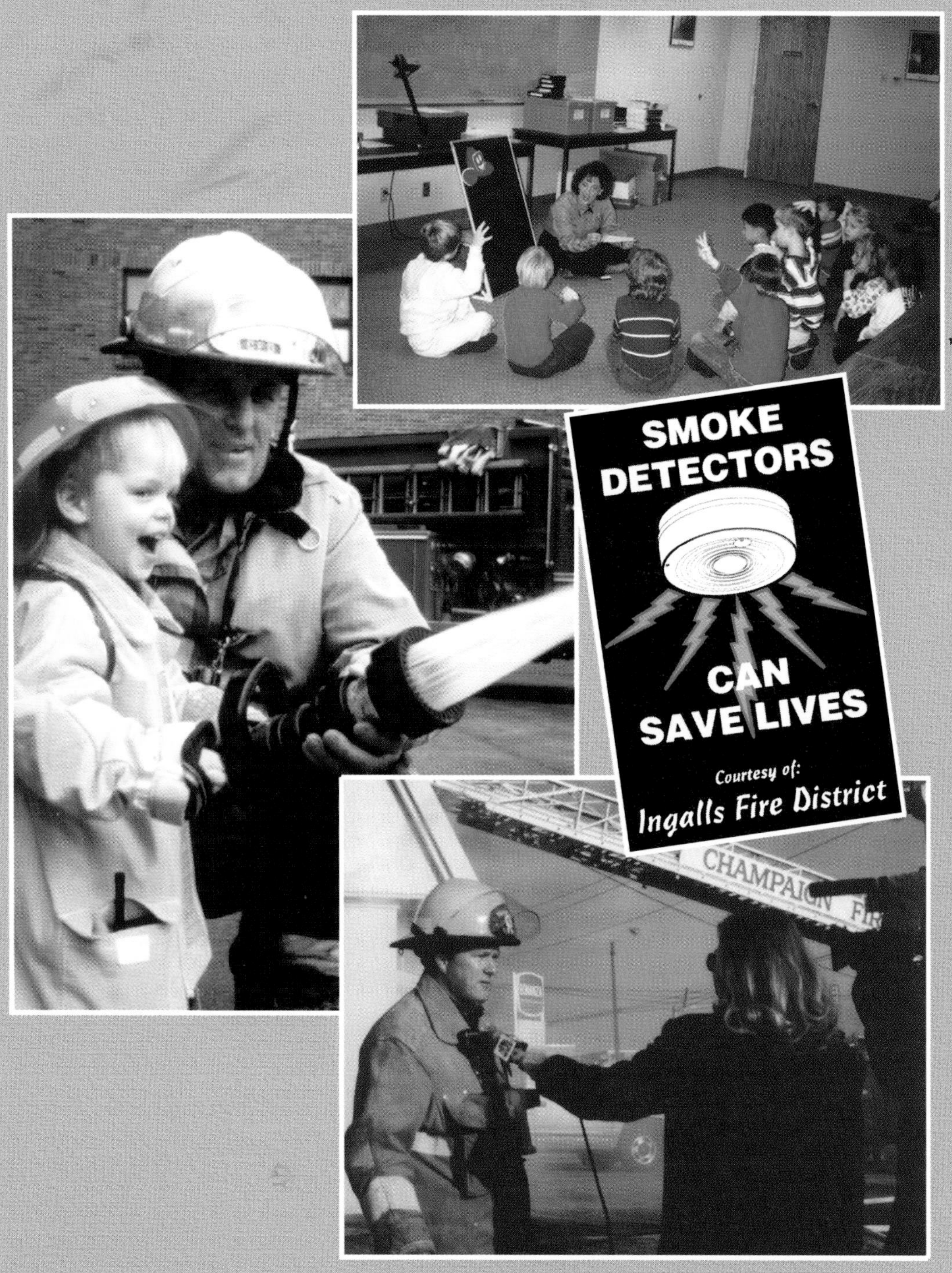
SMOKE
DETECTORS
CAN
SAVE LIVES
Courtesy of:
Ingalls Fire District
CHAMPAIGN

Selecting Educational Materials 15

LEARNING OBJECTIVES

This chapter provides information that addresses the following objectives of NFPA 1035, *Standard for Professional Qualifications for Public Fire and Life Safety Educator* (1993 edition):

Public Fire and Life Safety Educator I

3-4.1 Select instructional materials, given a subject, program objective, the intended audience, and related resources, so that the materials are appropriate to the audience and program objectives.

3-4.5 Distribute educational information, given material, specified audience, and time frame, so that information reaches the audience within the specified time.

Public Fire and Life Safety Educator II

4-4.1 Develop informational materials, given an identified issue, so that information provided is accurate, relevant to the issue, and comprehensible to the audience.

Public Fire and Life Safety Educator III

5-4.1 Create original resource materials, given an identified issue, so that material created is accurate, relevant to the issue, and comprehensible to the audience.

Chapter 15
Selecting Educational Materials

INTRODUCTION

The materials used by the fire and life safety educator play a key part in all fire and life safety education programs. When the fire and life safety educator uses these materials effectively, the audience can actually see the effects of fire, burns, and unsafe practices, as well as learn the specific steps to take to avoid them.

Fire and life safety educational materials must compete for the attention of the audience. Effective materials are very important tools in getting and keeping the attention of the audience. Today's children and adults are bombarded with information from books, magazines, and newspapers; from network and cable television; from radio; from telephones (even in the car!); from videos and compact discs; and from computer programs and games.

However, as important as they are, *materials alone do not make an education program*. An effective fire and life safety education program also must include specific measurable objectives and evaluation instruments and must use instructional methods that match the stated or written objectives. The materials used by the educator help the learner accomplish the objectives and the educator reinforce instructional methods.

In general, materials used by the fire and life safety educator fall into three broad categories, based on their intended purpose:

- Awareness materials
- Informational materials
- Educational materials

Awareness materials attempt to make the audience more aware of a problem or situation. For example, bumper stickers that say "Firefighters still make house calls" promote awareness about the fire service. A poster of Smokey Bear with a caption "Only you can prevent forest fires" increases awareness of an individual's responsibility in preserving the forest (Figure 15.1).

Informational materials suggest an action or provide facts and figures. Bumper stickers that

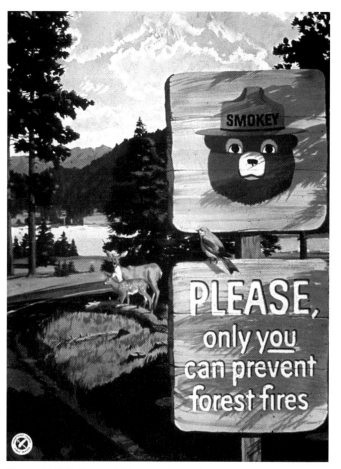

Figure 15.1 The intent of this poster is to make the audience more aware of a problem — forest fires. *Courtesy of U.S. Forest Service.*

say "Fire sprinklers save lives"[1] are informational materials: They state a fact and suggest an action (that is, install sprinklers) (Figure 15.2). For all practical purposes, awareness materials and informational materials are the same. Awareness and informational materials are sometimes called *promotional materials*.[2]

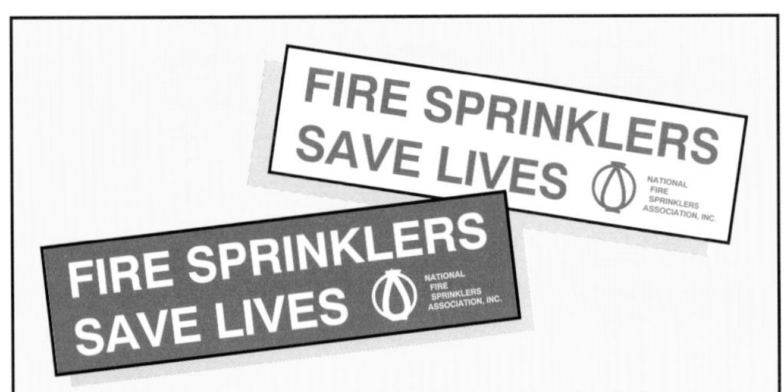

Figure 15.2 These bumper stickers are examples of informational materials. *Used with permission of the National Fire Sprinkler Association.*

Educational materials are designed to educate the audience. As defined in Chapter 13, *education is the process of training, teaching, or instructing students in new fire and life safety skills*. In other words, education requires a change in skills or behavior (Figure 15.3). Bumper stickers that say "Change your clock; change your battery" or "Stop, drop, and roll if your clothes catch fire" expect a change in behavior and are educational materials. Promotional materials, by contrast, do not change skills.

Educational materials are any physical teaching aids — printed matter, audiovisual materials, and "props" — that the educator uses to teach new fire and life safety skills to the audience. This chapter discusses the need for educational materials, lists and discusses types of educational materials, explains how to evaluate and choose the appropriate educational materials for the audience and subject, and shows fire and life safety educators how to create their own educational materials. This chapter does not cover tips for using audiovisual materials. That topic is included in Chapter 17, "Using Public Speaking Techniques."

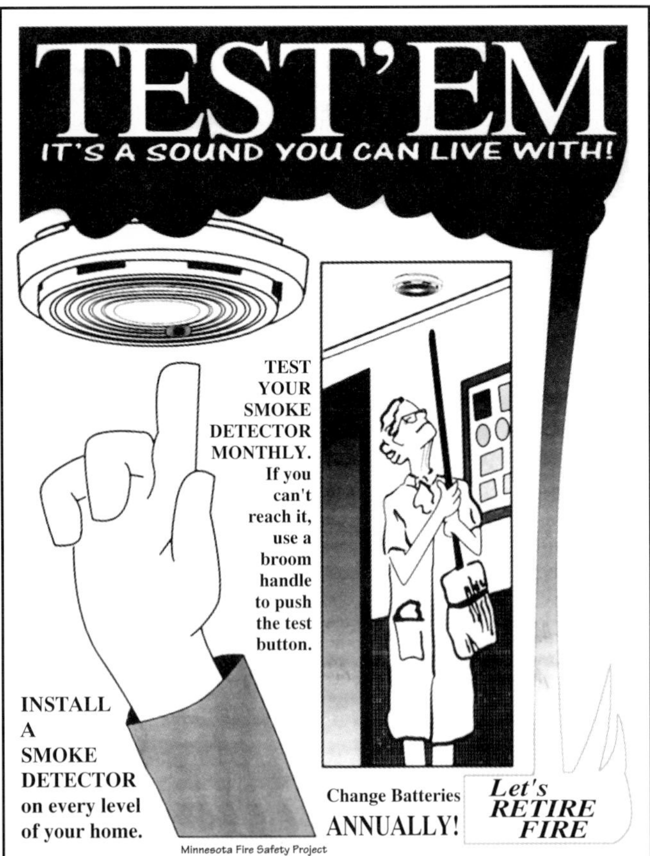

Figure 15.3 Educational materials are designed to train, teach, or instruct students in new fire and life safety skills. *Courtesy of Minnesota Fire Safety Project.*

The Need for Educational Materials

The need for educational materials is based on how people learn and remember. According to some estimates, 75 percent of what people learn comes to them visually. An estimated 13 percent of all human knowledge is gained through hearing, and the remaining 12 percent of knowledge comes from a combination of smell, taste, and touch. Because people are sensory learners, fire and life safety educators need to teach to the senses — especially to the sense of sight. Comprehension increases threefold when a picture replaces words and sixfold when pictures and words are used together.

> **About 2,500 years ago, Confucius said:**
> "I hear and I forget
> I see and I remember
> I do and I understand."

Basic Kinds of Educational Materials

The three basic kinds of educational materials are print matter, audiovisual materials, and props.

Print materials include brochures (also called *flyers* or *folders*); posters; fact sheets, coloring books, and activity sheets; educational card or board games; and pretests/posttests. Print materials are usually less expensive than audiovisual materials and can be handed out for the audience to take home. Print materials are sometimes called *consumables* because they are usually limited to one-time use.

The variety of audiovisual materials is expanding and now includes films and filmstrips, videotapes and audiotapes, 35 mm slides and slide-tape combinations, transparencies (sometimes called *overheads*), and computer simulators (Figure 15.4). Flipcharts, chalkboards, and mark-and-wipe boards are also sometimes considered audiovisual materials (even though there is no audio), just as audiotapes are included (even though there is no video).

Props are objects that the audience can see, touch, smell, or hear. A burned remnant from a home fire, a piece of melted glass, a manual fire alarm pull station, or a smoke detector — any of these could be an effective prop during a fire and life safety presentation (Figure 15.5).

Props are extremely effective teaching aids because they make the subject appear very real. Because they often involve several of the senses, props are also an excellent memory aid. Two questions, however, are helpful in deciding whether or not to use a prop.

- Does the prop help the audience learn how to perform a fire and life safety behavior or how to understand the need for the behavior? (**NOTE**: If the prop is more for the sake of "show and tell" or "believe it or not" than for showing a behavior or need, the prop may distract the audience from the educational message.)
- Does the prop help illustrate behavior or need tastefully and in a way that is nonthreatening? (**NOTE**: A prop that is shocking or frightening may distract the audience.)

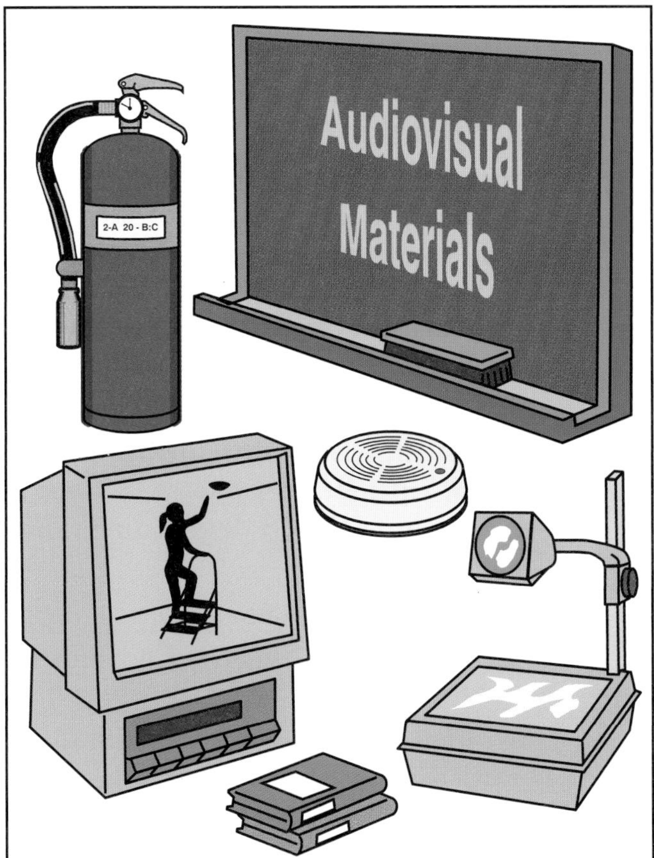

Figure 15.4 The educator selects the training aids that best contribute to learning.

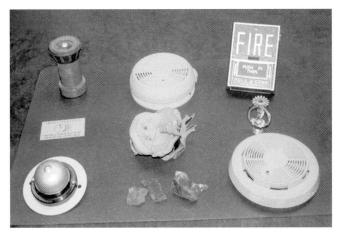

Figure 15.5 Props should be appropriate to the lesson being taught.

EVALUATING EDUCATIONAL MATERIALS

There are vast differences in the quality of fire and life safety education materials. Whether purchased commercially, borrowed or adapted from another educator, or created in-house, all educational materials should be evaluated.

When should this evaluation happen? At a minimum, educational materials should be evaluated before their first use. Once materials are integrated into fire and life safety education programs, the materials should be re-evaluated every year or so. The purpose of the follow-up evaluation is to make sure that what was acceptable at first still is. As a result, the follow-up evaluation can be simpler than the first evaluation.

The techniques for evaluating materials range from asking a few simple questions to using sophisticated testing. The amount of evaluation needed depends on (1) how much money the fire and life safety educator has to invest, (2) how many people the material is expected to reach, and (3) how long the material will be used.

The kinds of evaluation techniques for educational materials can also vary greatly. Evaluation techniques can be either *qualitative* or *quantitative*. Qualitative approaches do not use numbers, are fairly subjective, and rely on the fire and life safety educator's experience, judgment, and interpretation. Quantitative approaches use numbers to compare different materials and methods, are likely to be more sophisticated than qualitative methods, and involve formal testing. *In evaluating educational materials, the key point is to evaluate all materials being considered in the same way.*

Qualitative evaluations:

"I feel good today."

"I like this brochure."

Quantitative evaluations:

"My temperature is down to 98.6°F."

"The brochure scores a 6 on the Flesch Index."

Qualitative Approaches

Evaluating educational materials can be as simple as reviewing the material against a standard checklist. Several questions should be asked during the qualitative review:

- How well does the material match the specific educational objectives of the fire and life safety program?
- Does the material provide the information that is needed to bring about educational change? Does the material explain action that the learners must take?
- Is the material technically accurate?
- Has the material been produced by a reputable organization?
- Can the information presented be clearly understood by members of the potential audience?

  The only way to answer this question is to ask one or more members of the potential audience! Rather than ask, "Do you understand what this video is saying?" invite your sample audience to tell you what the key points were. Invite them to describe or demonstrate skills that the material is trying to teach. If the sample audience is unclear about the key points or cannot describe or demonstrate the skills, the material will probably not be understood by the audience at large!
- Is the material age-appropriate?

  With 3- to 4-year-old children, for example, are stories or activities limited to the 5-minute typical attention span for that age?

  Does material for 4- to 5-year-olds avoid showing unsafe behaviors (which the children will copycat)?

  With 5- to 6-year-old children, are stories or activities limited to the 15- to 20-minute typical attention span for that age? Do materials take advantage of this age group's interest in using large muscles ("Stop, drop, and roll," for example) and in coloring?

  NOTE: For additional examples of how to link fire and life safety education to human development, see Chapter 13, "Learning Fire and Life Safety Educational Theory."
- Is the material free of bias? Does it objectively reflect how people in the audience really live and work?

  Only a few years ago, fire and life safety education materials were largely developed by and for white Anglo-Saxons. Until very recently, materials depicted children as living in two-parent families and retired adults as using canes and living in nursing homes.

Audiences are increasingly sensitive about being typecast or stereotyped. As a result, fire and life safety educators need to make sure that their educational material is free of bias that could turn an audience away.

Differences in race, gender, age, weight, accent, style of hair or dress, religion, social/economic background, education, job, family structure, or disability can lead to bias.

The audience may be offended by a phrase or illustration that the educator thinks is bias-free. For example, the term *handicapped* has been replaced by the term *disabled*. But educators who refer to their audience as "the disabled" may well cause offense — the preferred form of reference is now "people with disabilities" or even "differently able."

The acceptable terms change often. *The only way to make sure that material is bias-free is to invite (and accept) comments from a few members of the potential audience.*

NOTE: For a refresher on how today's audiences for fire and life safety education live and work, see Chapter 8, "Knowing Your Audience."

When responses to these questions are all "yes," the educator can feel fairly comfortable with the quality and usability of the materials. Questions that receive "no" answers indicate problems and signal the need for adjustment or abandonment of the educational materials.

The Pan-Educational Institute has developed a more sophisticated approach to evaluating materials as part of its *Practical Criteria and Instruments for Selecting and Implementing Sound Fire and Burn Education Programs in School and Community*.[3] The package includes work sheets for assessing posters and print visuals, written informational materials (brochures, stand-alone handbooks, storybooks, coloring books and workbooks/work sheets), and audiovisual materials (media campaigns, public service announcements, and audiovisual presentations).

By completing the work sheets, fire and life safety educators rate materials on a scale of 1 to 5 in each of eight categories. (**NOTE**: Although the ratings use numbers, the ratings are subjective and qualitative.) The listing below outlines the eight areas of evaluation:

- Program goals and objectives
- Organization and format
- Appropriateness to age and experience of the learners
- Completeness of presentation materials (is extra work needed?)
- Quality of print and graphics
- Clarity and precision of printed and/or audio presentation
- Adaptability to local needs, interests, audience capabilities
- Fire service involvement as a resource (does the fire service help develop the materials or teach the classes?)

When the scoring is complete, a material is found to fit within one of five categories: limited quality, below average quality, medium quality, high quality, or comprehensive high quality.

Quantitative Approaches

Quantitative approaches use numbers to compare different materials and methods, are likely to be more sophisticated than qualitative methods, and involve formal testing.

READABILITY INDEXES

Reading ease is a major consideration in selecting written fire and life safety education materials. A seventh- to eighth-grade reading level is typical for adults in the United States. Daily newspapers are often written at about that reading level.

Follow simple guidelines when checking the readability of print materials:

- Look for sentences written in the active voice. Active sentences are shorter and easier to read than passive sentences.

  Active: Steve taught the audience how to test smoke detectors.

  Passive: The audience was taught how to test smoke detectors by Steve.

- Look for short sentences with straightforward subject/verb construction. Short sentences are easier to read than long sentences. Dependent clauses or phrases make reading more difficult.

  Easy: The local smoke detector ordinance requires interconnected units. The ordinance took effect on January 1.

  Difficult: The local smoke detector ordinance, which requires individual devices to be interconnected, became effective on January 1.

- Look for a majority of one- and two-syllable words. Generally, words of one or two syllables are easier to read (and comprehend) than words of three or more syllables.

Several indexes measure how easy (or difficult) a passage is to read. Commonly used indexes include a passive-sentence index (a simple percentage of passive sentences within a passage), the Flesch Reading Ease/Flesch Grade Level Index, and the Gunning FOG Index.

The Flesch Index is based on a 100-word passage of the written material. This index counts the average number of words per sentence and the average number of syllables in the passage. Grade level and reading ease are matched to each other, as Table 15.1 shows.

The Gunning FOG Index, on the other hand, combines the overall sentence length with the number of words containing more than one syllable per sentence.

TABLE 15.1
Grade Level And Reading Ease

Flesch Grade Level	Reading Ease*
4	Very easy
5	Easy
6	Fairly easy
7 to 8	Standard
Some high school	Fairly difficult
Some higher education	Difficult
Higher education	Very difficult

*With the Flesch Index, 17 words per sentence and 147 syllables per 100 words is "Standard" reading ease.

To establish a FOG Index, perform the following steps:

Step 1: Select three 100-word passages from the material. Include the entire sentence that contains the 100th word.

Step 2: Calculate the average sentence length of one passage by dividing the number of words in the sample passage by the number of sentences.

Step 3: Count the number of words having three or more syllables. Do not include proper nouns (those that are capitalized), words that are a combination of short words (such as *chairperson* or *firefighter*), or words in which the third syllable is -ed or -es (such as *expanded*).

Step 4: Add together the average sentence length and the number of difficult words.

Step 5: Determine the average grade level of the passage by multiplying the sum of the average sentence length and the number of difficult words (computed in Step 4) by 0.4.

Step 6: Repeat Steps 2-5 for the remaining two passages.

Step 7: Find the average for all three passages by adding the grade levels for each passage and then dividing that answer by 3.

These indexes can be used manually or through some word processing programs. Whether the indexes are used manually or through the word processor, *the important point is to check whether sample materials are harder or easier to read than some standard that reflects the audience.* A highly precise test is not necessary as long as the fire and life safety educator knows whether written materials are "in the ballpark" for readability.

What happens when a 100-word passage (see sidebar, "FOG Index Application") from a fire and life safety brochure is examined according to readability indexes?

FOG Index Application

Number of words:	100
Number of sentences:	11
Average sentence length:	$\frac{100}{11} = 9.09$
Number of difficult words:	13
Average sentence length plus number of difficult words:	9 + 13 = 22
Average grade level:	22 x 0.4 = 8.8

Changing only a few words can lower the FOG Index. For example, changing "additional" to "more" and "significantly" to "greatly" and replacing the word "detector(s)" with "alarm(s)" six times reduces the number of difficult words from 13 to 5. The FOG Index then becomes —

Average sentence length plus number of difficult words:	9 + 5 = 14
Average grade level:	14 x 0.4 = 5.6

PURCHASE
A SMOKE DETECTOR
A smoke detector is a fire alarm that buzzes when it detects smoke, warning you in time to escape.
WHAT KIND?
• Smoke detectors can be either house-current or battery operated. Either kind can do a good job.
• Make sure the model you choose has been listed by a nationally recognized testing laboratory.
HOW MUCH?
• A smoke detector may be purchased at most retail stores for about $8.00-$30.00
HOW MANY?
• There should be at least one smoke detector on every floor of the house except attics, unless the attic space is used for sleeping. Additional detectors will significantly increase your chances of survival.

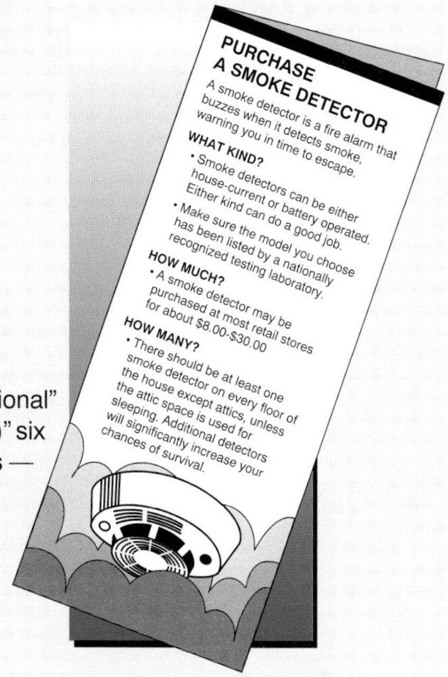

- Passive sentences

  Only 1 sentence out of 11 ("A smoke detector may be purchased...") was passive. This yields an active sentence percentage of more than 90 percent.

- Flesch Reading Ease and Grade Level

  The average sentence had 9 words (much lower or easier to read than the standard of 17). The 100-word passage contained 155 syllables, just slightly higher than the standard seventh- and eighth-grade level of 147.

  The tested passage would be rated between sixth-grade level (fairly easy) and eighth-grade level (standard).

- Gunning FOG Index

  The average sentence had 9 words; the passage included 13 difficult words.

  The passage would be rated between eighth-grade level and ninth-grade level.

Preproduction Testing of Materials

In some cases, fire and life safety educators may need to test materials before going into full production. The purpose of preproduction testing is to make sure that the intended message is reaching the intended audience. The educator should ask several questions when determining whether or not to test materials prior to production:

- Could someone get hurt if the educational message is misunderstood?
- How widely will the material be distributed?
- How difficult or expensive will it be to change the material once it is produced?

After considering questions such as these, the Learn Not to Burn® Foundation decided to test a planned television public service announcement (PSA). The results are published in *Pre-Production Evaluation of the "Tell a Grown-Up to Put It Away" Public Service Announcement for 3-6 Year Olds.*[4]

In that test, 50 children aged 3 to 6 saw the preproduction version of the 30-second PSA twice. The children were then interviewed, one at a time, after each viewing to determine the following:

- How well they understood the story line (a grandfather puts away the lighter and matches)
- How well they understood the message ("Tell a grown-up to put matches and lighters away.")
- How well they understood the visual part of the PSA (a lighter used as a prop and the grandfather's action as he puts lighters in a cupboard)

The test results influenced the Learn Not to Burn® Foundation's decision *not* to produce the PSA. Among the test results were these findings:

- The children did not grasp the basic message.
- The children had trouble following the story, especially after the first viewing.
- Age was important — 3- and 4-year-olds found it more difficult than 5- and 6-year-olds to follow the story and to restate the basic message.
- Older and younger children had difficulty identifying the lighter that was used as a prop in the PSA.
- Children from middle-income families were more able to understand the story and restate the message than children from lower-income families.

The Learn Not to Burn® Foundation experience offers some lessons for all fire and life safety educators. The preproduction test had a set interview procedure and questions — so the results compared "apples with apples." The test evaluated how well the target audience responded: If only middle-income children had been in the study, the results would have been different. Perhaps the most important lesson was that the material was tested before it was produced.

In other cases, it may be possible to change the material, rather than discard it. Illustrations or text in printed material, for example, can be changed relatively easily before the material goes to press.

CREATING EDUCATIONAL MATERIALS

Create or Purchase?

Many fire and life safety educators like to prepare their own educational materials rather than buy them from a business or nonprofit organization. Others like to adopt and adapt what other educators have already created. The interest in developing materials often is related to saving money ("Those other materials are too expensive for me") or the desire to give materials a local flavor.

Developing educational materials is something like fire fighting: It is more complicated than it appears to the casual observer. Before deciding to create their own materials, fire and life safety educators can use this checklist:

- How much will it really cost to develop materials?

  Production costs may be lower than a purchase price. However, production costs do not include the *time spent* in creating the material and coordinating production. The educator's time has value. The cost of time and overhead must be included in a budget, even though the educator is on the payroll.

  Production costs do not include the *cost of mistakes*. Mistakes happen all too easily and range from factual errors to typos (leaving out the word "not," for example) to picking an unreadable combination of paper and ink. Mistakes cost both time and money to fix.

- How important is local flavor? How can it be added at the lowest possible cost?

  Local flavor, while desirable, may be a luxury that fire and life safety educators simply cannot afford.

  Options for adding a local feeling to materials include stamping the name of the fire department or other local sponsor on printed material and supplementing more expensive commercial material (such as videotapes) with low-cost, locally developed material (such as flyers or handmade posters).

- What is the motivation to create the materials?

  Are locally created materials really needed and cost-effective? Or does the educator just prefer to create materials?

- Does the fire and life safety educator have the technical knowledge, experience and equipment to create materials?

  How will the educator assess his or her ability to create materials? Who will provide backup for technical questions, review, and proofing?

Developing Print Materials

There are five basic elements of any print material: the text, the illustrations, the white space on the page, the paper, and the ink. Together these elements make up the design of the print material (Figure 15.6).

Design is much more than whether or not the print material "looks good." The object of the design is to create material that the audience will read and remember. As a result, design must appeal to today's busy reader.

Today's readers share a few characteristics:

- People tend to scan written material, rather than read word for word.
- People expect short written pieces.
- People prefer visual to print materials. Today's readers are visually oriented. They rely on illustrations, headlines, captions, pie charts, graphs, and subheads for print information.

Educational materials design needs to take these characteristics of the modern reader into account. For instance, use subheads and captions to impart information to those who scan. Be concise and provide specific examples. Shorten sentences and paragraphs for those who would rather read several short messages than one long one. Use appropriate color and illustrative design to reach visually oriented readers.

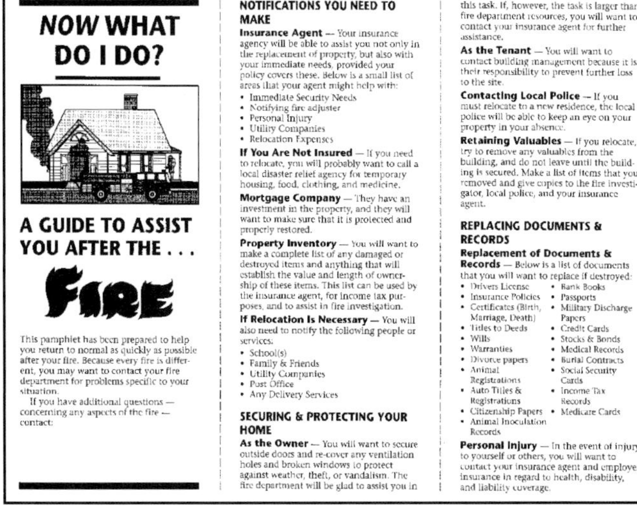

NOW WHAT DO I DO?

A GUIDE TO ASSIST YOU AFTER THE . . . FIRE

This pamphlet has been prepared to help you return to normal as quickly as possible after your fire. Because every fire is different, you may want to contact your fire department for problems specific to your situation.

If you have additional questions — concerning any aspects of the fire — contact:

NOTIFICATIONS YOU NEED TO MAKE

Insurance Agent — Your insurance agency will be able to assist you not only in the replacement of property, but also with your immediate needs, provided your policy covers these. Below is a small list of areas that your agent might help with:

- Immediate Security Needs
- Notifying fire adjuster
- Personal Injury
- Utility Companies
- Relocation Expenses

If You Are Not Insured — If you need to relocate, you will probably want to call a local disaster relief agency for temporary housing, food, clothing, and medicine.

Mortgage Company — They have an investment in the property, and they will want to make sure that it is protected and properly restored.

Property Inventory — You will want to make a complete list of any damaged or destroyed items and anything that will establish the value and length of ownership of these items. This list can be used by the insurance agent, for income tax purposes, and to assist in fire investigation.

If Relocation Is Necessary — You will also need to notify the following people or services:

- School(s)
- Family & Friends
- Utility Companies
- Post Office
- Any Delivery Services

SECURING & PROTECTING YOUR HOME

As the Owner — You will want to secure outside doors and re-cover any ventilation holes and broken windows to protect against weather, theft, or vandalism. The fire department will be glad to assist you in this task. If, however, the task is larger than fire department resources, you will want to contact your insurance agent for further assistance.

As the Tenant — You will want to contact building management because it is their responsibility to prevent further loss to the site.

Contacting Local Police — If you must relocate to a new residence, the local police will be able to keep an eye on your property in your absence.

Retaining Valuables — If you relocate, try to remove any valuables from the building, and do not leave until the building is secured. Make a list of items that you removed and give copies to the fire investigator, local police, and your insurance agent.

REPLACING DOCUMENTS & RECORDS

Replacement of Documents & Records — Below is a list of documents that you will want to replace if destroyed:

- Drivers License
- Insurance Policies
- Certificates (Birth, Marriage, Death)
- Titles to Deeds
- Wills
- Warranties
- Divorce papers
- Animal Registrations
- Auto Titles & Registrations
- Citizenship Papers
- Animal Inoculation Records
- Bank Books
- Passports
- Military Discharge Papers
- Credit Cards
- Stocks & Bonds
- Medical Records
- Burial Contracts
- Social Security Cards
- Income Tax Records
- Medicare Cards

Personal Injury — In the event of injury to yourself or others, you will want to contact your insurance agent and employer insurance in regard to health, disability, and liability coverage.

Figure 15.6 The size and type of the text, the illustration, and the amount of white space in this design work together to make an attractive brochure.

THE TEXT

Fire and life safety educators need to write for today's reader. Follow these simple guidelines for the text of your print materials:

- In general, follow the KISS acronym: **K**eep **I**t **S**hort and **S**imple.
- Use small words, short sentences, short paragraphs, and active voice.

  Explaining complex subjects, such as fire safety, in simple language can be difficult. One technique is to start by getting complex information on paper and then editing the draft for simplicity. Several drafts may be needed. The willingness to edit and redraft, though, is the sign of a good writer.
- Assume that the reader will only read part of the written material. In fact, most people do not read main text.

  Put the most important information first. Use headlines, subheads, and captions. Supplement the text with illustrations.

Fire and life safety educators will make several decisions on how to present the words so that they will be read. These decisions involve the typeface and type size (or font), the line length, and whether or not the type is justified (spaced so that lines of text come out even at the margin).

Readability is the prime consideration in picking a font (typeface). Familiar fonts are generally more readable than unfamiliar ones. Serif fonts — those in which the letters rest on small horizontal lines called *feet* — are generally more readable than sans serif fonts — those without feet. There are many popular fonts used in printing materials. The font not only should be readable but also should reflect the purpose and complement the design of the printed piece.

A very easy test is available to compare the readability of fonts. Cover a sample of type with a plain piece of paper, and slowly pull the paper down, revealing the top of the letters. The sooner the partially revealed sample can be read, the more readable that typeface is.

More About Fonts

Which of the fonts below do you find most readable, the serif or the sans serif?

This sentence is set in a serif font.

This sentence is set in a sans serif font.

Each of the popular typefaces below has a different appeal and readability.

Baskerville	Optima
Bodoni	New Century Schoolbook
Souvenir Demi	Times Roman
Helvetica	Stone Serif
Garamond	Kabel Medium

Too many typefaces clutter written material, making it difficult to read. As a rule of thumb, use one typeface for main text and another for headlines, subheads, and captions.

Type size also influences readability. Type is measured in points (and line lengths are measured in picas). There are 72 points to the inch, 6 picas to the inch, and 12 points to the pica. Therefore, the higher the point, the larger the type size. The minimum size is 10-point type, with 12-point type becoming more common (Figure 15.7).

When selecting type, it is often helpful to see the type in the specified size because some fonts look larger than others — even though they are the same size. For example, compare the following two sentences:

This is Times 12 point.

This is New Century Schoolbook 12 point.

The ideal length of a line of type is related to how much material the eye can see without moving. The ideal length is 40 to 50 characters per line. Lines between 35 and 55 characters are within the acceptable range. Many publications designers choose to err on the narrow side.

Type can be aligned in four ways: left justified (also called *ragged right*), centered, right justified (also called *ragged left*), or justified. Although headlines, subheads, and captions may be aligned in any of these ways, body text is usually left justified (ragged right) or justified.

This sample paragraph has a ragged right margin. This sample paragraph is ragged right. This sample paragraph is ragged right. This sample paragraph is ragged right. This sample paragraph is ragged right. This sample paragraph is ragged right. This sample paragraph is ragged right.

This sample paragraph has justified margins. This sample paragraph is justified. This sample paragraph is justified. This sample paragraph is justified. This sample paragraph is justified. This sample paragraph is justified. This sample paragraph is justified. This sample paragraph is set justified.

Justified type is formal and traditional. Ragged-right type is informal and friendly. Ragged text holds the reader's attention and is

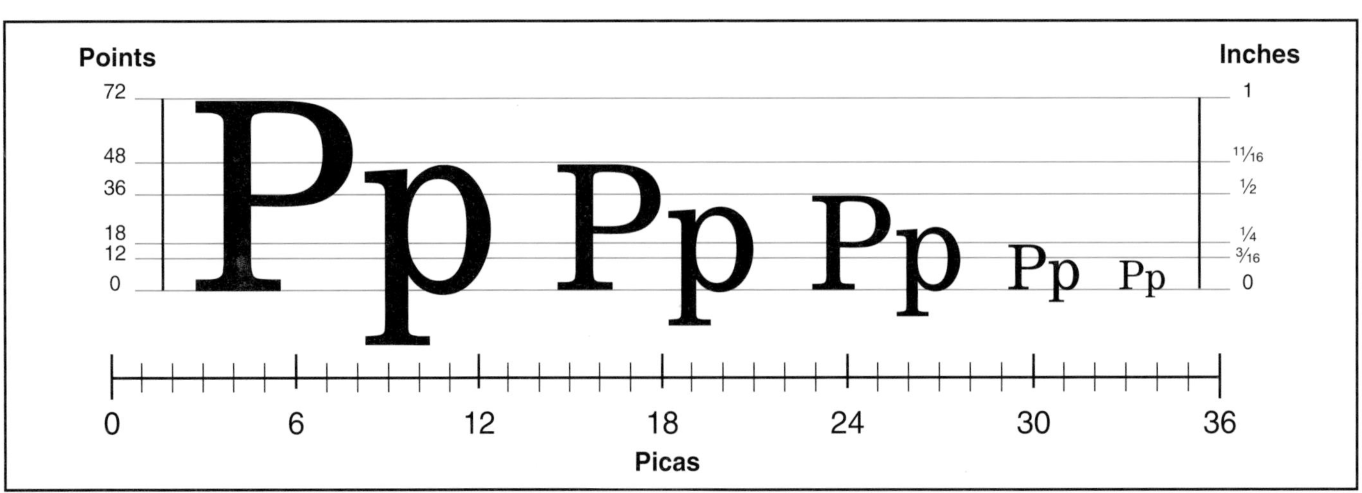

Figure 15.7 Type is measured in points, while line length is given in picas.

Educational materials can be one-color, two-color, or four-color (sometimes called *full-color*) printing. The numbers refer to the number of colors of inks, which corresponds to the number of times the item must go through the press. Each press run increases the price. Increasing the number of inks from one to two raises the printing costs by about a third.

Creating Audiovisual Materials

Audiovisual materials range from the simple — flipcharts, 35 mm slides, and transparencies — to the very sophisticated, including films and filmstrips, videotapes and audiotapes, slide-tape combinations, and computer simulators. (**NOTE**: The techniques for creating very sophisticated audiovisual materials are beyond the scope of this manual.) Each of these audiovisual materials has its advantages and disadvantages (Table 15.2).

Flipcharts, 35 mm slides, and transparencies can be very effective audiovisual educational materials. *The key points are to limit the text, to use visuals, and to keep the visual image as simple as possible.* Large-size or projected words are simply words — not visuals.

FLIPCHARTS

Flipcharts are very often used to record ideas from meetings (Figure 15.11). They can also be used as educational materials — especially if illustrations (such as escape diagrams) are added. Flipcharts are inexpensive, easy to change or adapt for reuse at different presentations, and effective with small groups. Although the paper is always white, marking pens come in a wide variety of colors. Prepared flipcharts can be reused a few times, but they will need to be replaced when they become battered.

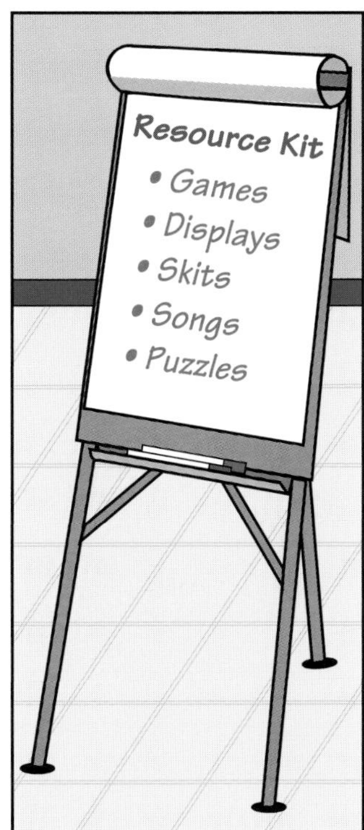

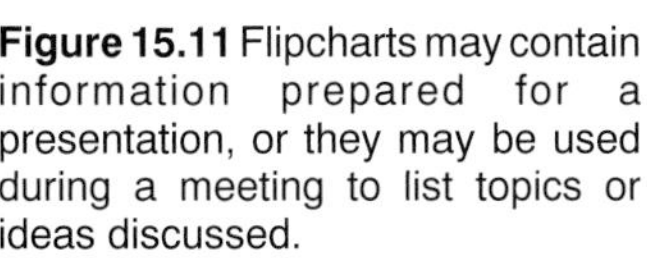
Figure 15.11 Flipcharts may contain information prepared for a presentation, or they may be used during a meeting to list topics or ideas discussed.

When using flipcharts as educational materials, educators should observe the following guidelines:

- Recognize that handwriting is critical. Fire and life safety educators who are worried about the legibility of their handwriting can get someone else to print the flipcharts for them.

  NOTE: If your department or jurisdiction has a poster printer, type your flipchart information on 8Z | x- by 11-inch paper and run it through the printer. Then add underscores, boxes, checks, simple visuals, and color. This technique is easier than handwriting the flipcharts and creates professional and legible flipchart pages.

- Prepare the flipcharts ahead of time. Place a lined piece of flipchart paper underneath to use as a writing guide.
- Before making flipcharts, test to see whether the marker will bleed through the paper. If it does, place a blank sheet under the page you are creating.
- Lightly, and in small print, pencil in information or desired responses that will be added during the classroom session.
- If you are creating several flipcharts on one tablet, be sure to leave a blank sheet after each chart so that the writing on the page does not show through the page on top of it.
- Select (and maintain) a format for capitalization and punctuation. *The most readable format is what people are most used to reading*: a capital at the beginning of a sentence or line, followed by all lowercase letters.

  Punctuation can clutter the image, so keep punctuation to what is really needed. A question mark, for example, is needed. A period, on the other hand, may not be

TABLE 15.2
Advantages And Disadvantages Of Different Audiovisuals

Medium	Advantages	Disadvantages
Overhead transparencies	Can be created in-house	Commercially developed overheads on fire and life safety are rarely (if ever) available.
	Can be rearranged for different presentations	
	Are inexpensive to create	May lack excitement
	Can be used for large groups	Are static; lack movement
	Can be marked on during presentation	Are subject to keystoning
35 mm slides	Can be created in-house	May lack excitement
	Commercially developed slides on fire and life safety are widely available.	Are static; lack movement
	Can be rearranged for different presentations	
	More expensive to create than overheads	
	Can be used for large groups	
Filmstrips	Some commercially developed filmstrips on fire and life safety are available.	Cannot be created in-house
		Cannot be rearranged for use in other presentations
	Offer movement	
	Commercially available materials may be older.	
Films	Offer movement and excitement	Cannot be created in-house
	Commercially developed films on fire and life safety are widely available.	Cannot be rearranged for use in other presentations
	Can be used for large groups	
	Are extremely durable	
Videotapes	Closely resemble the popular medium of television	Cannot be rearranged for use in other presentations
	Offer movement and excitement	May be expensive
	Can be created in-house	
	Commercially developed films on fire and life safety are widely available.	
	Can be used for large groups	
	Are extremely durable	

needed at the end of each line if phrases, rather than sentences, are used.

- Test legibility to make sure that the lettering on the flipchart is large enough to be read. Complete one flipchart, and make sure it can be read from as far away as the farthest member of the audience will be.
- Keep the first page blank, or use it for a welcome message or the name of the presentation. Begin the presentation on the second page.
- Add visual interest. Use two or three colors consistently (green ink for information and red ink for action, for example). Add illustrations: Enlarge small illustrations on the copier, place them under the page where they will appear, and trace over them.
- Keep flipcharts simple. Limit each flipchart page to one idea. State that idea in as few words as possible — 12 to 15 words per page is a good target. Use bullets to keep words to a minimum. Limit illustrations to one per page.
- Use flags or paper clips to mark pages that will be repeated.
- Practice turning the pages until the technique is smooth and quiet.

35 MM SLIDES

35 mm slides are a very popular medium for do-it-yourself audiovisuals (Figure 15.12). They are far superior to flipcharts in illustrating concepts (the extensive damage caused by a home fire), emotions (the face of a firefighter after a rescue), and objects (the parts of a smoke detector). Personal computers have vastly improved the quality of text slides — making slides made of transfer letters obsolete.

Slides are also easy to rearrange into different presentations. They are effective with large groups. In addition, they are more durable than flipcharts or transparencies.

There are, though, several disadvantages with using slides. The lights must be down or off, making eye contact with the audience difficult or impossible. Once the presentation has started, it

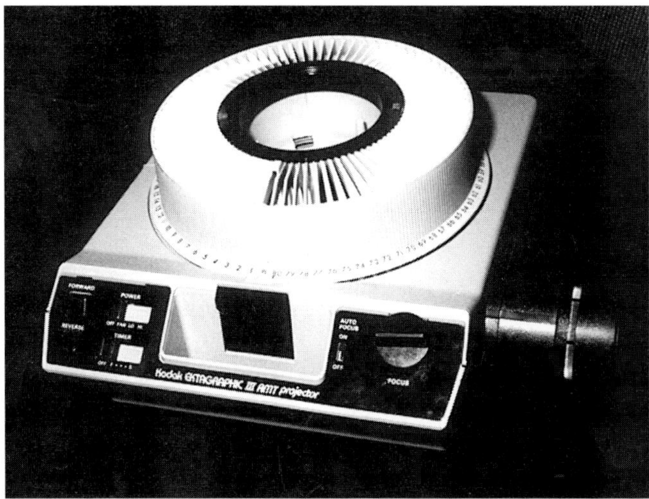

Figure 15.12 35 mm slides are compact, are convenient to manage, and give clear, detailed images.

is very difficult to revise it — to adjust the length of the presentation, for example. Also, the fan on the slide projector may be noisy.

The following are guidelines to follow when creating 35 mm slides:

- Insist on excellent photography — clear, sharply focused crisp colors. Fire and life safety educators would not consider distributing a blurry handout and likewise should not show fuzzy or faded slides.

  Some fire and life safety educators gained their photographic skills as fire investigators. *Documentary photographs that a fire investigator shoots are not necessarily good teaching tools.* Educational materials need to involve the audience and to have strong visual impact. Taking a community-college-level photography course is a good investment for anyone who creates 35 mm slides for teaching.
- Maintain a style for capitalization and punctuation.
- Keep the visual image as uncluttered as possible. The visual subject of the slide should be clearly evident. A pointer should not be needed to highlight what the slide is about!
- Make all slides either horizontal or vertical. (**NOTE**: Because the projections of slides in the vertical format often con-

tinue off the top or bottom of the screen, the horizontal format is preferred.)

- Keep slides simple. Limit each slide to one idea. State that idea in as few words as possible. Use bullets to keep words to a minimum. Limit illustrations to one per slide.

A number of personal computer programs are available to assist the fire and life safety educator in creating 35 mm slide presentations. The fire and life safety educator can choose a standard format (with or without a frame, for example) for text slides, choose from a menu of typefaces, and import clip art. Especially at first, there may be a temptation to use too many features. Remember: Keep the image simple and the message clear.

A final word on 35 mm slides: equipment. Educators must be absolutely sure they know how to use the projector and that the equipment is working. Trying out equipment *before each presentation* is as important for the experienced educator as for the novice.

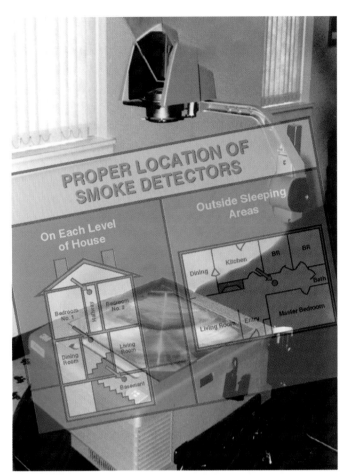

Figure 15.13 Transparencies of drawings, written material, and photographic reproductions can be projected onto a screen.

TRANSPARENCIES

"Overheads" are among the most popular teaching aids of all time — for good reason (Figure 15.13). They are durable, inexpensive, and fast to make. Transparencies (unlike flipcharts) can be used in rooms ranging in size from that of a classroom to that of an auditorium. They show text and line art (tables, charts, graphs, diagrams, and icons) to good advantage. Also, the user can mark on them (unlike slides) to underscore a point during a presentation. The lights can be on full or almost full. Transparencies can be rearranged for use in several presentations.

Like flipcharts and 35 mm slides, though, transparencies do have some disadvantages. Plain paper copiers do not reproduce photographs well on transparencies; commercial copy centers may provide better results.[5] Also, like the slide projector, the transparency projector can be noisy.

Follow these guidelines when creating transparencies:

- Follow the guidelines for flipcharts and slides:
  - — Limit the concept to one per transparency.
  - — Use bullets to keep the number of words low.
  - — Use symbols, icons, and graphics to transform an idea into a picture that the audience will remember.
- Decide on a horizontal (preferred) or vertical format.
- Maintain a style for capitalization and punctuation.
- Just as you would never use handwritten handouts, never use handwritten transparencies.
- Test for legibility. A quick way to test legibility is to put the transparency on the floor and try to read it while standing on a chair. If it can be read, it will be legible when shown. Typewriter type — even

"Orator" or similar typewriter type — will rarely pass this test. As a general rule, the main text should be in 30- to 36-point type. Lesser text can be in 18- to 24-point type.

- Use overlays and colored markers to add color and to highlight especially important information.
- Explore using a commercial software package to generate transparencies. Several excellent packages provide a choice of borders, font, and art.

CONCLUSION

Fire and life safety educators rely on their educational materials a great deal. The materials literally give shape and color to the information and skills that the educators teach.

Materials are also important from the standpoint of resources. Next to the educator's time, materials are the most expensive item in the public educator's budget.

For these reasons, fire and life safety educators should take special care in selecting or creating their materials. Recognizing that educational materials are tools (rather than a program) and matching the material to the educational objective and to the audience are the keys to selecting and using educational materials.

Chapter 15 Notes

1. These bumper stickers are available from the National Fire Sprinkler Association, 4 Robin Hill Corporate Park, Patterson, New York 12563, Telephone: (914) 878-4200.

2. For a good discussion of the differences between purposes of materials, see "Unit 5: Applying Analysis Skills to Educational Methods and Materials," *Instructor Guide for Developing Fire and Life Safety Strategies*, National Fire Academy.

3. *The Practical Criteria and Instruments* document is informally known as "The Stillwater Standard." The package is available from the Pan-Educational Institute, 10922 Winner Road, P.O. Box 520347, Independence, MO 64052; telephone 816-461-0201; fax 816-461-0210.

4. Gary Pretsfelder, Ed.M., for the Learn Not to Burn® Foundation, December 1990.

5. The technology for reproducing photographs onto transparencies is improving. However, the quality of the reproduction is poor: The images are often not very clear, and the color is faded. The technology is still more expensive than slides or text transparencies. When deciding to use photographs on transparencies, it is recommended that only one or two be done initially to test the quality.

Chapter 15 Review

Directions

The following activities are designed to help you comprehend and apply the information in Chapter 15 of **Fire and Life Safety Educator**, second edition. To receive the maximum learning experience from these activities, it is recommended that you use the following procedure:

1. Read the chapter, underlining or highlighting important terms, topics, and subject matter. Read the sidebar material, study the photographs and illustrations, and read the captions with each.
2. Review the list of vocabulary words to ensure that you know the chapter-related meaning of each. If you are unsure of the meaning of a vocabulary word, look up the word in the glossary or a dictionary, and then study its context in the chapter.
3. On a separate sheet of paper, complete all assigned or selected application and review activities before checking your answers.
4. After you have finished, check your answers against those on the pages referenced in parentheses.
5. Correct any incorrect answers, and review material that was answered incorrectly.

Vocabulary

Be sure that you know the chapter-related meanings of the following words:

- [print] character *(284)*
- consumables *(277)*
- font *(283)*
- [print] justified *(283)*
- pica *(284)*
- [print] point *(284)*
- ragged *(284)*
- typeface *(283)*

Application of Knowledge

1. Choose an educational material from the **Fire and Life Safety Educator Resource Kit** or from your own department. Perform a qualitative evaluation of the materials by asking and answering the questions on page *278*. If any of the questions receive a "no" answer, explain what you would do to make that aspect of the material meet "yes" qualifications.
2. Obtain a copy of *Practical Criteria and Instruments for Selecting and Implementing Sound Fire and Burn Education Programs in School and Community*. Complete the work sheets to qualitatively assess two educational materials used in your department.
3. Analyze the readability of a single 100-word passage in one of your department's educational materials. Apply the passive sentence test, the Flesch Reading Ease and Grade Level evaluation, and the Gunning FOG Index. Compare your results.
4. Write five passive and five active voice sentences.

Review Activities

1. Distinguish among *awareness materials*, *informational materials*, and *educational materials* used by the fire and life safety educator. *(275, 276)*
2. Explain the need for educational materials. *(277)*
3. Briefly explain the three different kinds of educational materials. *(276, 277)*
4. List questions that the fire and life safety educator should ask before using a prop as a teaching aid. *(277)*
5. Distinguish between qualitative and quantitative evaluation techniques. *(278)*
6. Provide several specific examples of qualitative and quantitative evaluation techniques. *(278)*
7. Explain the materials evaluation system outlined in *Practical Criteria and Instruments for Selecting and Implementing Sound Fire and Burn Education Programs in School and Community*. *(279)*
8. List the general guidelines that the fire and life safety educator should use when checking the readability of print materials. *(297, 280)*
9. Explain the purposes of preproduction testing of fire and life safety educational materials. *(281)*

10. Compile a list of guidelines for designing fire and life safety educational print materials. Include information on page design, font selection, point size, line length, justification, and readability. *(282, 283)*

11. State the four purposes of illustrations in written materials. *(285)*

12. State two improper reasons for using illustrations or photographs in fire and life safety educational materials. *(285)*

13. State the rule of thumb for white space on pages of printed materials. *(285)*

14. Discuss the considerations facing the fire and life safety educator when choosing paper and ink for educational materials. *(286)*

15. Discuss the advantages of flipcharts, transparencies, and slides. *(288)*

16. List guidelines for creating each of the following fire and life safety educational materials:
    - flipcharts *(287)*
    - 35 mm slides *(289)*
    - transparencies *(290)*

17. Identify the following items:
    - active sentence *(279)*
    - passive sentence *(279)*
    - flipchart *(287)*
    - flyer *(277)*
    - full-color *(287)*
    - grid *(285)*
    - justified *(284)*
    - KISS *(283)*
    - overhead *(277)*
    - overlay *(291)*
    - promotional materials *(276)*
    - props *(277)*
    - serif/sans serif font *(284)*
    - simulator *(277)*
    - white space *(285)*

Questions and Notes

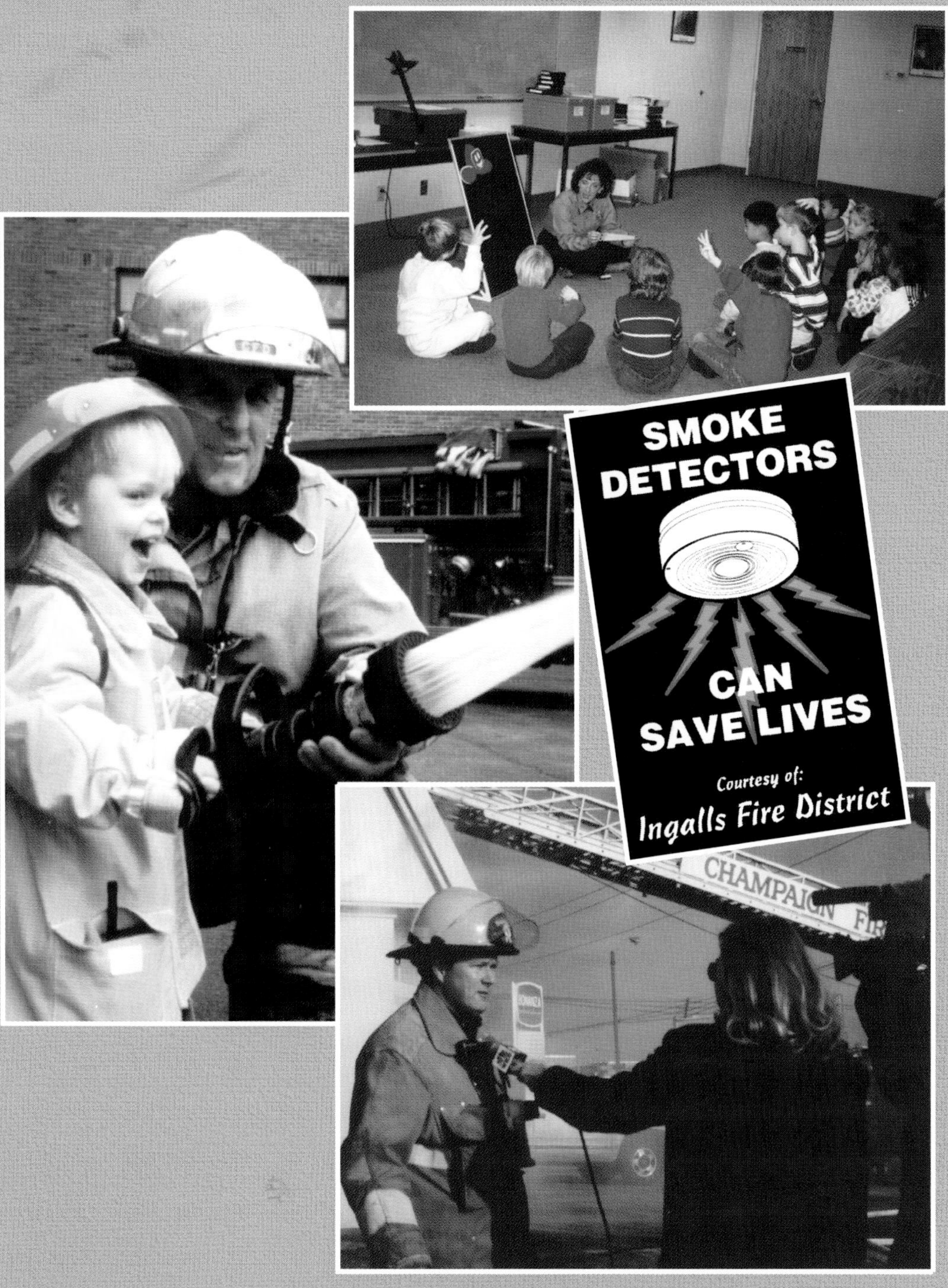
SMOKE
DETECTORS
CAN
SAVE LIVES
Courtesy of:
Ingalls Fire District
CHAMPAIGN

16 Working With the Media

LEARNING OBJECTIVES

This chapter provides information that addresses the following objectives of NFPA 1035, *Standard for Professional Qualifications for Public Fire and Life Safety Educator* (1993 edition):

Public Fire and Life Safety Educator I

3-4.4 Notify the public, given a scheduled event, so that the location, date, time, topic, and sponsoring agency are included.

3-4.4.1 *Prerequisite Knowledge:* Local media resources.

3-4.4.2 *Prerequisite Skills:* Written and oral communication.

3-4.5 Distribute educational information, given material, specified audience, and time frame, so that information reaches the audience within the specified time.

3-4.5.1 *Prerequisite Knowledge:* Legal requirements for the distribution and posting of materials.

Chapter 16
Working With the Media

INTRODUCTION

Mentioning the word *media* in the fire station brings about mixed reactions. Today, the department chief delights in the positive impression caused by a particularly complimentary news article and so thinks highly of the media. Yesterday, however, the fire and life safety educator thought poorly of the media after being misquoted by a reporter at the scene of a fire. Similarly, a signboard with fire safety tips may receive much positive attention from community members (Figure 16.1), yet a feature article on the money needed for a station-relocation project may rile citizens into protesting the action. There is no question that the media plays a powerful role in today's society.

This chapter introduces the fire and life safety educator to today's media resources. The chapter helps the educator understand what makes news, discusses how various media fit the needs of the fire service as well as the needs of other injury prevention agencies, explains how to match the medium with the message, and details how and why the fire and life safety educator must work at building communication bridges within the department and across the community. Covered also are techniques for working with reporters at an emergency scene as compared with providing fire facts for a feature story to be run later. Legal issues such as the Freedom of Information Act and Sunshine Laws are addressed. And, finally, the chapter explains where publicity, promotions, and public relations fit into the picture and suggests ways that fire and life safety educators can provide pertinent promotional information to the public.

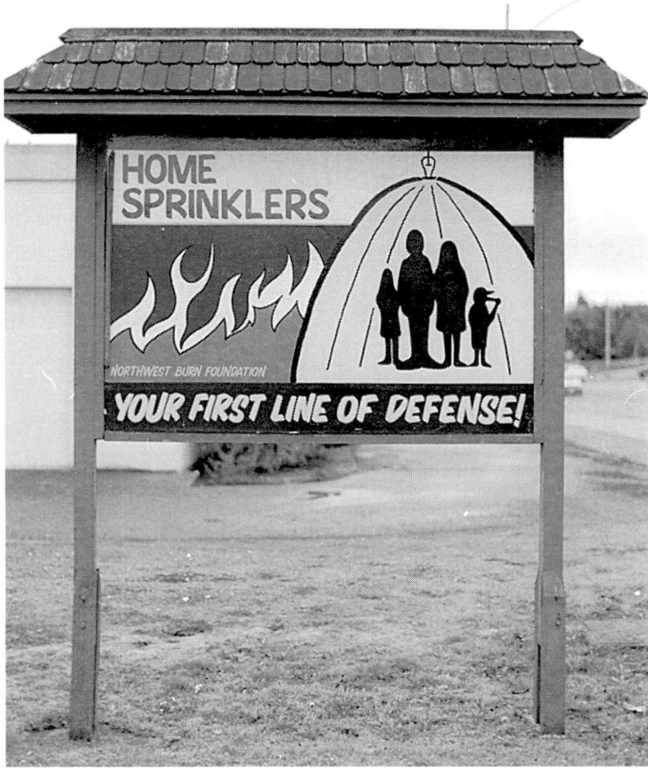
HOME
SPRINKLERS
NORTHWEST BURN FOUNDATION
YOUR FIRST LINE OF DEFENSE!

Figure 16.1 Fire and life safety educators want to receive community attention through positive means such as this signboard. *Courtesy of the City of Bremerton (WA) Fire Department.*

DEFINING MEDIA AND COMMUNICATIONS

Communication, as defined in Chapter 14, "Applying Fire and Life Safety Educational Theory," is the ongoing process that educators and their audiences use to complete the exchange of information and attitudes about fire and life safety. For the purposes of this chapter, it can be defined further as *the exchange of ideas and information that conveys an intended meaning in a form that is understood* (Figure 16.2). It is the process by which individuals interact to impart knowledge and to influence each other.[1] The

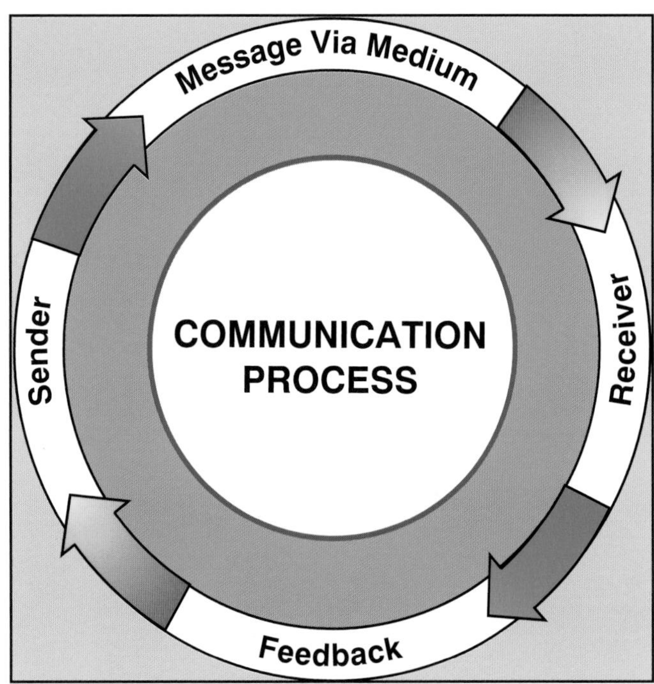

Figure 16.2 The components of communication.

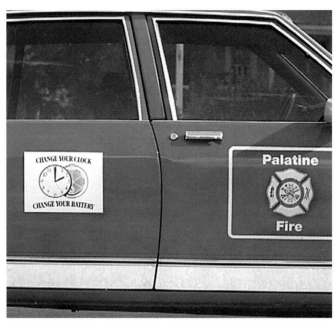

Figure 16.3 Having signs on the sides of fire department vehicles is one of many ways of communicating fire safety messages. *Courtesy of Palatine (IL) Fire Department.*

ideas or information that people exchange is often called the *message*. The channel or system that a person uses to communicate the message is called the *medium* (plural *media*). (**NOTE**: Today, the term *media* is used commonly as a collective noun referring to "the mass media.")

Humankind's earliest communication medium was probably facial gestures (smile, frown, raised eyebrows, or bared teeth). Facial gestures were eventually incorporated into spoken language. Then the medium of visual communication through representational art evolved, and last of all, humankind devised a system of written language. Presently, there are a great many media through which people communicate: conversation, role-play, dramatizations, facial gestures and hand and body movements, song, dance, movies, letters, posters, books, pamphlets, billboards, computers, radios, televisions, newspapers, and magazines, to name a few. Today, we even use our clothes and vehicles as media to communicate both written and visual messages (Figure 16.3).

Mass media are publications, broadcasts, and visuals that are designed to reach large numbers of individuals[2] and usually carry advertising. The mass media was born thousands of years ago with the representational art of the first crude cave drawings. Prior to this, humans transmitted all messages face-to-face through gestures and language. They could reach only those within seeing and hearing distance. They could communicate effectively only with those who spoke their same language. Once their face-to-face messages had been transmitted, these messages were lost forever — except through the imperfect recall ability of human memory. With representational drawings, however, the sender of the message

Computers, a New Mass Medium?

Generally, when a person refers to "the" media, he or she is referring to one of the four primary mass media: newspapers, television, radio, or magazines. However, computers — particularly with the advent of Internet — are rapidly moving into position to serve as a prime mass medium (Figure 16.4). Computers allow audience interaction and provide instant feedback. Messages can be geared to our senses of sound and sight. These messages incorporate realistic simulations, video clips, calendars, bulletin boards, music, cartoons, etc.

Like the television and VCR, the computer has joined the ranks of standard household appliances. It is reasonable to think that in the near future, educators will rely on electronic mail rather than on the exchange of telephone and hard copy messages when communicating news stories and information to the media. It is time for fire and life safety educators to determine how this medium will enhance the delivery of fire and life safety messages.

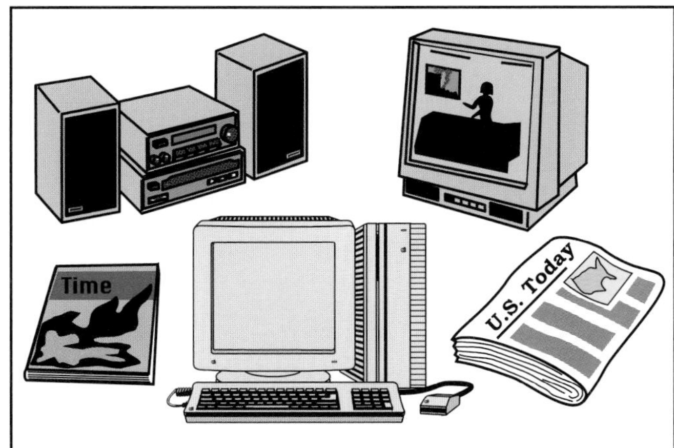

Figure 16.4 Along with the four primary mass media, the computer is also rapidly becoming a prime mass medium.

did not need to be present for a message to be transmitted. Further, messages could be received by numerous others over long periods of time — even after the sender was dead. This ability to communicate with the masses is most evident today in the four primary mass media worldwide: newspapers, television, radio, and magazines.

Using one or another of the mass media to communicate a message is not as simple as it would appear. Communication is much more than sharing an idea with another person or persons. Effective communication does not take place unless the receiver of the message provides the sender with appropriate *feedback* (a response that demonstrates understanding) (Figure 16.5). It is one thing for the fire and life safety educator to know what information must be provided to the public. It is a totally different matter to elicit appropriate feedback — to have the public receive, understand, and then act upon that information.[3]

Children's Television Network conducted a study on how television could be used to teach fire safety to preschoolers. The study found some safety messages inappropriate for television broadcast for preschoolers.

Notorious imitators, young children hold a limited understanding of the world around them. Television, being an impersonal mass medium, sends the same message to millions — with no opportunity for feedback. Feedback is necessary to ensure that the children are indeed receiving

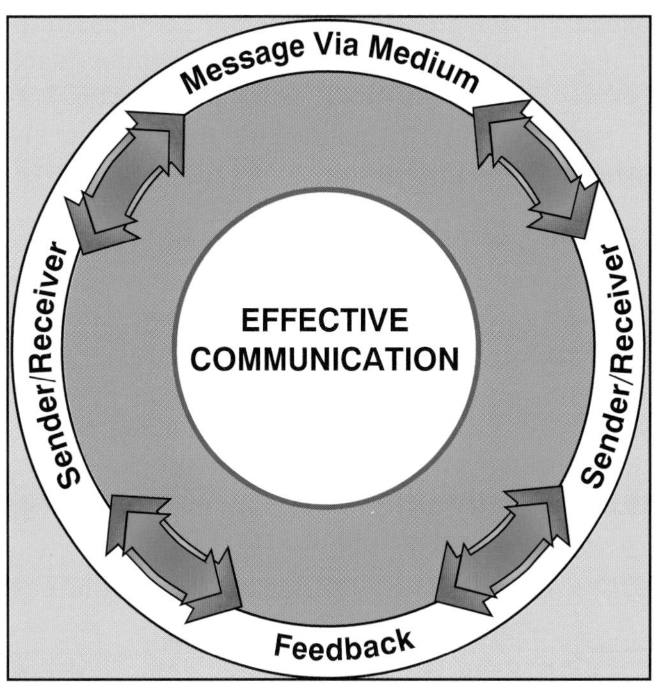

Figure 16.5 Communication is accomplished when the receiver confirms that the intended message has been received.

the message that the sender intended. If the verbal message sent is "Don't touch electrical outlets; you can be hurt," but a picture of someone touching the outlet is shown, then there is a good chance that the child will imitate what he or she sees rather than the voice-over of what he or she hears. Children are great imitators.

Among the messages *inappropriate for television* because they required an adult to ensure that the child received the correct fire safety messages were the following:

- Matches are for grown-ups.
- Put a burn in cool water.
- Stop, drop, and roll if your clothes catch fire.
- Crawl low under smoke.

Poorly planned education and publicity campaigns may rely on media to get the message out but neglect to build feedback into the process. Today, fire and life safety educators are rejecting this one-way model in favor of more interactive views of communication. One example, the "co-active" approach explained by Professor James F. Evans of the University of Illinois in his course "Education Campaign Planning," treats communication an as "interaction among participants, an exchange in which each participant brings something vital to the process. Each is a sender. Each is a receiver. The message flows back and forth as participants figuratively move toward one another in communication."[4]

UNDERSTANDING WHAT MAKES NEWS

Patricia Calvert, editor of *The Communicator's Handbook: Techniques and Technologies*, defines news as "any piece of information that will affect your head, heart or pocketbook."[5] Obviously, news is also a report of something new. News editors decide whether or not information provided them is indeed newsworthy by looking at several news values or news pegs (Figure 16.6):

- **Timeliness** — Is the story immediate or near the present?
- **Proximity** — How close is the information physically or psychologically to the audience? (Local news is preferred.)
- **Conflict** — Are there opposing sides?
- **Progress** — Has an operational change occurred because of this event?
- **Consequence** — How significant or important is the idea, event, situation, or person? What impact will this have?
- **Uniqueness** — Is the story rare, odd, unusual, or bizarre?
- **Human interest** — Does the story possess ideas, events, or situations that touch human emotions?[6]

At least three-fourths of all news stories fall into the general categories of consequence (impact, importance, significance), uniqueness (unusual, strange, bizarre), or human interest (touches human emotions).[7]

News editors also categorize news by its urgency. In this system, news falls into one of two categories: hard news or soft news. *Hard news* is news that has a time value.[8] It must be delivered immediately, or it becomes stale and is no longer newsworthy. Hard news may be considered news today but may not be news at all tomorrow. Most hard news hangs on the "consequence" news peg. Fires and emergency disasters fall under the category of hard news (Figure 16.7).

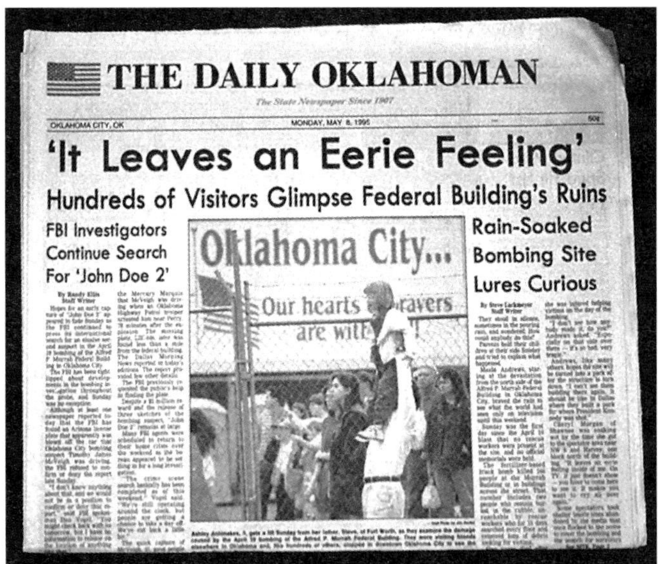

THE DAILY OKLAHOMAN

OKLAHOMA CITY, OK — MONDAY, MAY 8, 1995

'It Leaves an Eerie Feeling'

Hundreds of Visitors Glimpse Federal Building's Ruins

FBI Investigators Continue Search For 'John Doe 2'

Rain-Soaked Bombing Site Lures Curious

Figure 16.6 Whether or not information is deemed newsworthy is determined by its value to the reader.

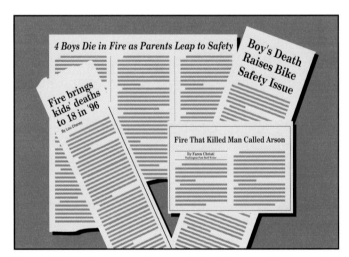

Figure 16.7 Hard news may be news today but may not be news at all tomorrow.

Just because the situation does not fit the *emergency* model does not mean that the story is not newsworthy. Unlike hard news, soft news has little urgency. *Soft news* is news that can be printed or broadcast today, tomorrow, or next week. It does not have to be delivered on a particular day. Most soft news hangs on the "human interest" news peg. (Figure 16.8). Maybe a 35-year veteran of the department is retiring. Perhaps an Eagle Scout has completed his project by building a garage to house the department's robotic fire truck. Perhaps a new life safety program is being introduced in a local school.

The fire and life safety educator must also remember that news is relative. Every day a

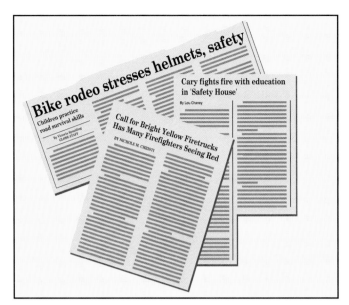

Figure 16.8 Soft news can be printed or broadcast today, tomorrow, or next week.

different set of dynamics defines the news. These may include the volume of hard news, advertising pressures, the type of medium (newspaper, television, radio, etc.), and the medium's audience.

The fire and life safety educator creates a lot of newsworthy information. The big four mass media — television, radio, newspaper, magazines — are often interested in the news that the public fire and life safety educator can provide, especially if that news is formatted according to the particular medium's standard guidelines. These media cannot afford to have reporters at every door. Educators may serve as eyes and ears for the reporters, and the medium may serve as the voice.

So, in that pile of work for the week — aside from tours and community education programs — the fire and life safety educator has several opportunities to create newsworthy stories to communicate with the community. For example, in a single week, the public fire and life safety educator may let the community know about upcoming activities for Fire Prevention Week, may provide statistics showing an increase in drowning accidents, may send the daily fire-calls log to the local newspaper, and may deal with an emergency hazardous material spill or other emergency incident that occurs in the area.

While most local fire service stories lack the inherent hard news value of national events, there is generally ample community interest in the information to warrant sharing it. Therefore, many of these soft news stories are broadcast or printed locally. Local media and the community at large are usually interested in meetings, rallies, seminars, open houses, and educational activities such as public education programs and statistics. Public statements on local affairs, awards given and received, fund drives, calls for membership, promotions, new equipment acquisitions, and the appointment or resignation of local officials also generate considerable community interest. Announcements of the availability of speakers whose services are free, films for loan, and the findings of department reports and surveys all have community news value. The trick is letting the media know — in their terms — how the message or story can fit into their plan. The educator should find the *media's* news values in the *department's* story and use those as the news pegs on which to hang the story and sell the reporter. One fire and life safety educator reports that he keeps soft news stories prepared and available for "slow news days" — those days when the media is looking for stories to fill up a page or round out a broadcast.

WORKING WITH THE MEDIA TO DELIVER FIRE AND LIFE SAFETY EDUCATION MESSAGES

Fire and life safety educators must view their local media as partners. This takes an understanding of each medium's mission, as well as its guidelines. The educator must then possess the ability to fit fire service information into those media-dictated guidelines. To be able to deliver a wide variety of educational and publicity messages to different audiences, the educator must be able to work with a number of different local media.

There are several ways that educators can work with the media to deliver fire and life safety education messages. To lay the groundwork, the educator needs to be able to do the following:

- Know the community's media services.
- Build the department's reputation with the media.
- Identify key players.
- Match the medium to the message.

Knowing the Community's Media Services

In order to create a working relationship with the media, the educator must take time to understand the responsibilities and target audiences for each local mass medium. Each radio station, each television channel, and each newspaper has a particular audience and a particular area that it claims as listeners, viewers, or readers. The media in the area should be able to provide the educator with a good overview of those audiences they consider their own. A hazy notion of exactly who these media's audiences are may ease the fire and life safety educator's job, but this lack of knowledge will complicate all other parts of that process and may result in watered-down messages, weak delivery systems, and frustration with the way the message is delivered to the public. A hazy notion of audience also adds waste and clutter by forcing would-be communicators to fling messages at persons who have no need for them or interest in them.[9]

Only by knowing the community's media can the educator learn what the various media will cover in the way of stories, announcements, and news items (Figure 16.9). In addition to knowing local media audiences, the educator who wishes to use the local media to communicate fire and life safety messages to the community at large must also become thoroughly familiar with the format and preferences of each medium in the area. Generating media coverage requires that educators develop a reporter's sense of newsworthiness. Educators must be able to identify the news value of the message or story that they want the media to cover. If the educator can identify the headline, tell how the story affects the community, or tell what sets the story apart from the other 45 stories the news editor has to review or assign, then the educator improves the chances of getting the story aired, viewed, or printed.

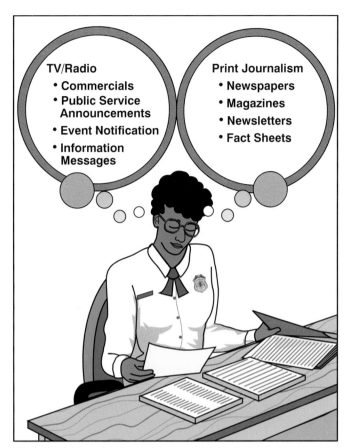

Figure 16.9 The educator must learn which media to use and must be familiar with the format that the various media use to cover stories, announcements, and news items.

Building the Department's Reputation With the Media

Building the department's reputation with the media is critical. After meeting with the fire and life safety educator the first few times, reporters, editors, and program directors form opinions about the educator's operating style. They look to see whether the educator can provide what they need. They want to know that the educator will give them accurate facts. They want to know that educators will keep their promises — that they will call back when they say, that they can be depended upon to provide all the details necessary for reporters to write the stories they are researching, and — especially — that they will consistently meet deadlines.

Deadlines are critical in the business of broadcasting and journalism. In professional communicators' minds, submitting complete and accurate stories on time is as critical as it is for firefighters to arrive on the fire scene within the first few minutes. It is inexcusable to be late. Reporters run a fast-paced, competitive, and deadline-driven business. Does that sound familiar?

Identifying Key Players

To get fire and life safety messages to the media, the educator must also identify the key players at the local newspapers, television stations, and radio stations (Figure 16.10). What are their names? their titles? What are their usual working hours? What specifically does each of them do? What are their specialty areas? When are their daily deadlines? When are they most receptive to calls? to submittals? How do they prefer information be transmitted to them — by fax? computer? hard copy? telephone?

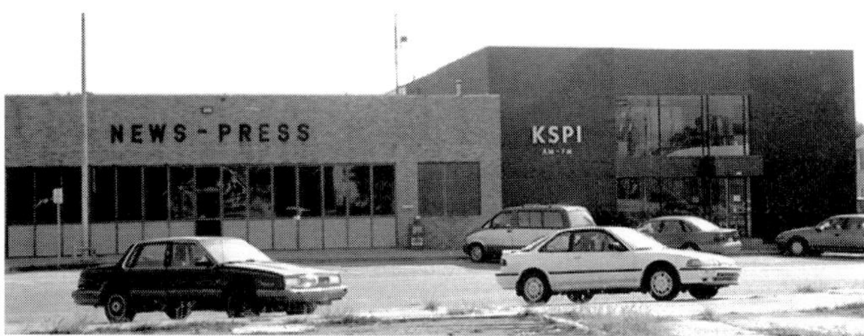

Figure 16.10 In order to receive needed media support, the educator must become very familiar with the people at the local newspapers, television stations, and radio stations.

Not now. . .I'm busy!

Take the time to find out exactly what time each local medium will be rushing to meet its daily print or broadcast deadlines. Whether you are contacting radio, television, or newspaper, *avoid approaching media personnel near these deadline times*. For television, avoid the hour just before a news show. If the radio station has an hourly news program, the best time to talk with the news director would be just after the show. Do not call newspaper editors or submit releases in person during the time when personnel are frantically rushing to "put the paper to bed."

If educators expect reporters to understand their roles as fire service information resources, then they, too, must make an effort to understand the job duties and roles of various media positions. This is only common courtesy and respect for another's profession. The more effort an educator puts into communicating — sharing information — the more understanding that takes place, and the more effectively communication efforts are met. The fire and life safety educator should make every effort to become acquainted with at least one area reporter, editor, and station manager at each of the local mass media. The educator should get to know these persons, not necessarily as friends, but as professional colleagues. The educator should talk with these contacts face-to-face. In this way the educator has "inside" contacts (key players) to whom news items and public service announcements can be sent directly.

Maintaining these important contacts is an ongoing process and one not easily accomplished. Turnover in the media is high. Often, just when the educator becomes familiar with one reporter, editor, photographer, or manager, that person moves away or assumes different responsibilities, and a new person takes his or her place.

Fire and life safety educators can heed the following guidelines to identify and maintain contact with important local media personnel:

- **Make a list of local media**. Try not to limit the list to big city dailies and prime broadcasters. Balance the media list to include neighborhood, ethnic, and suburban media, as well as urban ones. Public fire and life safety educators in rural areas should also make a list of their media resources.
- **Read the newspapers on the media list**. Study mastheads, bylines, and photo credits. Find out and write down the names, titles, phone numbers, and fax numbers of those reporters, editors, and photographers who seem most skilled and who would be most helpful as contacts.
- **Listen to and watch the radio and television stations on the media list**. Become familiar with each station's programs and schedules. Study the various types and times of broadcasts to determine which would best serve your needs. Find out and write down the names, titles, phone numbers, fax numbers, and E-mail addresses of the people in charge — the station managers, program directors, and broadcasters (Figure 16.11).
- **Create a flowchart for each organization listed on the media list** so that you will know whom to call for a variety of situations.
- **Talk with your contacts**. Know exactly who they consider their target audiences to be.

Media File Aid							
Station	**Channel/ Affiliate**	**PSAs**	**Public Affairs**	**News**	**Contacts**	**Telephone Number**	**Fax**
WDQP	6/CBS	10, 30 sec	Community Calendar	6 a.m.	Henry Rohl, News		
			Speak Out	12 p.m.	Sue May, Public Affairs		

Figure 16.11 A media file aid can assist the educator in maintaining important information concerning radio and television stations.

- **Talk to other public educators and other public relations personnel in the community**. Who are *their* contacts?
- **Browse through the Yellow Pages** of the telephone directory.
- **Look at media directories**. If a media directory is unavailable, check the local library for a regional directory. One such directory, *Gale Directory of Publications and Broadcast Media*, provides a wealth of information. This annual guide to publications and broadcasting stations includes newspapers, magazines, journals, radio stations, television stations, and cable systems. It provides names of people in charge, telephone numbers, and audience numbers.

Once fire and life safety educators have identified key local media personnel, they may want to assemble a media kit to introduce themselves and to help key media players know them and their organization better. Media kits (packets of information about the educator's own organization) may be sent out for a variety of reasons. They are useful when the educator first meets the media and may be useful later to jog the contact's memory when the educator wants a special activity publicized.

Matching the Medium With the Message

How do I know which medium I should choose to send my message? This is a common question. The answer depends very much on what is needed at the time. In terms of media, each has its own

Assembling a Media Kit

Media kits help key media players get to know you and your organization. When assembling the kit, be well aware of its color, layout, and design. The unwritten messages sent are often far more revealing than the actual written words. For instance, if you are a nonprofit organization urging the media and the public to support a fund-raiser and your media kit is slick, slick, slick, then the message sent is that you already have enough money to spend. On the other hand, if you send out a poorly written or sloppily edited release, the message sent may be that you are not worth the organization's time or energy.

Based on their initial impressions of your first media kit, reporters, producers, and editors will decide whether your request for space or time should receive serious consideration. Include a document in the kit *only* when a specific purpose is served. Not every document listed below needs to be in every media kit. Use professional judgment.

Media release — The media release should provide an overview of your service, the event, and its significance to the public. Keep it to a single sheet announcing the event. Use a strong opening sentence or *lead* to capture the attention of the editor or producer.

Event schedule — Send a schedule on a separate page when handling a complex event with a variety of activities occurring over a period of time — such as Fire Prevention Week activities. Time restrictions must always be considered when dealing with the media. Reporters appreciate notes that warn of special circumstances. For example:

Fire chief due to cut ribbon at 10:05

(He's off to another meeting at 10:15)

The parenthetical note signals reporters that they have available only ten minutes to cover the chief's appearance.

Fact sheet — Use this component to explain in more detail the significant points of your service. Highlight the aspects that set your department or activity apart from similar services. Perhaps the city has had a significant decrease in injuries to senior citizens receiving hot-liquid burns. This decrease can be attributed to a new program presented by the department. Share the local as well as county, regional, state, and national statistics pertinent to the point being made.

Photograph — Include photographs in the media kit, but remember: A picture is worth a thousand words — only if it is high-quality and in focus.

Previous articles — Perhaps include one or two recent articles written about the department. The information must be relevant to your current activity. Avoid, at all costs, sending a very recent article featuring your story but written by a competitor.

Biography — The biography should be a briskly written one-page document that weaves facts about your education and background into a scenario centered on the chosen topic.

Briefing or background sheet — Use this sheet to explain any information sent in the kit. This information may also be combined with the biography.

unique features that make it the best in a given situation. Basically, all communication channels have distinguishing features, each situation is different, and each requires a fresh look.[10]

RADIO

Radio is the medium of the mind.[11] It is cost-effective, and it is local. According to the Arbitron radio rating service, over 95 percent of all people 12 years and older listen to radio at least once a week, and two out of three listeners tune in to FM stations.[12] People like radio because it is an intimate medium. It is far less intrusive than television and requires less concentration than the newspaper. People also like radio because it is portable. It can be listened to while doing almost anything else (Figure 16.12).

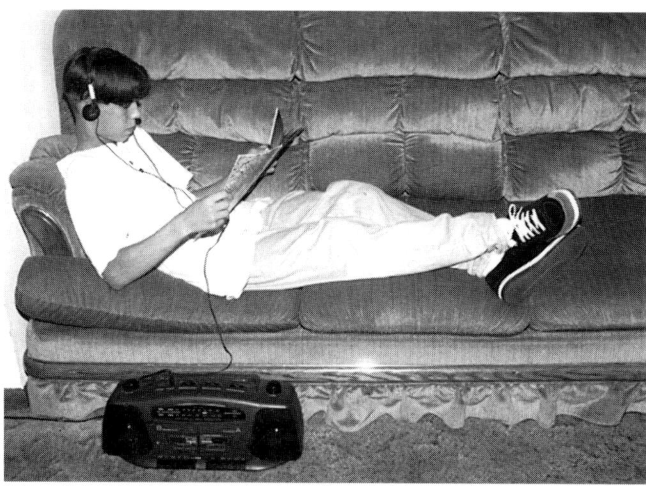

Figure 16.12 Radio messages reach audiences of all ages.

Writing radio PSAs. For the public fire and life safety educator, radio works best when used to notify, remind, or tell uncomplicated messages, such as brief public service announcements (PSAs), that are easily remembered. A listener cannot fold up a radio program and take it along to other places; therefore, radio messages must be simple and to the point. Broadcasters appreciate 60-, 30-, even 20-second messages, sprinkled with a few 90-second, "in-depth" items. Eight to nine typed lines of information will equal about 30 seconds of airtime.

Radio Public Service Announcements

[10-Second Announcement]

Don't let electricity in the bathroom shock you. Keep electrical appliances away from wet floors and counters, and put your home *On the Safety Circuit.* This message from your local fire department and the United States Fire Administration.

[30-Second Announcement]

Most fatal fires take place at night, when you and your family are asleep — when seconds can make the difference between life and death. Are you protected? If you have one or more working smoke detectors in your home, you double your chances of surviving a fire! That's protection! And smoke detectors are inexpensive and easy to install. Smoke detectors — they're real protectors. A message from this station and your local fire department.

[60-Second Announcement]

When was the last time you tested your smoke detector?...or changed the battery in your smoke detector? Did you know that most fatal fires occur at night, when you and your family are asleep — when seconds can mean the difference between life and death? Smoke detectors double your chances of surviving a fire. But, like any other home appliance, they must be properly maintained. Smoke detectors should be checked monthly — by depressing the alarm's test button or lighting a candle and fanning the smoke under the detector. Also, the battery should be changed at least once a year. Pick a day — your birthday, perhaps — and mark your calendar. And remember, never disconnect the battery if it sounds off from cooking smoke or the fireplace. Instead, simply fan the smoke away from the detector and the alarm will stop. Smoke detectors — they're real protectors. A message from this station and your local fire department.

(**NOTE**: See Appendix B, "Public Service Announcements," for more PSAs.)

Generally there are two types of public service announcements that a radio or television station receives. The first is an event notification — open house, prevention activity, retirement receptions, safety house time schedules, etc. The second type of public service announcement includes the informational reminders that fire and life safety educators want people to remember — smoke detector testing, carbon monoxide dangers, and hot liquid burns. Each station handles the copy a bit differently. Check with the local stations to see whether they prefer live copy or written copy that they can edit and change to meet their needs.

Radio station organization. The size of a radio station usually dictates the title of the person whom the fire and life safety educator contacts. In the radio broadcast business, the station manager (general manager) is the person in charge of all operations. Frequently, at smaller stations, the station manager will be the owner, the program director, and the chief engineer all rolled into one. Therefore, at small radio stations, the fire and life safety educator's contact generally is the station manager. At larger stations, however, the station manager may be too high on the organizational chart to use as a contact (Figure 16.13).[13] At these large stations, the fire and life safety educator would probably contact the program director. The program director is in charge of the station's news and sports. The program director may be the person with whom the fire and life safety educator works most frequently when using radio as the medium for fire and life safety messages.

TELEVISION

Statistics supporting the power of television continue to be impressive. In April 1994, the Roper Organization for Television Information Office reported that 72 percent of the U.S. population depends on television as its primary source of news. That is an increase of 7 percent in less than ten years.[14]

Additionally, a 1985 *Wall Street Journal* study found that daily the U.S. population spent varying amounts of time with the four primary mass media. However, they spent the greatest amount of time watching television — nearly twice as much time as they spent listening to the radio, and a whopping eight times more than they spent reading a newspaper[15]:

Television	252 minutes
Radio	124 minutes
Newspapers	31 minutes
Magazines	15 minutes

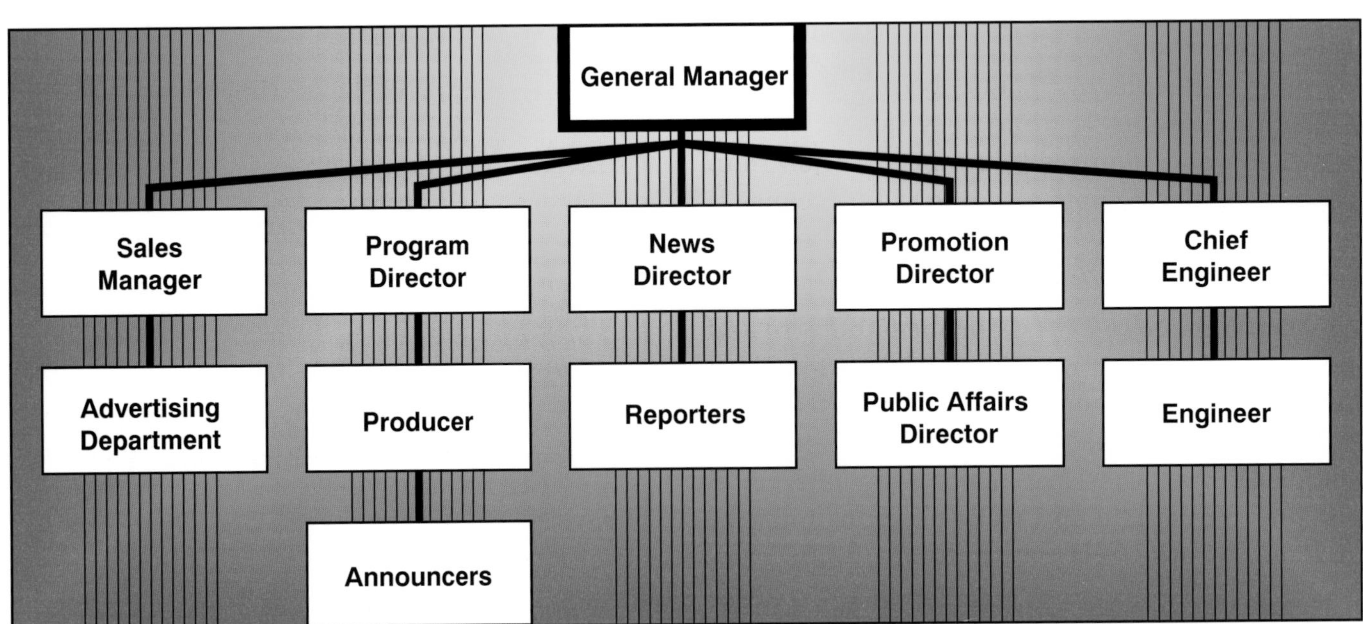

Figure 16.13 Understanding the organizational structure of the media can help the educator determine appropriate contacts for assistance. *From* Practical Publicity *by David Tedone. Published by The Harvard Common Press, 535 Albany Street, Boston, MA 02118. Used with permission.*

With the advent of cable and public access television, these television viewing minutes will continue to climb.

For all this television watching, television tends to be under-used for educational purposes. In the emerging information age, when the trend is to move "from institutional help to self-help," television and videotapes can be the fire and life safety educator's forum to reach millions of people in the places where they live, study, work, and play. The equipment is in place. The channels are open. The medium is available and waiting for educational fire and life safety messages.[16]

Knowing television delivery formats. Most often, fire department information on a nightly newscast focuses on emergency situations — a fire, a horrible wreck, or a child poisoned. Emergencies fill all the news pegs and are, thus, the prime format for television news programs. However, sharing fire department emergency information with television reporters is primarily the responsibility of the Public Information Officer (PIO) or his or her designee. (**NOTE**: The role of the PIO is discussed in more detail later in this chapter.)

What television formats are available to the fire and life safety educator? The format for delivering emergency news is only one of several television formats available for delivering fire and life safety messages. Other formats include public affairs programming, public service announcements (PSAs), and newscasts.

The same news pegs — newsworthiness values — that help determine the newsworthiness of emergency situation news also help educators format soft news so it will receive television attention. Perhaps the department just spent $20,000 on a fire safety house to teach the "crawl low under smoke to escape" concept. Citizens might appreciate learning of the tax expenditure. A simple fact sheet and picture sent to local television stations may jog an editor to send a reporter and camera operator to the new fire safety house to create a story for the nightly news.

The station's public affairs and public service directors are the first people to contact. These two contacts will keep the educator up to date on the format and procedures used for the station's public affairs programming. Often there is someone in the programming department who is in charge of working with the community. If the station does not have a public affairs director, the educator should establish several key contacts in the news department: the news director, who oversees the news staff and broadcast; the assignment editor, who ensures that major stories and beats are covered and assigns reporters to stories; the news producer, who determines what reports will be aired; and the reporters who may cover stories relevant to the educator's cause.

Know the area stations' formats, audiences, and needs *before* approaching with a plan to televise a story on or an aspect of a fire service education program. Careful analysis of the audience and the message is critical. Be sure to match the message with the medium *and* with the station's viewing audience.

As is readily recognized, television provides information in a visual, action-oriented way. Because of this, and in order to maximize a story's value for television, it is necessary to provide something interesting for the camera to show. Messages in which a person simply stands or sits before a camera and speaks to the audience are unproductive. In the industry, these types of poorly planned television or video messages are jokingly called "talking heads." Television editors appreciate movement and action. Fire and life safety educators should highlight the movement sections of the story idea provided or suggest ways in which action can be shown.

For nonemergency stories, advanced notification is critical. Television stations must schedule the use of a limited number of busy camera crews.

Fire and life safety educators who successfully arrange for television coverage must prepare for it. They should formulate concise answers to expected questions in advance. Television reporters generally work on a tight deadline and are often in a hurry. There is no time for groping words when the reporter arrives. If the educator's response is not short (1 to 15 seconds) and to the point, it will not be aired. There may be only 30 seconds to present the life safety message. Rule of thumb: Pare answers to essentials.

> **The Best Answer**
>
> *Question*: Why did the City help fund this safety house?
>
> *Inconcise answer* (ends up on the editing room floor): It took years for us to convince city officials that we needed the money. I had to go to every official personally and tell about those poor, sweet children. Then we formed a committee and met every week...
>
> *Concise answer*: Numbers speak for themselves. Practiced safety skills save lives. After one year of operating our safety skill trailer, our pretest and posttest skills show that the people who practice know what to do.

Even if the educator is unable to provide film, he or she can send written PSAs or fact sheets to television news editors and reporters to alert them to potential stories. If it is a timely matter, the editors may pick up on the idea and create a news story of their own. Then again, the ideas may not be used immediately. They may be tucked into the file for future reference — or they may never see the light of day. It is the chance the educator takes.

Many television stations provide talk shows or call-in formats to allow community members to share information. During these programs, fire and life safety educators may share information on a variety of topics: alerting citizens to hazardous wastes at home, educating parents on the dangers of hot-liquid burns, and teaching campus students about electrical fire safety.

In Oregon, Tualatin Valley Fire and Rescue produces professional-quality videos for a video library that is used by the media as well as by educators to train business and industry clients. The first titles in the lending library include *Fire Extinguisher Usage*, *Disaster Preparedness at the Work Place*, *Basic Emergency Medical Response*, and a Spanish version of *Smoke Detectors Save Lives*.

Another example of public affairs programming would be a two-minute spot on the noon news offering citizens a chance to talk about upcoming events. Perhaps the educator seizes that opportunity to highlight the department's juvenile firesetter program or to talk about bicycle safety. (**NOTE**: See Chapter 18, "Addressing Fire and Life Safety Behaviors and Special Topics," for more information on program topics.)

Another creative use of television aired in Maine. In the mid-1990s, *Operation Firebusters* aired on televisions throughout Portland, Maine, during Fire Prevention Week. Modeling an Oregon Firebusters program in use for nearly a decade and a half, Maine fire department personnel worked with a local CBS affiliate to implement its own program. The fire department distributed questionnaires to grade-school children, who took the questions home with instructions to listen for the answers on the evening news. In conjunction with the fire department, the station created five short educational film segments that ran on separate nights during Fire Prevention Week. At the end of the week, names of the children who answered all the questions correctly were placed in a drawing for prizes to include bicycles, toys, and clothing. All participants received a free meal from a local fast-food restaurant.

Public access television provides another excellent and inexpensive format for exposing the community to fire and life safety concerns. In the U.S., there are 2,000 public education or government-access channels that are either city-supported, member-based, or franchised through a cable company.

Creating television PSAs. The public service announcement (PSA) is another common type of educational format used on television (Figure 16.14). The Federal Communications Commission (FCC) defines a PSA as ". . . any announcement . . . for which no charge is made and which promotes programs, activities, or services of federal, state, or local governments . . . or the programs, activities, or services of non-profit organizations . . . and other announcements regarded as serving community interests."[17] Federal standards no longer require stations to provide a minimum amount of public affairs programming. However, some stations are required by city codes to provide airtime for public service programming and announcements.

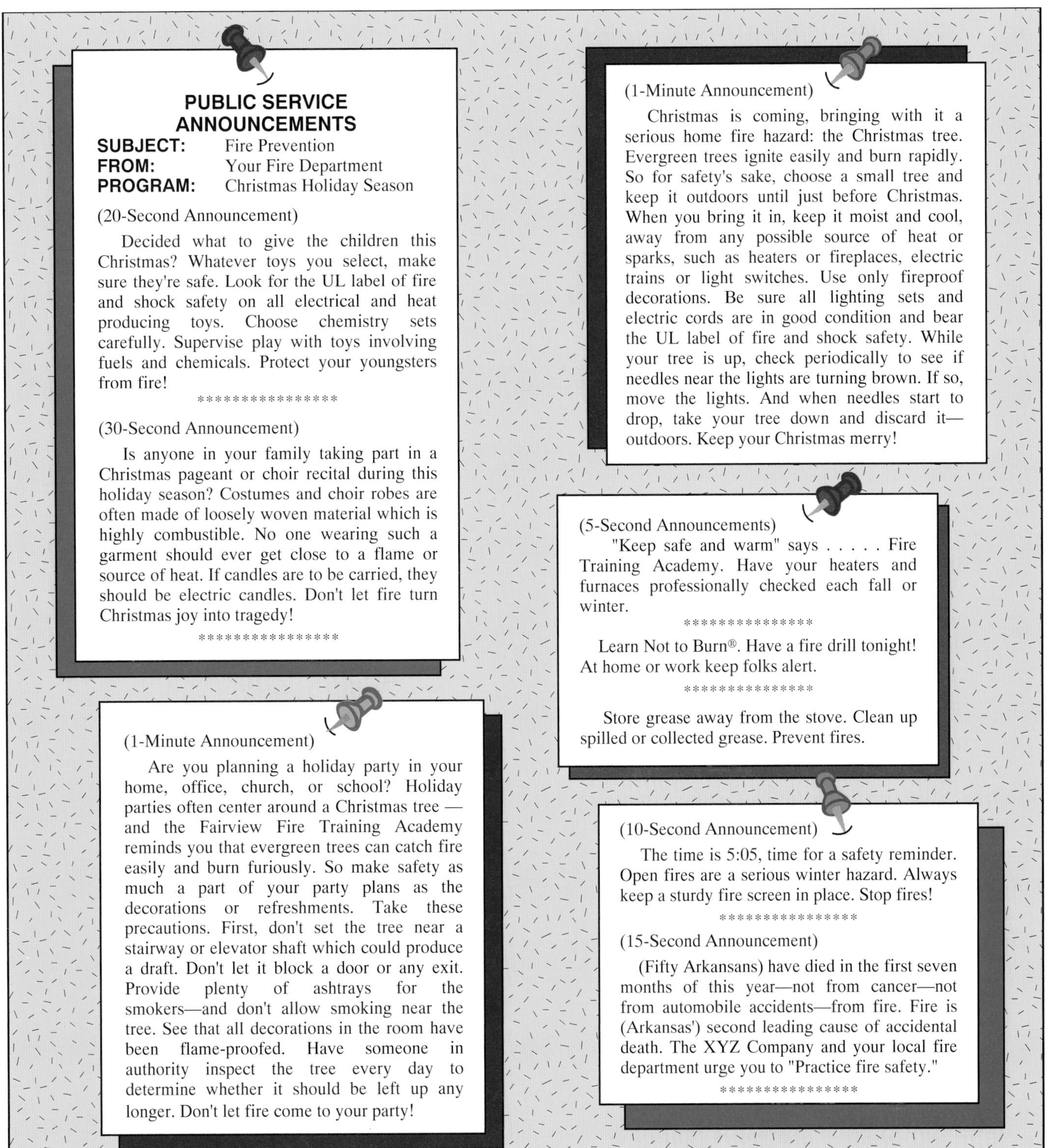

PUBLIC SERVICE ANNOUNCEMENTS

SUBJECT: Fire Prevention
FROM: Your Fire Department
PROGRAM: Christmas Holiday Season

(20-Second Announcement)

Decided what to give the children this Christmas? Whatever toys you select, make sure they're safe. Look for the UL label of fire and shock safety on all electrical and heat producing toys. Choose chemistry sets carefully. Supervise play with toys involving fuels and chemicals. Protect your youngsters from fire!

****

(30-Second Announcement)

Is anyone in your family taking part in a Christmas pageant or choir recital during this holiday season? Costumes and choir robes are often made of loosely woven material which is highly combustible. No one wearing such a garment should ever get close to a flame or source of heat. If candles are to be carried, they should be electric candles. Don't let fire turn Christmas joy into tragedy!

****

(1-Minute Announcement)

Are you planning a holiday party in your home, office, church, or school? Holiday parties often center around a Christmas tree — and the Fairview Fire Training Academy reminds you that evergreen trees can catch fire easily and burn furiously. So make safety as much a part of your party plans as the decorations or refreshments. Take these precautions. First, don't set the tree near a stairway or elevator shaft which could produce a draft. Don't let it block a door or any exit. Provide plenty of ashtrays for the smokers—and don't allow smoking near the tree. See that all decorations in the room have been flame-proofed. Have someone in authority inspect the tree every day to determine whether it should be left up any longer. Don't let fire come to your party!

(1-Minute Announcement)

Christmas is coming, bringing with it a serious home fire hazard: the Christmas tree. Evergreen trees ignite easily and burn rapidly. So for safety's sake, choose a small tree and keep it outdoors until just before Christmas. When you bring it in, keep it moist and cool, away from any possible source of heat or sparks, such as heaters or fireplaces, electric trains or light switches. Use only fireproof decorations. Be sure all lighting sets and electric cords are in good condition and bear the UL label of fire and shock safety. While your tree is up, check periodically to see if needles near the lights are turning brown. If so, move the lights. And when needles start to drop, take your tree down and discard it—outdoors. Keep your Christmas merry!

(5-Second Announcements)

"Keep safe and warm" says . . . . . Fire Training Academy. Have your heaters and furnaces professionally checked each fall or winter.

****

Learn Not to Burn®. Have a fire drill tonight! At home or work keep folks alert.

****

Store grease away from the stove. Clean up spilled or collected grease. Prevent fires.

(10-Second Announcement)

The time is 5:05, time for a safety reminder. Open fires are a serious winter hazard. Always keep a sturdy fire screen in place. Stop fires!

****

(15-Second Announcement)

(Fifty Arkansans) have died in the first seven months of this year—not from cancer—not from automobile accidents—from fire. Fire is (Arkansas') second leading cause of accidental death. The XYZ Company and your local fire department urge you to "Practice fire safety."

****

Figure 16.14 Typical public service announcements.

Across the nation, few departments are equipped to create their own television PSAs. Professional know-how, equipment, and much time and money must flow into creating quality television PSAs. Presently, few fire and life safety educators have the resources to create such educational aids. However, one easy way to provide professional-quality fire service PSAs is to provide the local television media with PSAs produced by reputable associations such as the National Safety Council, Learn Not to Burn® Foundation, and SAFE KIDS® Coalition. In the early 1980s, NFPA public service announcements starring Dick Van Dyke successfully showed positive ways to protect oneself from fires.

Another way of creating television PSAs is to hire freelance video professionals to help the department produce its own videos. This method often proves to be cost-prohibitive, however. PSA production also can be done on a volunteer or paid basis by television stations if a script or idea is provided. The educator might work with the person in charge of station public relations for the advertising sales staff. After checking on departmental and city policies, the educator might try working with station sales staff to find advertisers to pay for safety PSAs.

Those fire departments that are able to produce their own television PSAs are often innovative. For instance, in Illinois, the audiovisual department of the City of Springfield provides video services to the fire department. The city department creates 20- to 30-second spots using scripts the firefighters create. Fire personnel act in these productions and also help distribute the spots to be run on local television stations.

Creating television news releases. A *news release* is a short, factual description of an event or an issue. Fire and life safety educators may either write their own news releases, just as they would like them read on air, or they may provide the information in outline form and allow the television station's news director to craft the release. To write effective news releases that can be easily and quickly understood, educators should heed the following guidelines (Figure 16.15):

- Follow the K-I-S-S acronym: **K**eep **I**t **S**hort and **S**imple.
  - Use everyday language.
  - Write short sentences that follow the standard subject-verb-object pattern.
  - Use only one idea to a sentence.
- Use present tense and active verbs as often as possible. (For example, "Cynthia won the Fire and Life Safety Educator of the Year Award" *not* "The Fire and Life Safety Educator of the Year Award was won by Cynthia.")
- Round figures when possible (for example, change 788 to "nearly 800").
- Phonetically spell out names that are difficult to pronounce, and place in parentheses directly after the name (for example, Paul Walkiewiecz [Walk-a-wits]).
- Be sure to include all necessary reference information in each news release.
  - Writer's name and organization's name and address or phone
  - Date
  - Name and telephone number of writer's story source or sources
  - Reading time in seconds
  - Notation of release time (such as, "For Immediate Release" or "For Release 8 a.m. Monday, August 1)
- Use accepted format.
  - 8½- by 11-inch plain white paper
  - Typed one item per sheet
  - Double-spaced
  - One side of page only
  - Wide margins on top, bottom, and both sides of page
- Keep background information to a minimum.
- Test the release by reading it out loud.

PRINT JOURNALISM

Newspapers and newsletters are two common types of print media that work well for communicating fire and life safety information. However, even well-prepared articles written by professional communicators are not necessarily ensured a place within the pages of a newspaper or newsletter. There may be other more timely information vying for the same space as the article or idea the safety educator has presented. For this reason, it is critical for educators to know their own media outlets and what these media expect. They can help themselves by making certain their copy (the story, press release, and letter to the editor) provides local information and is correct, neat, and to the point.

Wide margins at top and sides of page

FIRE DEPARTMENT
Public Information Office

CITY OF COLORADO SPRINGS *Your organization's name*

NEWS RELEASE

DATE: April 29, 199-

SUBJECT: Two residential fires: 1054 Fontmore & 841 S. Corona St.

CONTACT: Ed Kirtley, Public Information Officer
661-5153 *Your name and phone number as story source*

RELEASE: For immediate release *Notation of release time*

READING TIME: 90 seconds *Reading time in seconds*

****

Typed double-spaced

Two overnight fires caused over $50,000 damage and displaced several families.

The first fire occurred at about 8:30 pm at 1054 Fontmore Road, Unit A ***Short sentence format.*** The first-arriving firefighters found large amounts of smoke in two apartments and smoke coming from the eaves of the four-plex condominium building. Battling heavy snow and rain, firefighters cut ***Present tense, active verb*** into the eaves and roof of the building to contain the fire.

According to Fire Investigator, John Worchester (Wooster) ***Name spelled phonetically,*** the fire began in a firewood storage area of Unit A. Apparently the resident had cleaned out the fireplace and placed a smoldering log outside in the firewood storage area. The smoldering log ignited the dry firewood, spreading fire up through the wall into the eaves and attic, filling two other apartments with smoke, and causing $50,000 in damage to the building and the contents of the three apartments.

There were no injuries, but because of fire and smoke damage, three residents of Units A, C, and D were unable to stay in their apartments. The local chapter of the American Red Cross coordinated lodging for the residents.

The second fire occurred about 3:00 am at 841 S.Corona Street, Apartment 843. On arrival, firefighters found fire shooting from the front window of the apartment. A quick attack contained the fire to the front room of the apartment ***Simple subject-verb-object sentence pattern.*** Damage was limited to $5,000 ***Rounded figure.*** Due to properly operating smoke detectors, all occupants escaped and no injuries occurred.

-end-

Figure 16.15 A typical news release.

Writing press releases. A *press release* is nothing more than a written news release for a newspaper. The most important part of a press release is the information it communicates. Often — and particularly if released to a small newspaper — the release will be printed in the newspaper exactly as the educator has written it. Because of this, writing good press releases requires the fire and life safety educator to learn the following basic journalistic guidelines:

- Start by summarizing the story in the first sentence. Answer the questions Who? What? When? Where? and Why?
- Use the inverted pyramid style putting the most important facts first and the least important facts last (Figure 16.16). This helps the reader get the most important information first and helps the editor to shorten a story without eliminating essential information.

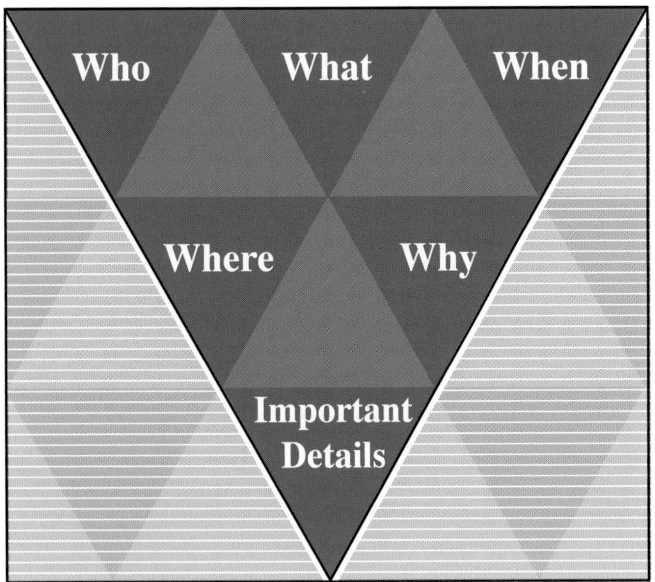

Figure 16.16 The inverted pyramid style is used for writing press releases.

Journalism's Five Ws

Most Important Facts First

[*When*] On Tuesday, August 2, at 9:00 a.m. [*where*] in Champaign Fire Department's main station training room, [*who*] two representatives of Telephone Pioneers of America [*what*] will demonstrate and present to CFD a working telephone system that allows young people to practice calling 9-1-1. *Every Word Counts*

Short Paragraph

[*Why*] Created especially for the public education division of Champaign Fire Department, the system may be used across the county to enhance awareness and understanding of the 9-1-1 system. Its practical applications could include use in schools, fairs, public displays, or even neighborhood programs. METCAD personnel will provide *Active Voice* validation suggestions and aid to the project.

Telephone Pioneers is a group of 350 active retired employees of Champaign-Urbana telephone companies.

- Limit sentence length. Rarely make them longer than 20 words.
- Write no more than four or five lines per paragraph; one-sentence paragraphs are common practice. (**NOTE**: One-sentence and very brief paragraphs are used in print journalism because they create white space within the standard narrow column layout and thus make reading easier.)
- Make every word count.
- Use the active voice. For example, write "Fire Chief Corbly announced..." instead of "It was announced by Fire Chief Corbly..."
- Write clearly and concisely; leave out fancy phrases and technical terminology. For example, rather than write "haz mat," use "hazardous materials" or "chemicals and other items that might cause harm to the public." Also, use a name, and possibly a brief description, rather than an acronym —write "International Fire Service Training Association" in place of "IFSTA."
- Make sure that all quoted and paraphrased information is attributed to its proper source. (**NOTE**: Failure to properly attribute sources can lead to charges of plagiarism or libel and protracted lawsuits.)

Creating fact sheets. Suppose Fire Prevention Week has arrived again and the fire and life safety educator wants to issue a press release on a new program to alert homeowners to the dangers of carbon monoxide poisoning and the importance of CO detectors. The educator has a lot of materials to provide the press and knows that releases should be limited to one page. How can the educator get all the facts to the reporter?

Use a fact sheet. While a press release quickly provides reporters and editors with the essence of a message, a fact sheet provides material that will allow the reporter to write an in-depth article. A fact sheet can be several pages long. It may include a historical perspective, anecdotal material, statistics, and local data.

Providing Media Interviews

During any interview (television, radio, or print media), the educator provides the link between the fire department and the community. The interview can either strengthen or weaken that critical link. If the goal is to have viewers watch or hear the interview and process and use the information received, then it is essential that the educator does not distract the viewer from the message by his or her personal verbal mannerisms, dress, or actions. A national survey indicates that two of the biggest interview faults in educational or informational radio and television programs are lack of enthusiasm and poor voice characteristics.

Even though one needs to be conversational and pleasant, an interview is not simply a conversation. Instead, the interview is a formal exchange of information. The educator is not just talking to a person with a pad of paper or a camera. The message conveyed goes to all the readers, all the listeners, and all viewers to whom that reporter provides information.

Use the following guidelines to improve media interviews:

- **Be prepared**. Review all pertinent information before the interview. Have reference notes. Inquire about what questions will be asked.
- **Act in a professional manner**:
  - — Dress appropriately.
  - — Be aware of your body language. Sit with feet on the floor, rather than crossed or on a nearby desk.
  - — Avoid chewing gum, smoking, or eating.
  - — Act confident.
  - — Look the reporter in the eye.
  - — Use appropriate language.

  (**NOTE**: Language is not neutral. For instance, calling a female reporter "Missie" or "Honey" is demeaning, whether it is intended that way or not.)
- **Use inclusive language**. For example, use "firefighter" (not fireman), "staffing" (not manning), and "mom or dad or the persons that live with you" (not families).
- **Be newsworthy, factual, and correct**. Check and double-check information before releasing it to the media.
- **Give the same story to all news stations**, but if a news reporter comes to your department with a story, don't give his or her station's story to another station.
- **Plan the points you want to make**. State the most important points or conclusions at the start of the interview. Single-sentence summaries are helpful.
- **Choose your words carefully**. Use language everyone understands; avoid fire service jargon and technical terms. Ask yourself what you would say if you were trying to explain the incident to an acquaintance unfamiliar with your job. Your audience simply wants to understand the situation. You are not there to impress people with big words.
- **Avoid acting stuffy or self-important** under the mistaken idea that these characteristics will make the interviewer or the audience take you more seriously. The fact that the reporter has chosen to talk with you is enough.
- **Project an image of credibility that will reflect well on your department**. As you communicate, try to create the headlines you ultimately want the audience to see, hear, or read.
- **Always assume that you are "on record."** Anything you say can (and probably will) be used.
- **Avoid saying "No comment."** It invites speculation. Instead you might say, "I don't have enough information to properly answer that question" (Figure 16.17).
- **Do not repeat a reporter's negative or leading words in your answer**. To a hostile or inaccurate remark, say something such as this: "First let me correct a misconception that was part of your question."
- **Hold your composure**. Some interviewers try to provoke angry responses in order to get additional information. If you remain calm and courteous, you short-circuit this practice.
- **Simply restate your policy or position, rather than attempting to answer hypothetical questions**. You may want to preface your restatement with a gentle reminder to the interviewer: "Here's the situation we are focusing on . . ."
- **If you do not know the answer to a question simply respond, "I don't know."** You might also include, "As soon

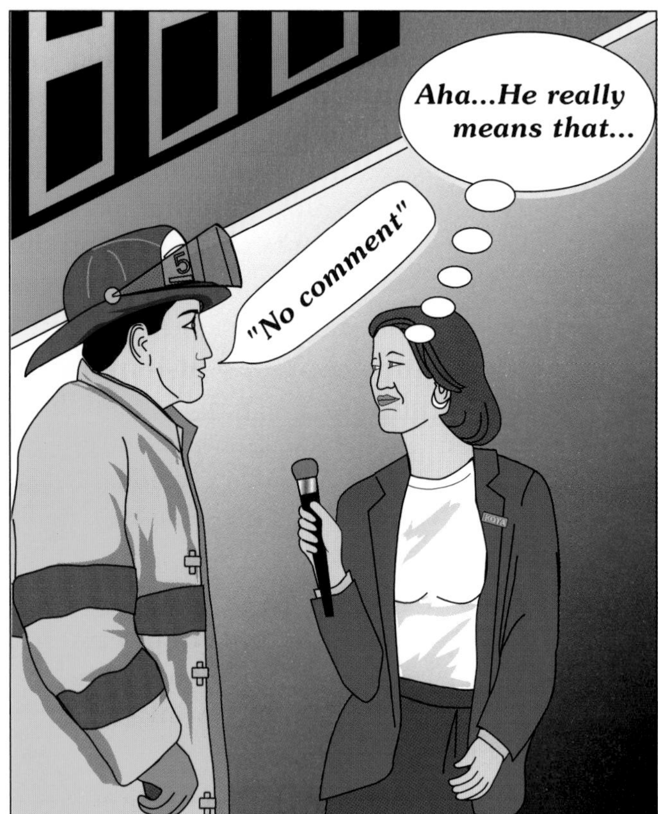

Figure 16.17 Saying "No comment" leaves the media guessing what you really mean.

as I get the information, I'll get right back to you." Then make a note of the question and diligently track down the answer.

- **Keep the interview on track**. Control the interview: Do not digress or allow the interviewer to move away from the subject at hand.
- **Avoid criticism of other agencies or educators**.
- **Assign no blame**. Avoid criticism, and do not take potshots at your competition.
- **Know the department's position**.
- **Be available for follow-up questions** after the completed interview. Let the interviewer know that you definitely want to clarify any questions that may come up as the story is written.
- **Keep control of a television interview**. If it is not live and you think that you can say what you just said more concisely, ask to redo the interview. Often during the second time, the wording is more concise.
- **Above all, be honest**. Never lie. Say what you know, not what you think (Figure 16.18).

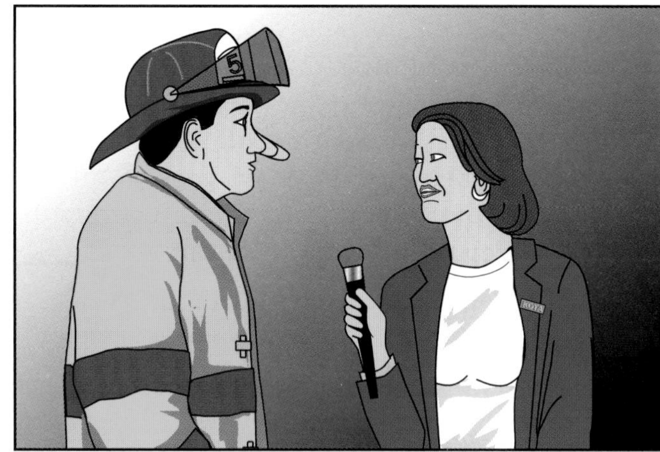

Figure 16.18 Be honest when communicating with the media.

More Interview Suggestions...

The National Association of Broadcasters provides more suggestions to enhance a person's television and radio appearances.

Television

- Avoid unnecessary movements and gestures. Move more slowly than you normally would.
- If you are being interviewed, look, listen, and speak to the person talking to you.
- Resist the temptation to look at yourself on the television monitor in the studio. It will distract both you and the viewers.

Radio

- Check the microphone. Tiny lapel clip-ons are no problem. However, old-fashioned mikes that sit on stands have a limited pick-up range. Stay within that range to avoid fading out.
- Remove jingling jewelry, as well as keys and pocket change.
- Avoid words containing the letters B, P, and S. These letters tend to pop, explode, and hiss when pronounced over the air.
- Assume that all microphones are live.

Adapted from *The Publicity Handbook*, by David R. Yale, Lincolnwood, IL: NTC Business Books, 1991, p. 245.

Assuming the Role of PIO

Often the fire and life safety educator assumes the role of public information officer (PIO) at the scene of an emergency (Figure 16.19). It should be made clear that in such cases, the

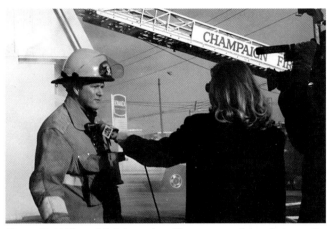

Figure 16.19 The public information officer acts as a liaison between the incident commander and the media. *Courtesy of Champaign (IL) Fire Department.*

educator is assuming a role (and its responsibilities) rather than a rank.[19] The educator, when acting as PIO, provides information to community reporters for a hard news story — one the media needs to provide to the public immediately.

As in every other aspect of the educator's job, the PIO function runs more smoothly if planning and thought have been put into practice ahead of time — before the inevitable emergency arises.

USING PIO TOOLS

Just as the veteran firefighter would not approach flames without a hose in hand, the PIO needs essential tools when facing reporters at the scene of an emergency. If the department does not have a PIO tool kit, the fire and life safety educator can put together a kit to include the following items:

- **Radio**. The PIO needs a radio to communicate with fire command and other suppression personnel.
- **Two sharpened pencils and a notepad**. Simple things such as addresses, names of persons injured, and telephone numbers can easily be forgotten in the adrenaline rush of a large emergency. Write it down.
- **Small tape recorder and tape**. Taping conversations allows for self-critique later. Also, if inaccurate reporting has become a problem, the tape recorder may show reporters that the PIO expects them to provide correct information.
- **Media quick-call list**. In the event of an escalating emergency, the PIO must be prepared to notify media sources or to update them as the situation changes. The quick-call list — a shortened version of the media address and phone list — provides up-to-date phone numbers of key media personnel. The list includes the news reporters most often dealt with: the local ABC, NBC, CBS radio and television reporters and the city reporters and editors for the local newspapers (Figure 16.20).
- **Mobile telephone**. A mobile phone is used for updating the news media and for communicating with others involved in the situation.
- **Basic question list**. This is a media work sheet. The Colorado Springs Fire Department offers its company officers and PIOs a "Company Officer PIO Guide" which is a laminated card that folds to wallet size (Figure 16.21). This handy guide includes interview tips; reminders of questions to ask for fire, EMS, and haz mat; and rescue information and phone numbers. (**NOTE**: See example in the **Fire and Life Safety Educator's Resource Kit**.)

Another reminder technique may be to keep several copies of basic questions easily obtainable so that the PIO does not have to think about what questions the reporters will ask.

Media Quick-Call List

	Contact Person	Phone Number	Fax Number
Print Organizations			
Radio			
TV			

Figure 16.20 The media quick-call list provides the PIO with a ready reference for local media contacts.

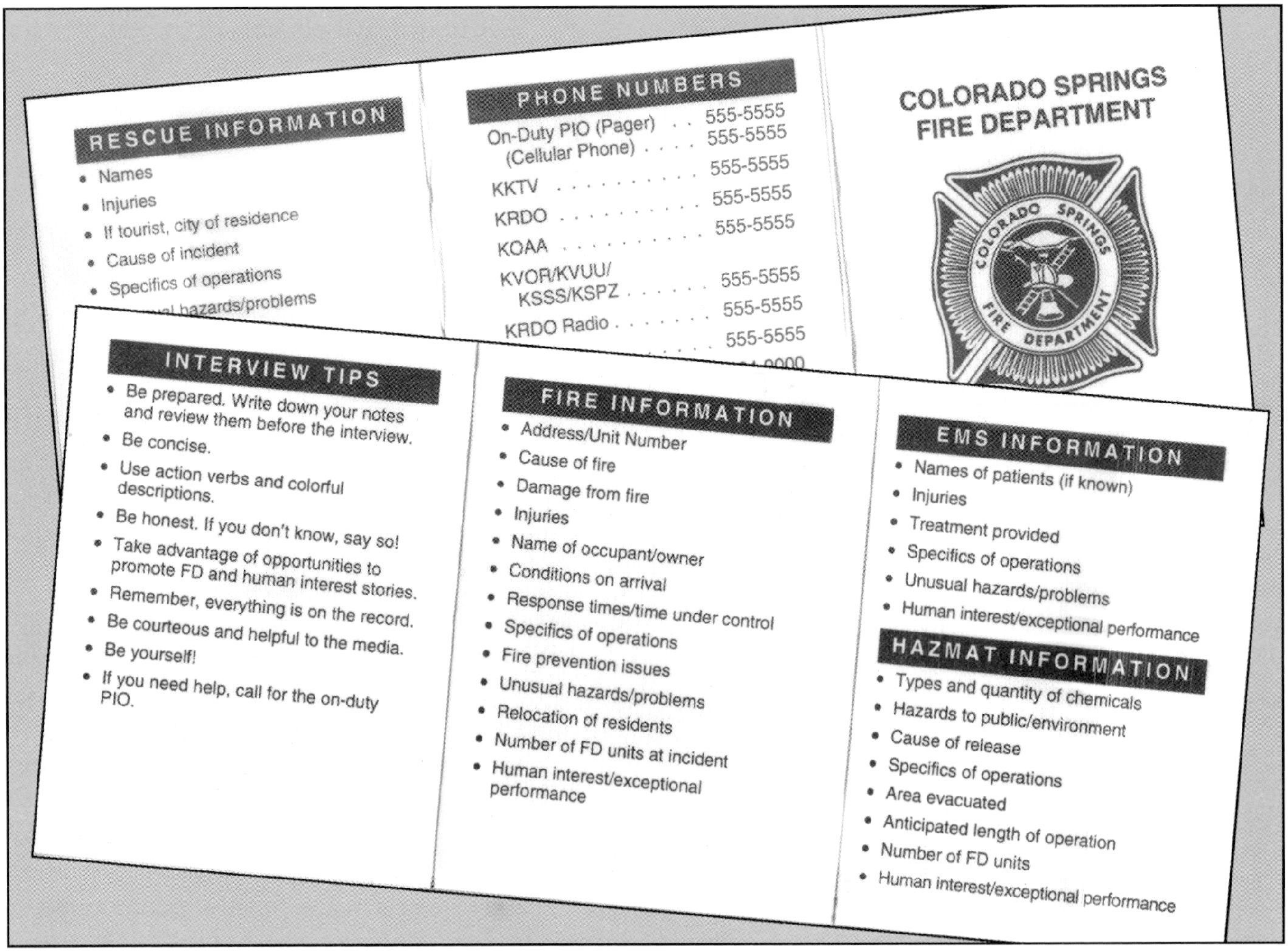

RESCUE INFORMATION

- Names
- Injuries
- If tourist, city of residence
- Cause of incident
- Specifics of operations
- ... hazards/problems

PHONE NUMBERS

On-Duty PIO (Pager) . . 555-5555
(Cellular Phone) 555-5555
KKTV 555-5555
KRDO 555-5555
KOAA 555-5555
KVOR/KVUU/
KSSS/KSPZ 555-5555
KRDO Radio 555-5555
. . . . 555-5555

COLORADO SPRINGS FIRE DEPARTMENT

INTERVIEW TIPS

- Be prepared. Write down your notes and review them before the interview.
- Be concise.
- Use action verbs and colorful descriptions.
- Be honest. If you don't know, say so!
- Take advantage of opportunities to promote FD and human interest stories.
- Remember, everything is on the record.
- Be courteous and helpful to the media.
- Be yourself!
- If you need help, call for the on-duty PIO.

FIRE INFORMATION

- Address/Unit Number
- Cause of fire
- Damage from fire
- Injuries
- Name of occupant/owner
- Conditions on arrival
- Response times/time under control
- Specifics of operations
- Fire prevention issues
- Unusual hazards/problems
- Relocation of residents
- Number of FD units at incident
- Human interest/exceptional performance

EMS INFORMATION

- Names of patients (if known)
- Injuries
- Treatment provided
- Specifics of operations
- Unusual hazards/problems
- Human interest/exceptional performance

HAZMAT INFORMATION

- Types and quantity of chemicals
- Hazards to public/environment
- Cause of release
- Specifics of operations
- Area evacuated
- Anticipated length of operation
- Number of FD units
- Human interest/exceptional performance

Figure 16.21 Company Officer PIO Guide. *Courtesy of Colorado Springs Fire Department.*

HANDLING ON-SCENE MANAGEMENT RESPONSIBILITIES

In the event of an emergency, reporters do not care whether a fire department handling the emergency is large or small. They simply need accurate, timely information. Big stories can occur in small places. If the department experiences infrequent contact with the press, it is all the more important to have a plan prepared. Busy departments tend to stay prepared. Do not be lulled into a false sense of complacency.

During an emergency situation, the incident commander remains responsible for managing public information. When needed or designated in the department's SOPs, the incident commander may establish a Public Information Sector (Figure 16.22). This designated area helps reporters gather up-to-date information by knowing where to report to get information about the emergency. Some departments use special color lighting (green lights versus red or blue) to designate where they are. Others use the IC vehicle as a meeting place for reporters or tape off a

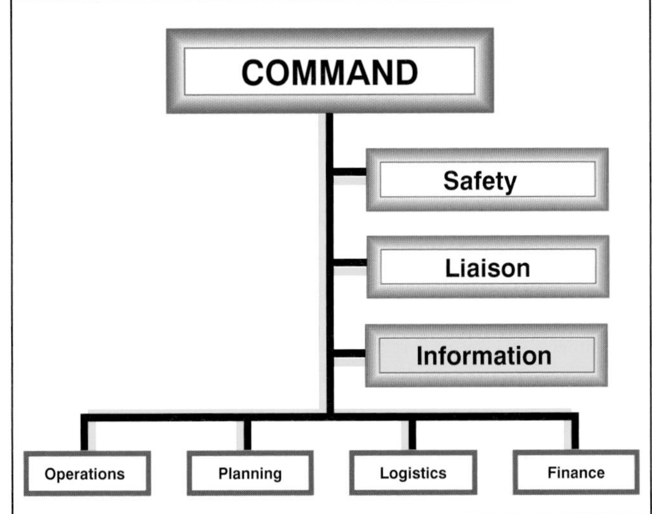

Figure 16.22 The PIO falls under the direct command of the incident commander during an emergency operation.

quadrant specifically for providing media updates. For further identification, some PIOs wear vests or special shields on their helmets.

It becomes the PIO's responsibility to gather, prepare and provide information to the media. The PIO sees that the media can get the story it needs safely, quickly, and efficiently. The PIO serves as a point of contact between the incident commander and the media. The goal is to help the media put together an accurate, understandable, fact-filled account of the emergency and to make certain that reporters are safe and not in the way of those who are attempting to secure the scene.

The following is an action plan. It tells the fire and life safety educator what to do and when to do it when assuming the role of PIO at an emergency scene:

Step 1: Report to the Incident Commander (IC) for a briefing on the situation. Receive instructions. Use a media work sheet to record the observed and gathered information about the incident. This work sheet basically anticipates questions the media will ask.

Step 2: Establish a media area for release of information. Choose an area fairly close to the IC, yet away from danger. Inform the IC of the location of the media sector. Identify it clearly.

Step 3: Alert the media to your location. Let the reporters know when to check back for updates of the breaking story — perhaps on the quarter hour or the half hour. Once you determine the meeting times, stick to them, whether you have new information or not. Tell reporters the ground rules up front. Where is it safe to be? Where is it unsafe or inappropriate?

Step 4: Prepare a news release.

Step 5: Gather the media and release your news. Note any questions that you could not answer. Attempt to find the answers to these questions.

Step 6: Coordinate photography with the media. Make every effort to help the photographer get the best shots that can safely be obtained. Identify for the photographer firefighters and situations in the photos.

Step 7: Continue to check in with the Incident Commander. Solicit updated information and listen to the emergency radio for any changes in status.[20]

CREATING AND FOLLOWING SOPS

The PIO links the fire department with the community it serves. Often those in the community do not understand the day-to-day operations and activities of the fire department. They may not understand how the modern fire service operates or the variety of tasks fire personnel perform. In most jurisdictions, the percentage of citizens calling the fire department for emergency assistance is low. Even with widespread public education and community service activities, a high percentage of most communities receive their information of fire department activities only from the media. Obviously, providing clear,

Remember...

- Report only facts. Rumors are not facts.
- Do not release personal information on victims or losses until names have been checked, double-checked, and cleared by the incident commander. The PIO generally does not release the identities of fire fatalities until all appropriate next of kin have been notified of the death.

  Reporters recognize that this type of information must be delayed. They will, however, need the identities as soon as possible.
- Show human concern and empathy when talking about sensitive issues such as property loss, injury, and death. Do not appear uncaring or distant by simply rattling off the cold, hard facts. Let your compassion show on your face.
- Ask for help if you are swamped. It is vital to everyone concerned that the information be presented accurately as well as professionally.
- Be courteous. Be professional. Be brief. If you follow these instructions, you will make a positive impression for the department you represent.

concise, and timely information to the media benefits everyone.[21]

The fire and life safety educator should create standard operating procedures (SOPs) for working with news media. SOPs can help answer questions such as who from the department may speak with the media and how the fire chief wants specific matters handled. (**NOTE**: See Appendix C for an example of an SOP for the Public Information Officer.)

Vital Statistics Vitally Important

When gathering information, *be certain* to get — and double-check — vital facts: the person's full name (including middle initial), the person's age, the hospital the person was taken to, and the physical condition of the injured person. This information will aid in putting together a departmental report. Do not release the information until the information has been verified and all appropriate persons have been notified.

USING ALTERNATIVE MESSAGES TO REACH THE PUBLIC

In contrast to media services, where the educator provides the media with information, in educational programming (publicity, promotions) the educator's focus is on the audience who will receive the message. The focus is not on the media service.

When working through educational programming to provide practical publicity, the educator must first identify specific audience(s) for the program. The educator must also understand the identified audience well enough to perfectly tailor educational and informational goals and methods to fit it.

When seeking answers about how information should be presented, the fire and life safety educator must take time to develop a plan:

- Establish departmental priorities.
- Analyze the audience.
- Research the marketplace.
- Select the right medium.
- Test, evaluate, and critique.
- Prepare the department for publicity.
- Define the fire and life safety educator's authority.
- Know what sorts of decisions will need prior approval.
- Know who will review the fire and life safety educator's work.
- Make everyone at the department aware of what is happening.

Fire departments delight in coming up with alternative outlets and campaign strategies. The remainder of this chapter will discuss some of these alternative media for delivering the fire and life safety educator's messages. When determining whether or not to use one of these alternative media, remember that it is essential to know the local community and hometown fire department before deciding what is or is not appropriate.

Billboards

Billboards may provide an opportunity to share information. Hire a professional or use the artistic talents within the department to design the billboard. Listen to the expertise of the person from whom the billboard is rented.

Often departments have poster contests for school children. One common prize includes enlarging the poster for placement on a billboard. Here are some tips for students creating posters for billboards (and judges will need these criteria as well).

- Use bright, bold colors with strong contrast.
- Avoid pastel colors as they do not show up well.
- Use seven words or less.
- Use only one basic idea.
- Use positive messages.
- Use large letters with simple letter-styles. Do not make the letters too thin or too thick. Use capital letters and lower case letters instead of all capitals. Use large letters because the message should be readable from several hundred feet away.
- Draw the design on horizontal paper.

Signboards

Talented firefighters at Bremerton Fire Department, Washington, created 4- by 6-foot outdoor signs to place in sign holders. These signboards, located in strategic areas of the community, alert the public to a variety of safety messages and activities. The signs are changed monthly. As specific problems are identified in the community, a corresponding prevention message is placed in local sign holders (Figure 16.23).

Hot-Air Balloons

Plano (TX) Fire Department formed a not-for-profit corporation in order to purchase and operate a 70-foot-high hot-air balloon over the skies of Plano. The flight crew, made up of off-duty fire department personnel and others, work on a volunteer basis. Annually, free balloon rides are provided to community members, including Learn Not to Burn® teachers in the school district. The balloon serves as a reward and a motivation to keep the program and community partnership alive (Figure 16.24).

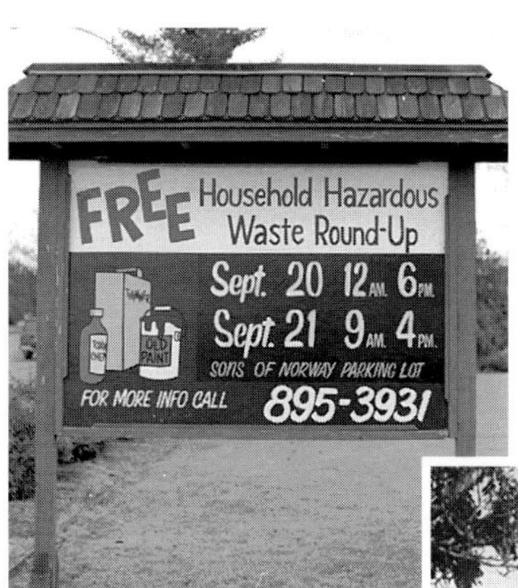

Figure 16.23 Educators can reach thousands of people each year with fire and life safety signboards. *Courtesy of the City of Bremerton (WA) Fire Department.*

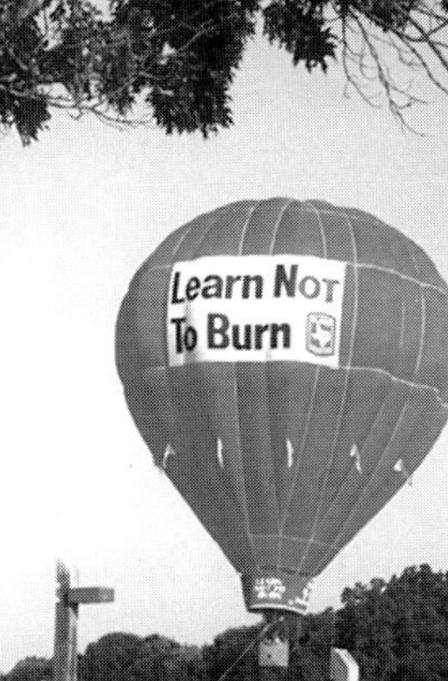

Figure 16.24 The Plano (TX) Fire Department uses a 70-foot-high hot-air balloon to promote fire and life safety education goals. *Courtesy of Plano (TX) Fire Department.*

Place Mats

Local fast-food restaurants may print fire safety messages on place mats for their food trays and distribute them in the weeks before, during, or after Fire Prevention Week.

Grocery Bags

Some grocery store chains may print fire and life safety messages on their bags. Check with store managers for details and deadlines (Figure 16.25).

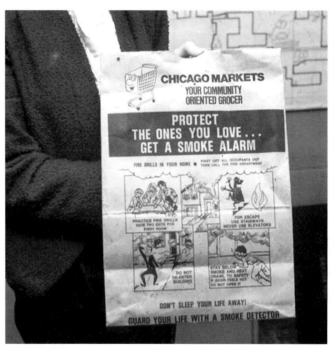

Figure 16.25 Grocery bags are an excellent item for a fire and life safety education message. *Courtesy of Glenn Rousey, Rock Island Fire Department, Rock Island, Illinois.*

Safety Trailers

Check state or county resources for a detailed list of smoke houses and safety trailers within the state or province. Often departments are willing to provide tips for building, and they will generally share their resources. The safety trailer can be used as a wonderful public relations tool and at the same time provide hands-on public education (Figure 16.26).

Newsletters

Newsletters can be a marvelous means of communication (Figure 16.27). The educator might create a newsletter for the fire department, or perhaps for the teachers of an area school system.

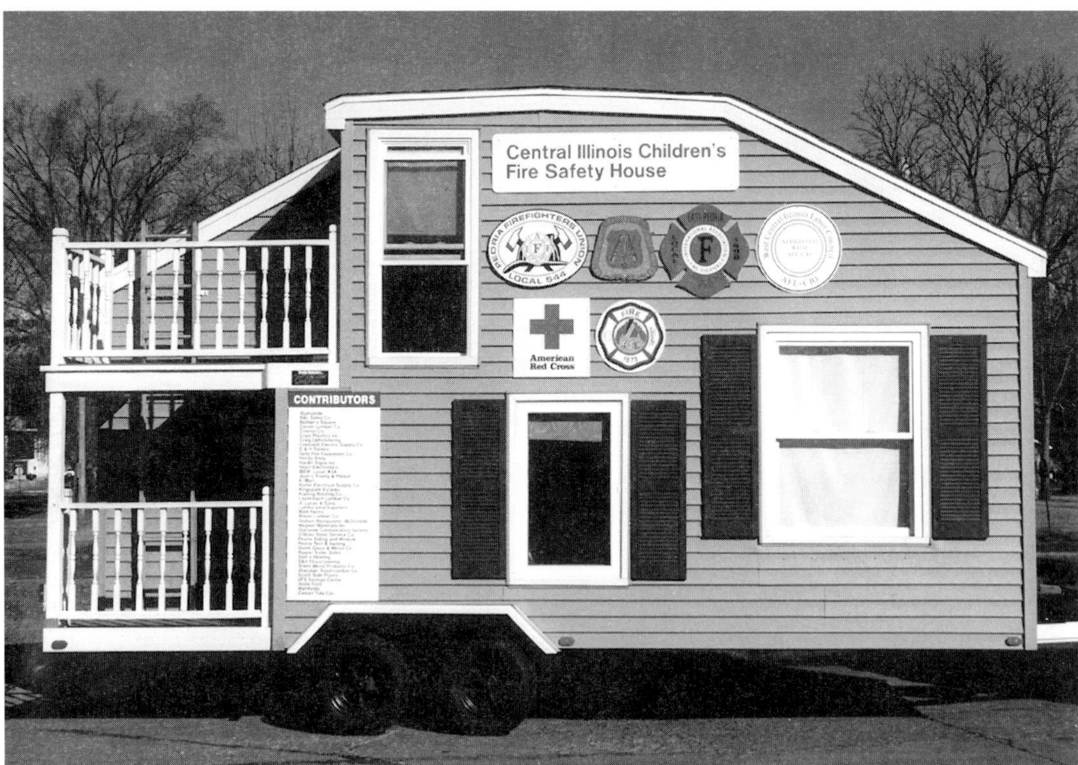

Figure 16.26 The safety trailer provides the audience with hands-on experience in fire and life safety behaviors. *Courtesy of Peoria (IL) Fire Department.*

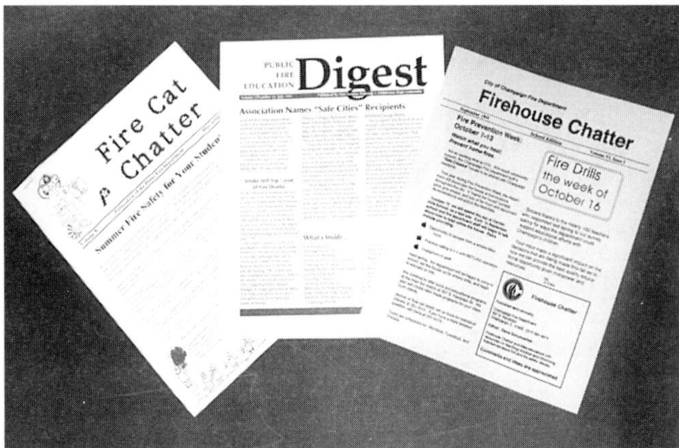

Figure 16.27 Fire and life safety education newsletters.

It pays — in terms of both time and money saved — to use a computer to produce a newsletter. The educator should investigate the many available computer software programs created to aid newsletter editors in designing and laying out their publications. Aside from providing a choice of column and headline sizes and formats, many of these programs contain clip art and noncopyrighted "filler" material for newsletter use. The beginning newsletter editor should talk to other newsletter editors and do some comparative shopping to find software that is right for the department's needs and budget.

Heed the following guidelines to create a polished piece of work.

- Know your audience.
- Define your purpose.
- Write so that the newsletter can be read quickly.
- Use familiar, short words.
- Keep your style informal.
- After the newsletter is written, let it sit for a day or two. This will provide the distance needed to be objective.
- After you have gained some distance, edit the newsletter: Delete extra words, check articles for clarity, and take time to get the headlines right. Headlines and first sentences are critical when writing newsletters. (See the **Fire and Life Safety Educator's Resource Kit** for an example of a newsletter.)

T-Shirts, Buttons, and Other Accessories

Today, fire safety messages and art can be inexpensively printed on T-shirts, buttons, key chains, bookmarks, bumper stickers, and many other mediums. Check with the local express copy service and T-shirt printer.

LEGAL ISSUES

Congress shall make no law . . . abridging the freedom of speech or the press reads the First Amendment to the Constitution. Journalists generally view the First Amendment as the cornerstone of free speech in our society. Fire professionals also recognize the importance of the First Amendment and the laws that govern our country.

The public information specialist is confronted by many legal issues: privacy law, copyright laws, lobbying, broadcasting regulations, to name a few. Although not a trained lawyer, the educator must understand the laws and how they apply to the fire and life safety educator's work.

Sunshine Laws

Sunshine laws address media access to records of public meetings. These laws are local, state, or provincial laws which require public notification and open attendance of government meeting. While varying from state to state, these laws generally cover the following points:

- The amount of notice required to hold a public meeting
- Whether or not a meeting is open to the public
- Requirements on meeting minutes or transcripts
- Executive session rules

Freedom of Information Act

The federal Freedom of Information Act was enacted in the mid-1960s and strengthened in 1974. It is a model for many state laws designed to make government information available to the public. In essence the government has 10 days to respond to a request and 20 days to respond to an appeal if records are denied.[22]

Libel and Slander Laws

Libel, slander, and privacy are related. Libel is written defamation. Slander is oral defamation. Libel is essentially a false or defamatory attack in written form on a person's reputation or character. Broadcast defamation is libel because there is usually a written script. Oral or spoken defamation is slander.[23] Laws of libel and slander protect the reputation of a person or institution.

Copyright Statutes

The copyright statute was revised in 1976 to take into account developments in photocopiers, videotapes, motion pictures, broadcasting, cable television, and other technologies that had arisen since the previous act was adopted in 1909. The copyright laws provide that copyright owners "shall have exclusive right" to reproduce, distribute and use original works of expression fixed in a tangible medium.[24]

As professional educators and role models in the fire service, it is critical to respect and follow copyright laws. For example, the NFPA has a

Grounds for Libel Suits

Matters that might be held libelous by a court would have to:

1. Imply commission of a crime
2. Tend to injure a person in his or her profession or job
3. Imply that a person has a disease, usually a loathsome disease that might lead to the individual's ostracism
4. Damage a person's credit
5. Imply a lack of chastity
6. Indicate a lack of mental capacity
7. Incite public ridicule or contempt

Here are some dangerous words that could be grounds for libel suits:

1. Thief, loan shark, shoplifter, gangster
2. Incompetent, failure, quack, shyster, slick operator
3. Wino, leper, has VD, AIDS
4. Unreliable, bankrupt, failure
5. Loose, seducer, B-girl, stud, immoral, mistress, hooker, streetwalker
6. Screwy, nutty, incompetent, strange, out-of-it
7. Phony, coward, hypocrite

From *News Reporting and Writing*, 4th ed., by Melvin Mencher, William C. Brown Publishers, Dubuque, IA, 1987, p. 557. Used with permission of the author.

copyright on Sparky® the Fire Dog. Permission must be obtained from NFPA for using the Sparky® character on newsletters, T-shirts, or other items (Figure 16.28).

To place a copyright notice on a written work, include the following information in the upper right-hand corner:

- ©, Copyright, or Copr.
- Date of publication
- Name of the owner of the copyright

Copyright varies from country to country. But registering a work with the U.S. Copyright Office in Washington, DC, is as simple as filling out a form, remitting a small fee, and sending two copies of the published work. Copyright forms can be obtained through the Copyright Office by calling (202) 707-9100 or writing to the following address:

Information and Publication Section LM-455
Copyright Office
Library of Congress
Washington, DC 20559

Registration is not necessary for the copyright to be valid, but if the author wishes to bring a suit against someone, the work must be registered. The registered copyright lasts the lifetime of the author, plus fifty years.

In addition to knowing how to copyright their own work, fire and life safety educators must know enough about copyright laws to avoid violating these laws when preparing public education materials and articles for the media. The law limits what the educator may copy, under what conditions the educator may copy, and for what purpose the educator may copy. This is not to say that any copying of materials is a violation of copyright law. The law permits educators access to information and permits them to copy materials under clearly defined guidelines.[25]

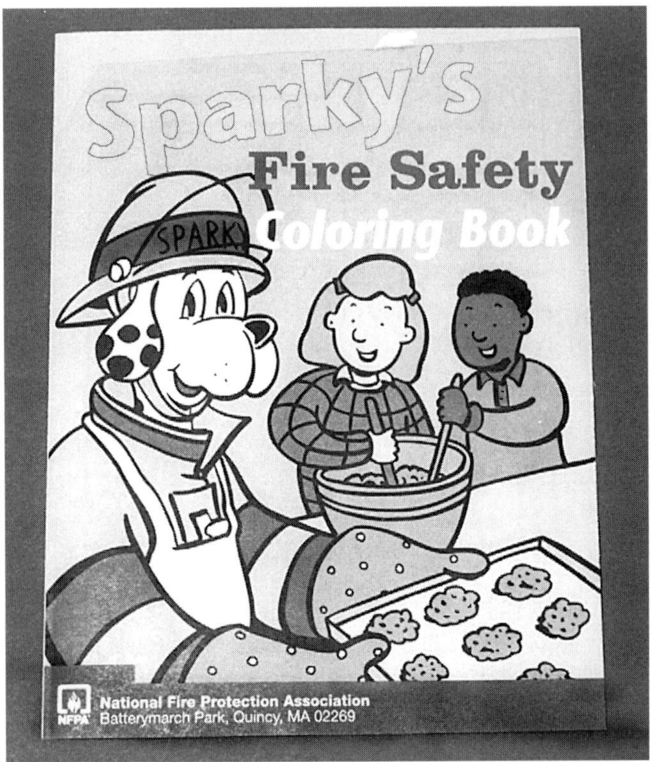

Figure 16.28 Anytime educators use other's materials, they must follow copyright laws. Sparky® *is a registred trademark of the National Fire Protection Association, Quincy, MA 02269.*

CONCLUSION

Effective communication takes time, patience, understanding, and emotional control. This task of communicating also involves hard work, skill, a sense of humor, and — at times — a pinch of luck.

The safety information the fire and life safety educator provides the media feeds vital knowledge to citizens who otherwise might not receive life-saving information. Linking the fire service, the media, and community provides enormous satisfaction to those skilled fire and life safety educators who strive to give their best.

Chapter 16 Notes

1. James F. Evans, "Education Campaign Planning," course reference, University of Illinios, 1985, p. 3-2.
2. Jess Stein (ed.), *The Random House College Dictionary*, rev. ed., Random House, New York, 1984, p. 830.
3. Evans, p. 3-9.
4. Evans, p. 3-3, 3-4.
5. Patricia Calvert (ed.), *The Communicator's Handbook: Techniques and Technologies*, Maupin House, Gainesville, FL, 1993, p. 119.
6. Ibid., p. 33. Used with permission. For ordering information, call 1-800-524-0634.
7. Melvin Mencher, *News Reporting and Writing*, Wm. C. Brown Publishers, Dubuque, IA, 1987, p. 58.
8. David R. Yale, *The Publicity Handbook*, NTC Business Books, Lincolnwood, IL, 1991, p. 67.
9. Evans, p. 3-9.
10. Evans, p. 3-17.
11. Calvert, p. 117.
12. Calvert, p. 118.
13. To order a copy of *Practical Publicity* by David Tedone, please send a check or money order for $11.95 (includes $3.00) shipping) to The Harvard Common Press, 535 Albany Street, Boston, MA 02218.
14. Mr. Dave Shaul, news director, WCIA-CBS, Channel 3, Champaign, IL, May 1995.
15. Mencher, p. 214.
16. Calvert, p. 139.
17. Yale, p. 237.
18. Calvert, p. 128.
19. Haberer, JoAnn B. (ed.), *The Public Information Officer: A Media Relations Training Program for the Fire Service*, Action Training Systems, Inc., Vancouver, WA, 1993, p. 4.
20. Ed Kirtley, Colorado Springs Fire Department, 1993.
21. Ibid.
22. Scott M. Cutlip, Allen H. Center, and Glen M. Broom, *Effective Public Relations*, Prentice-Hall, Inc., NJ, 1985, p. 140.
23. Carole Rich, *Writing and Reporting News: A Coaching Method*, Wadsworth Publishing Co., Belmont, CA, 1994, p. 337.
24. Cutlip, p. 143.
25. For information on such guidelines, see Stephen Fishman, *The Copyright Handbook*, 2nd ed., Berkeley, CA, Nolo Press, 1994.

Chapter 16 Review

Directions

The following activities are designed to help you comprehend and apply the information in Chapter 16 of **Fire and Life Safety Educator**, second edition. To receive the maximum learning experience from these activities, it is recommended that you use the following procedure:

1. Read the chapter, underlining or highlighting important terms, topics, and subject matter. Read the sidebar material, study the photographs and illustrations, and read the captions with each.
2. Review the list of vocabulary words to ensure that you know the chapter-related meaning of each. If you are unsure of the meaning of a vocabulary word, look up the word in the glossary or a dictionary, and then study its context in the chapter.
3. On a separate sheet of paper, complete all assigned or selected application and review activities before checking your answers.
4. After you have finished, check your answers against those on the pages referenced in parentheses.
5. Correct any incorrect answers, and review material that was answered incorrectly.

Vocabulary

Be sure that you know the chapter-related meanings of the following words and abbreviations:

- communication *(297)*
- fact sheet *(304)*
- FCC *(308)*
- feedback *(299)*
- mass media *(298)*
- medium *(298)*
- news release *(310)*
- PIO *(307)*
- press release *(311)*
- program director *(303)*
- PSAs *(308)*
- SOPs *(317)*

Application of Knowledge

1. Write a 30-second educational and informational public service announcement for each of the following topics:
   - safety
   - fire prevention
   - smoke detectors
2. Using the journalistic guidelines on page *xx*, write a press release for your retirement from the fire service.
3. Update or establish a list of frequently called media sources in your jurisdiction.
4. Assemble a media kit to include the following information:
   - media release
   - event schedule
   - fact sheet
   - photograph
   - previous articles
   - biography
   - briefing or background sheet
5. Obtain and review several of your department's SOPs for working with the media.

Review Activities

1. List the four primary mass media sources. *(298)*
2. Explain the importance of feedback to ensure that television messages are received as intended by young children. *(299)*
3. Name the three general categories into which three-fourths of all news stories are grouped. *(300)*
4. Distinguish between the terms *soft news* and *hard news. (300, 301)*
5. List several situations or opportunities that provide information for a soft news story. *(301)*
6. Identify the components for laying the groundwork with the media to deliver a fire and life safety education message. *(301)*
7. Summarize the importance of knowing the community's media services in order to establish a good working relationship. *(302)*

8. List guidelines to identifying and maintaining contact with important local media personnel. *(303, 304)*
9. Discuss the following documents in terms of organizing and assembling a media kit:
   - media release *(304)*
   - event schedule *(304)*
   - fact sheet *(304)*
   - photograph *(305)*
   - previous articles *(305)*
   - biography *(305)*
   - briefing or background sheet *(305)*
10. State reasons why people like to listen to the radio. *(305)*
11. List examples of the following public service announcements: *(306)*
    - event notification
    - informational
12. Explain in detail the importance of knowing televsion delivery formats for emergency and nonemergency situations. *(307, 308)*
13. Distinguish between PSAs produced by reputable associations and PSAs produced by freelance video professionals. *(309, 310)*
14. Describe the basic guidelines for the following releases:
    - news *(310)*
    - press *(311, 312)*
15. Name two interviewing weaknesses in educational or informational radio and television programs. *(312, 313)*
16. List several guidelines to follow for improving media interviews. *(313)*
17. List several suggestions for enhancing a person's television and radio appearances. *(313, 314)*
18. Describe PIO tools to use when facing reporters at the scene of an emergency. *(315)*
19. List ways to identify a Public Information Sector used during an emergency situation. *(316, 317)*
20. Identify the seven steps of an action plan used at the emergency scene by a PIO. *(317)*
21. Discuss the information that a fire and life safety educator would include in a SOP for working with the news media. *(317, 318)*
22. Summarize the procedure that should be followed when gathering a victim's vital statistics. *(318)*
23. Discuss the importance of developing a plan for using alternative messages to reach the public. *(318)*
24. Identify and give examples of various ways of reaching the public using alternative messages. *(318-321)*
25. Discuss the following legal issues as they apply to a fire and life safety educator: *(321)*
    - First Amendment
    - Sunshine laws
    - Freedom Information Act
26. Distinguish between the terms *libel* and *slander. (321)*
27. Explain in detail copyright statutes. *(321, 322)*

Questions and Notes

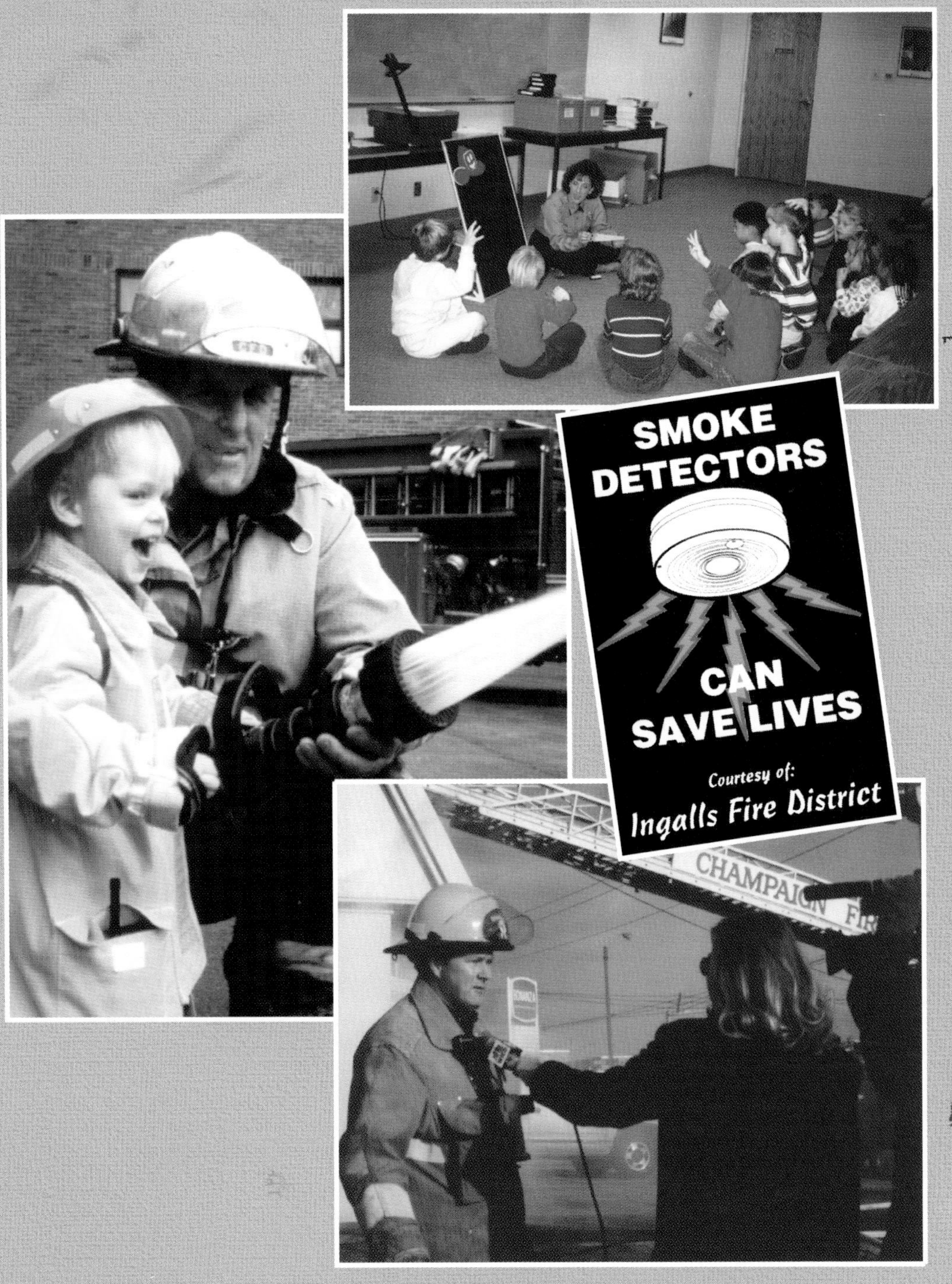
SMOKE
DETECTORS
CAN
SAVE LIVES
Courtesy of:
Ingalls Fire District
CHAMPAIGN

Using Public Speaking Techniques 17

LEARNING OBJECTIVES

This chapter provides information that addresses the following objectives of NFPA 1035, *Standard for Professional Qualifications for Public Fire and Life Safety Educator* (1993 edition):

Public Fire and Life Safety Educator I

3-4.1.2 *Prerequisite Skills:* Communication skills, use of prepared lesson plans with identified learning objectives, methods for active participation/involvement, methods of developing and maintaining a positive learning environment for the student including physical environment and student/instructor relationships, and proper use and care of audiovisual equipment and materials.

3-4.2 Present a prepared program, given lesson content, time allotments, and identified audience, so that program objectives are met.

Chapter 17
Using Public Speaking Techniques

INTRODUCTION

The difference between presentations that succeed and those that fail is usually not in how well fire and life safety educators know their subject. The difference is in how effectively they present the subjects they know so well.

Just what is a *presentation*? According to Ron Hoff, author of the popular book on presentations, *I Can See You Naked*,

> A presentation is a commitment by the presenter to help the audience do something. Simultaneously, throughout the presentation, the audience is evaluating the presenter's ability to deliver — to make good on the commitment.[1]

Fire and life safety educators make many different types of presentations, ranging from leading a tour and education session at the fire station, to speaking at a junior high school assembly, to speaking before the Kiwanis, to teaching a class at a local business during Fire Prevention Week. Information presentations, the educator should remember, do not require the audience to practice a technique. In each case, the educator is asking the audience to do something — to learn new fire and life safety skills.

Presentations are a central part of fire and life safety education programs. An education program (as discussed in Chapter 15, "Selecting Educational Materials") has specific measurable objectives and evaluation instruments, uses instructional methods that match the objectives, and uses appropriate materials to reach the objectives and reinforce the methods. Usually several presentations along with other program elements make up a fire and life safety education program.

This chapter provides general guidelines for planning presentations and describes how to build the three basic parts of a presentation. It also includes ways of keeping the audience's attention and lists "Ten Tips for Speakers." The effective use of audiovisual materials is also covered. The chapter closes with "Fifty Secrets of Success."

BEFORE THE PRESENTATION

Experienced presenters know that preparation is the key to success (Figure 17.1). Preparation has two basic parts: thinking about the audience and

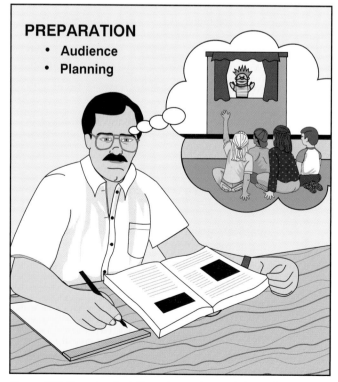

Figure 17.1 The educator tailors a lesson to match the audience.

planning a presentation that will help *that specific audience* do something (such as install a smoke detector or practice swimming safety) or learn something.

Consider the Audience

The members of the audience — not the presenter — are the most important people in a presentation. The audience must be foremost in the educator's mind throughout every step of preparation.

As fire and life safety educators prepare for every presentation, they can ask themselves these questions:

- Who is the audience?
- What does this audience need to learn from this presentation?
- What does this audience already know?
- How will their daily lives at home and at work influence their fire safety?
- How does this audience learn? (**NOTE**: See Chapter 13, "Learning Fire and Life Safety Educational Theory.")

> **Learning Characteristics: A Refresher**
>
> Educators design fire and life safety presentations to help the audience learn something. As you know from Chapter 13, "Learning Fire and Life Safety Educational Theory," a few characteristics are common to all learning.
>
> - Learning is a lifelong activity, beginning at birth and ending at death.
> - Learning can be very uncomfortable and stressful because it necessitates a change in attitude or behavior.
> - People learn at different rates.
> - People learn in a variety of ways.
> - To be effective, learning must be reinforced.
> - Effective learning requires support from the people who influence or control the students.
> - Learning is enhanced when the senses are stimulated.
> - Learning is most effective when it is focused on a specific behavior.
> - Learning is incremental.
> - Learners must identify with the importance or personal significance of the message.

Create the Presentation

Effective presentations have a clear beginning, a solid middle, and a strong ending. These three basic parts of a presentation are usually called the *opening*, the *body*, and the *close*. Use the following eight specific steps to creating such a presentation (Figure 17.2)[2]:

Step 1: Define the objectives.

Step 2: Design the close.

Step 3: Create the opening.

Step 4: Outline the body.

Step 5: Add "spice."

Step 6: Design visual aids.

Step 7: Create cheat sheets.

Step 8: Rehearse, rehearse, rehearse.

DEFINE THE OBJECTIVES

In defining the objectives for a presentation, the fire and life safety educator spells out what the audience can expect to learn how to do. The educational objectives for a presentation should be in the same format as objectives for an education program (**NOTE**: See "Chapter 10, Developing the Program Curriculum.") *The important point is that the educator clearly knows exactly what the audi-*

> **Sample Objectives for a Presentation**
>
> *Affective Objective*
>
> At the conclusion of the presentation to the Kiwanis Club on residential fire safety [*condition*], the Kiwanis participant will be able to relate two factors [*standard or criterion*] that illustrate the importance of testing and maintaining smoke detectors [*performance or behavior*].
>
> *Cognitive Objective*
>
> At the conclusion of the presentation to the Kiwanis Club on residential fire safety [*condition*], the Kiwanis participant will be able to describe three key steps [*standard or criterion*] in testing and maintaining smoke detectors [*performance or behavior*].
>
> *Psychomotor Objective*
>
> At the conclusion of the presentation to the Kiwanis Club on residential fire safety and given a smoke detector for demonstration purposes [*conditions*], the Kiwanis participant will be able to change the smoke detector's battery [*performance or behavior*] so that the detector alarm signals when tested [*standard or criterion*].

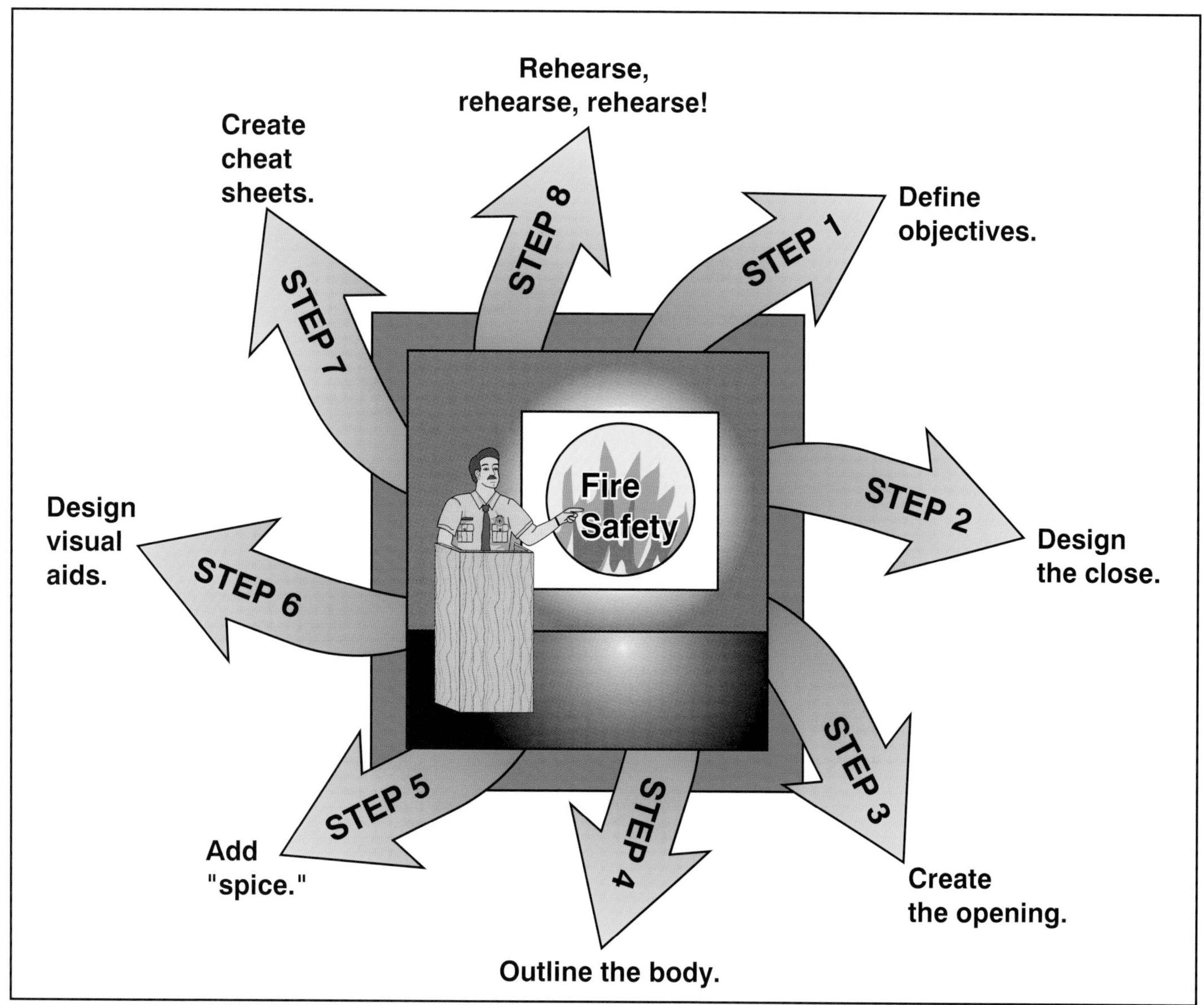

Figure 17.2 Eight steps to creating a presentation.

ence is expected to learn from the presentation. The rest of the planning activity is targeted toward fulfilling the presentation's objectives.

DESIGN THE CLOSE

The close is much more than just the end of the presentation; the close is the last two or three minutes of a presentation and is what the educator wants the audience to take away with them (Figure 17.3). For this reason, questions from the audience should come *before* the close. The close brings the entire presentation into sharp focus so that the audience will understand, remember, and act on what they have learned. (**NOTE**: In sales, the "close" is when the customer decides whether or not to buy.)

The close is the most important part of the presentation. As a result, experienced presenters spend as much time preparing for the close as for the entire presentation.

In designing a close, fire and life safety educators can ask themselves the following questions:

- What would I say if I had only two or three minutes with this audience?
- What do I most want this audience to understand, know, or do?
- Does the close summarize the information and motivate the audience?
- Does the close fulfill the objectives of the presentation?

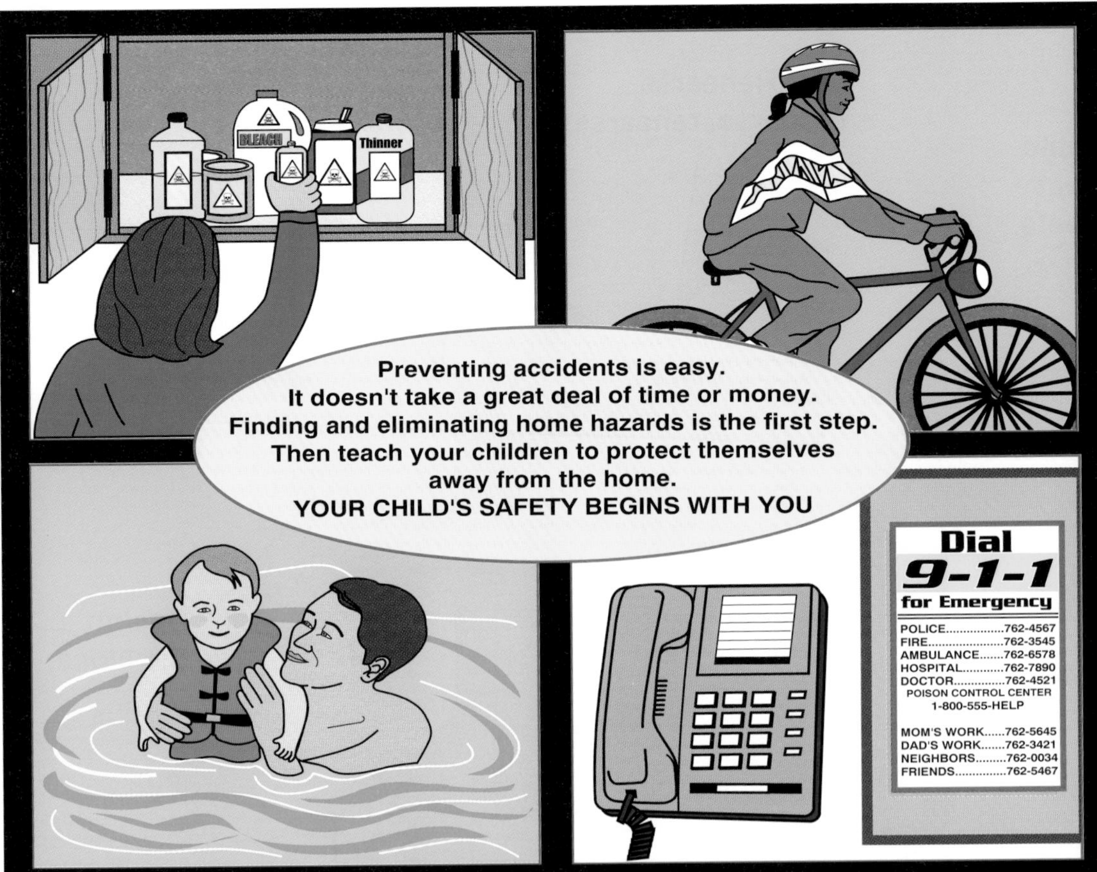
Thinner
BLEACH
Preventing accidents is easy.
It doesn't take a great deal of time or money.
Finding and eliminating home hazards is the first step.
Then teach your children to protect themselves
away from the home.
YOUR CHILD'S SAFETY BEGINS WITH YOU
Dial
9-1-1
for Emergency
POLICE.................762-4567
FIRE.....................762-3545
AMBULANCE.......762-6578
HOSPITAL...........762-7890
DOCTOR..............762-4521
POISON CONTROL CENTER
1-800-555-HELP
MOM'S WORK......762-5645
DAD'S WORK.......762-3421
NEIGHBORS.........762-0034
FRIENDS..............762-5467

Figure 17.3 The close contains the information that is most important for the audience to remember after the presentation.

Professional presenters often plan their closes word-for-word. The following is a sample close for a presentation to the Kiwanis on smoke detector testing and maintenance:

> "As you've learned in the last half hour, the single, most important thing you can do to make your family more fire safe is to have working smoke detectors in your home. Working smoke detectors alert you to a fire early enough to escape to safety and to call the fire department from the safety of a neighbor's home.
>
> What do you do to make sure that your smoke detectors will work when your family needs them? You test your detectors and you maintain them.
>
> Test your detectors monthly by pushing the test button or by using incense or cigarette smoke.
>
> Maintain your detectors by keeping their batteries fresh and by keeping them clean.
>
> These are easy steps to take for your family's safety, aren't they? Your family is worth it — can we count on you to do these few things for their fire safety?"

CREATE THE OPENING

The opening sets the scene for the entire presentation (Figure 17.4). Openings can be quite short — as little as two or three minutes. During the opening, the fire and life safety educator must accomplish three things:

- Take charge of the presentation.
- Capture the attention of the audience, and begin to establish rapport.
- Let the audience know what to expect — what is in it for them.

Through a series of small actions, the fire and life safety educator takes charge of the presentation in the first few seconds. These actions include starting on time, walking confidently to the front, making eye contact right away, pausing for a split second before beginning to speak, and speaking clearly — from the very first words.

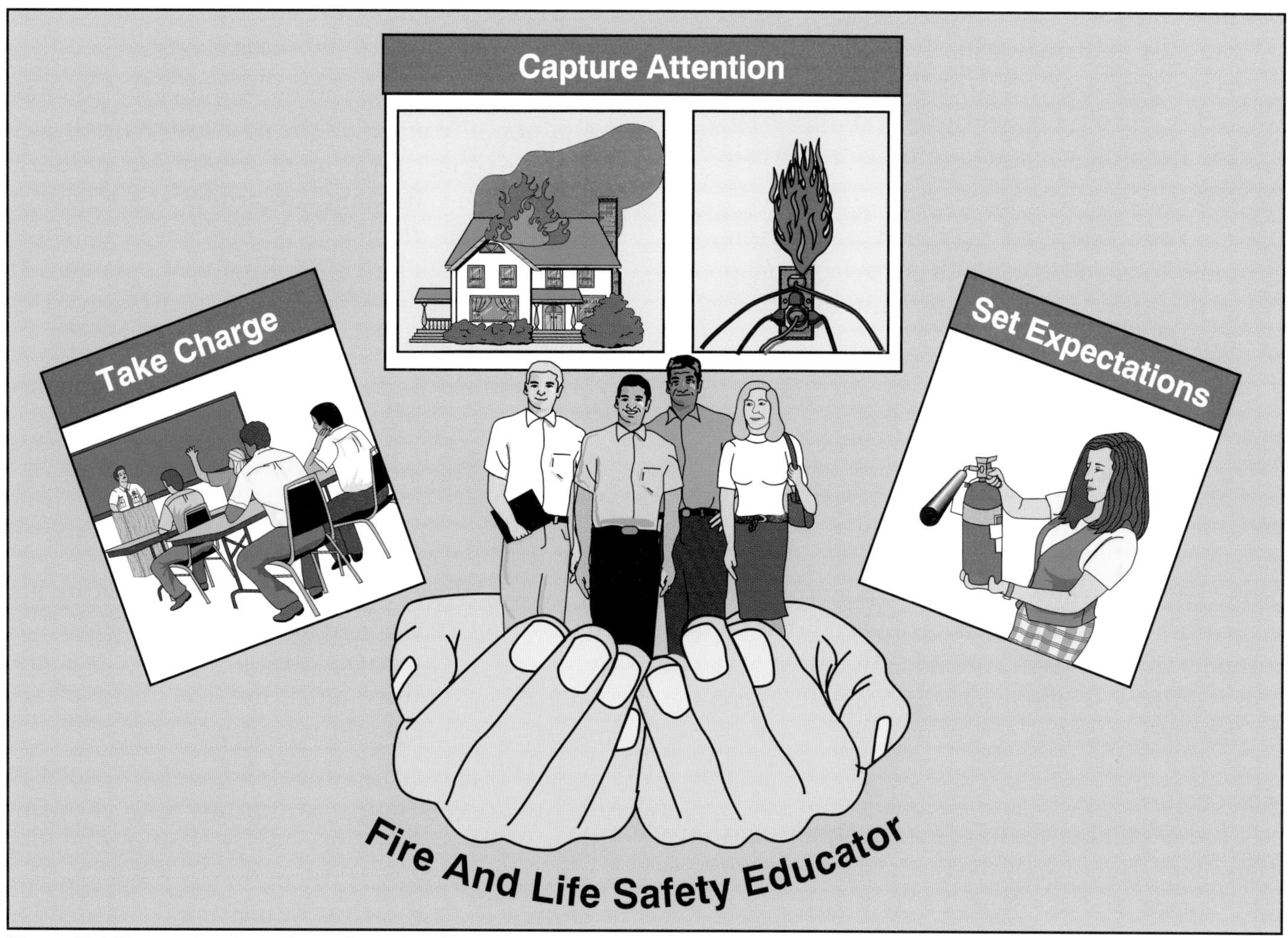

Figure 17.4 The opening draws the audience into the presentation.

Attention and rapport are related to each other: an attentive audience has established rapport with the speaker and vice versa. Connecting the audience and the presentation's topic is the most common way of gaining the audience's attention. Connecting the audience and the presenter is a common way of gaining rapport. Of course, smiling where appropriate helps establish rapport with the audience.

Opening a presentation also includes setting expectations. Most important, how can the audience expect to benefit from the presentation? What will they learn, and why does it matter to them? What solutions will be offered? How long will the presentation take? What format will be used? Will there be audiovisuals? Will there be breaks?

Professional presenters often plan their opening word-for-word. The following is a sample opening for the Kiwanis presentation on smoke detectors:

> "Thank you for inviting me to tell you about how to install and maintain smoke detectors in your homes.
>
> Just last week, an elderly couple who lived about two miles from here died during a fire in their home. Their smoke detector had no batteries in it. A working detector would probably have saved their lives.
>
> Do your elderly parents and neighbors have smoke detectors that work? Does your home have enough smoke detectors? Are they in good working order?
>
> At the end of the next thirty minutes, you'll know how smoke detectors sense fire in its earliest stages. You'll learn how to decide how many detectors your home

needs, as well as what to look for when you buy detectors. Finally — and this is a very important part of the presentation today — you'll learn the few simple steps for keeping your smoke detectors working.

You'll see some overhead transparencies, and each of you will get to look inside a detector. I'll welcome your questions anytime you have them.

Let's get started."

OUTLINE THE BODY

The body of the presentation begins with an outline of all *possible* key points. Often, the presenter is faced with more possible points than time. After listing all points, fire and life safety educators need to check themselves. Do the points support the objective and move the presentation toward its close? *Include only the points critical to this presentation.*

ADD SPICE

Today's audiences have extremely short attention spans. Because the body of the presentation is the longest and the most packed with information, it needs "spice" to keep the audience's attention.

Spice can take a number of forms: a change of pace or technique, the introduction of an attention-getting prop (such as a melted smoke detector that successfully alerted a family to a home fire), or an exercise that involves the participants. Such exercises are often called *energizers*.[3]

Energizers raise the energy level of the participants (and perhaps the educator as well!). At the same time, they promote readiness for learning, create excitement, overcome the effects of fatigue, and develop a sense of shared fun. Energizers are quick and often involve movement. In fact, the simplest energizer is to have participants stand and stretch.

Presenters find energizers and other splashes of spice most useful when a long session begins to drag, between long sessions, and after meals and breaks.

DESIGN VISUAL AIDS

So far, the fire and life safety educator has completed five steps in planning a presentation: defining the objectives, designing the close, creating the opening, outlining the body of the presentation, and adding spice.

At this point, the educator designs (or selects) visual aids for the presentation. Note that this approach is very different from grabbing a videotape on the way out the door for the presentation. Chapter 15, "Selecting Educational Materials," covers the characteristics of effective visual aids.

CREATE CHEAT SHEETS

Cheat sheets are the one or two pages or index cards that fire and life safety educators carry with them to a presentation. Individual

Adding "Spice" to Counteract the Short Attention Span

Did you know that the on-the-job attention span of a business executive is only six minutes? That the typical television network news story lasts only three minutes? That most television advertisements whiz on and off the screen in one minute or less? Both children and adults have short attention spans. To counteract short attention spans, try the following techniques:

- Think of a presentation as a series of scenes, and limit each scene to six minutes or less.
- Use phrases such as "Let me make a point here" or "Let's nail down this point" once in each scene.
- Segment the presentation with different audiovisual techniques.
- When team-teaching, change presenters every six minutes.
- Move throughout the entire room for the presentation; never stay in one place for the entire presentation.
- Think of a headline for each six-minute segment. Use this as shorthand for repetition, reinforcement, and summary.
- Use colors to mark segments in audiovisuals. Transparencies, posters, and flipcharts are especially easy to color code to match the segments of a presentation.

Reprinted from *"I Can See You Naked" A Fearless Guide To Making Great Presentations* by Ron Hoff.

people develop their own shorthand for cheat sheets, which often includes key points and phrases and times for major segments, along with instructor notes ("hand out brochure," for example). For precision and to aid recall, presenters often include numbers ("578 house fires last year") on cheat sheets.

REHEARSE, REHEARSE, REHEARSE

Rehearsal is the last — but not the least — step in preparing for a presentation. Rehearsal means speaking the actual words and using the audiovisuals. This run-through helps gauge the actual time needed. *There really is no substitute for rehearsal* (Figure 17.5).

Early in an educator's career, or when preparing for a new presentation, rehearsal will be fairly complete. A complete rehearsal will be word-for-word and may even be videotaped.

Even seasoned educators who are giving a presentation for the twentieth time will rehearse — maybe in the shower the morning of a talk and again in the car on the way to the presentation. Because the opening and closing are the most critical parts of a presentation, it is especially important to rehearse them.

Ten Tips for Speakers

- Tell the audience the presentation's objective — in their terms.
- Speak loudly and clearly.
- Be enthusiastic.
- Be confident.
- Use eye contact.
- Smile when appropriate.
- Pace and edit along the way.
- Watch for distracting mannerisms.
- Use AVs and handouts effectively.
- Begin and end on time.

USING AUDIOVISUALS EFFECTIVELY

Educators find audiovisual materials extremely useful supplements to fire and life safety education presentations. The educator must remember that audiovisuals are tools, not the presentation itself. Effective use of audiovisuals lets them serve as tools, rather than as a substitute for preparation.

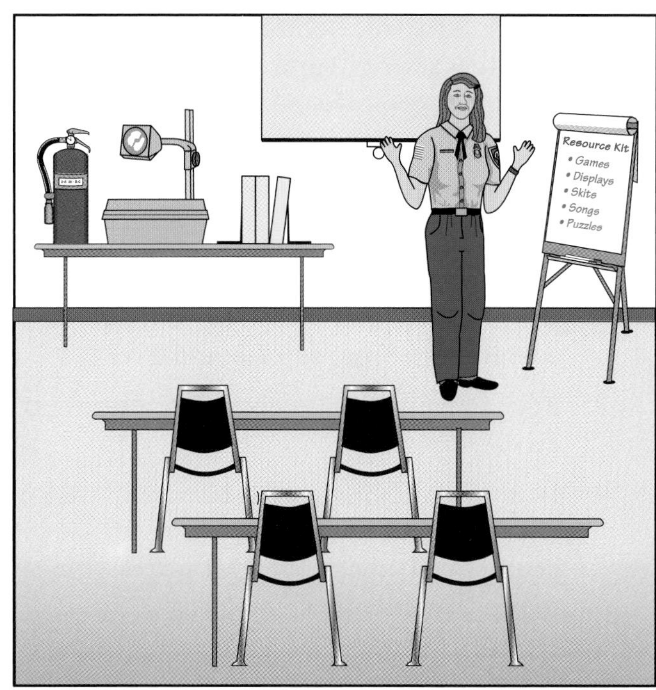

Figure 17.5 Practice is an essential part of preparing a presentation.

Among the dozens of techniques for using audiovisual materials effectively, the following suggestions are the most basic.[4]

Room setup

- Set up the room to locate the screen and projector 180 degrees away from any uncurtained windows.
- Check to see that no one in the audience is seated closer than twice the width of the screen and no farther away than six times the screen's width.

  Fire and life safety educators who routinely use the same screen can calculate the ideal seating arrangement.
- Before the audience arrives, sit in various areas of the room to make sure that the view of the screen is unobstructed.

Equipment

- Test all equipment before each presentation.

  If using 35 mm slides, test the projector and the remote advance. Check to ensure that all slides are loaded right side up and facing forward. Before using transparencies, test the light and clean the lens of the overhead projector. Also make sure that all transparencies are stacked correctly.

- Check for and correct keystoning.

  Keystoning is a distortion of the projected transparency image that happens when the projector and screen are not square to each other (Figures 17.6 and 17.7).

- Focus projectors before the audience arrives.

- If a microphone must be used, test it before the audience arrives. To check the sound level, speak the first few sentences of the presentation's opening.

- If using a wireless microphone or a long cord, test the sound level in several areas of the room before the audience arrives.

  One room may have "hot" areas (areas where the microphone is quite sensitive) or "dead" areas (areas where the microphone lacks sensitivity). As much as possible, avoid those hot spots and dead spots.

- Preset the volume on VCR monitors.

Audiovisual material

- Preview all material before using it the first time.

- Preview all material that someone else has used since your last use.

- After creating slides and transparencies, project and proofread them once before actually using them. (Mistakes are much more visible when projected!)

- Advance your own slides and overheads whenever possible — avoid needing to say "Next slide, please."

The educator/presenter

- Speak to the audience — never the screen.

- Cue videotapes before the audience arrives. Do not make the audience wait while you cue material.

- Rewind videotapes after the audience leaves.

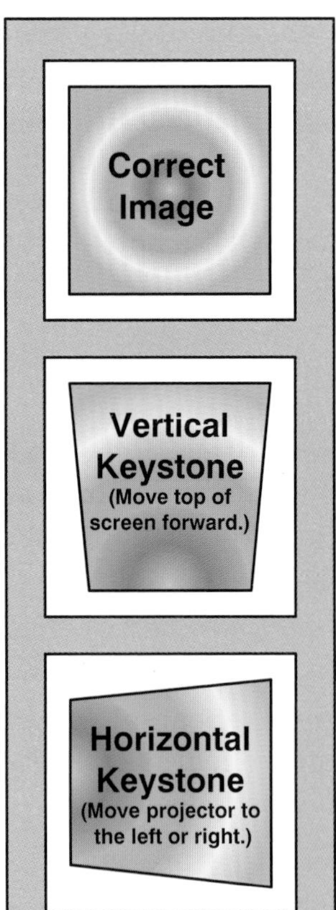

Figure 17.6 One of the problems encountered in using an overhead projector is a "keystoned" image.

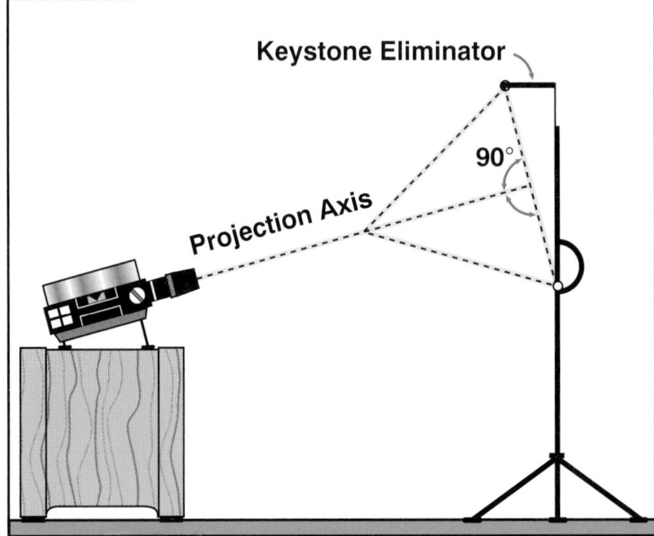

Figure 17.7 Keystoning can be eliminated by tilting the screen until it is perpendicular with the projector.

- Sort transparencies, remove them from any protective sleeves, and put them in order before the audience arrives.

- Rearrange and re-sort transparencies after the audience leaves.

By and large, audiovisual equipment is very reliable. However, equipment does occasionally

Specifically, this means explaining hazards and monitoring visitors. Station hazards to which to be alert include falling through the opening for a firefighter pole, slipping on a wet apparatus floor, fire vehicle traffic, or getting knocked down by firefighters hurrying to the apparatus. Being careful in the station house protects both the visitors and firefighters (Figure 18.9).

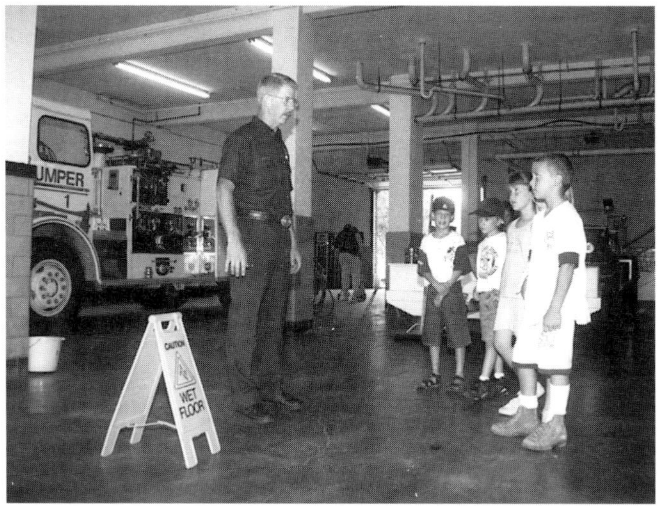

Figure 18.9 Safety is a primary concern when conducting station tours.

Safety is related to the number of people on the tour — and children will need more supervision than adults. Those in charge of station tours should check with local authorities on the number of adults required to supervise children.

Because children imitate what they see, live fire demonstrations are not recommended for children 10 years old or younger. Even for older children and adults, demonstrations have their own special hazards. Any live fire demonstration — even a small fire on a table top exhibit — is hazardous. The hazards of the demonstration should be discussed with the teacher or other group leader before the visit is scheduled. The educator should establish and enforce a clear line between the fire and the public (masking or duct tape on the ground or floor can mark the line). Ample fire fighting personnel and fire extinguishers should be on hand during the demonstration. The fire department attorney and building owner should approve any live fire demonstration and consider a rider on insurance policies.

Nonfire demonstrations can also be hazardous. For example, the weight of a shifting helmet broke the neck of a 5-year-old who was trying on the helmet. A child wearing firefighter boots may fall — and receive a head or facial injury. Educators (and those assisting) should be alert to such hazards, consider the age and size of the child, and share experiences and ideas with others.

GOOD PUBLIC RELATIONS PRACTICE

Guests in the fire station have a special interest in "their" fire station and "their" firefighters. So it is important for the fire and life safety educator to remember to "Put your best foot forward!"

- **Be friendly and courteous**. The visiting public is not an interruption — the public is why the fire service exists.

  Visitors may be shy or awkward and will appreciate a welcoming smile, "Hello!" or handshake. Spending time with children or foreign-born visitors (who may be uncomfortable with city officials or anyone in uniform) is especially important.

- **Be careful about conversation and language**. Voices carry in a fire station. The visitors will listen to everyone, not just the tour leader.

- **Respect the questions of visitors, and be prepared to answer them truthfully but appropriately for visitors' ages**. Visitors may be very curious about details of station life and fire fighting. Firefighters can also expect questions such as "How many smoke detectors do *you* have at home?" or "Do you *really* practice a home escape plan?"

  Questions reflect personal interest, and personal interest is the foundation of public support.

- **Stick to appropriate subjects**. Firefighters should never air their gripes — no matter how legitimate — about union contracts, pay scales, shift work, employment benefits, working conditions, or fire department operations during station tours or demonstrations.

Approaches to Juvenile Firesetting and Fire Play

> **Terms to Know**
>
> The fire and life safety educator needs to know the meanings of these terms:
>
> *Firesetting* is an intentional act that creates a disturbance or that harms people, animals, or objects. In children, firesetting often refers to repeated acts or to acts that happen during family or emotional difficulties.
>
> *Fire play* is other involvement with fire or fire materials, usually lighting matches or lighters without the approval or supervision of a parent. Fire play is often an isolated event that is motivated by curiosity. Fire play may result in accidental fire.
>
> *Arson* is a deliberate and malicious burning and is a crime. A fire does not become arson until a defendant is found guilty.

PROBLEM REVIEW

How big is the problem? Many fire prevention bureau personnel and others in the fire service have received an anguished call from a parent, "My child set a fire! What do I do?"

Until a generation or so ago, children who set fires or played with fire were often taken to the fire station for a stern lecture from a firefighter. The lecture was both the beginning and the end of "educational programs" or "treatment" for children who set or played with fire. More recently, trained members of the fire service have interviewed firesetters and their families, have worked on more sophisticated intervention strategies, and are working with mental health professionals to prevent future episodes of firesetting and fire play.

The increased emphasis on firesetter intervention programs was certainly needed. Fires set by children account for a surprising portion of the overall fire problem.[13]

- Child firesetting was responsible for 457 deaths in 1991 — nearly one out of every eight structural fire deaths.
- Child fire play accounts for more than one-third of fire deaths among preschool children.
- "Children playing" was the only fire cause to increase between 1980 and 1991.

Why are these numbers so high? Fire play is much more widespread than most parents — and firefighters — realize.

Children's interest in fire is "almost universal," according to researcher Dr. Ditsa Kafrey.[14] In fact, in her landmark study of 99 elementary school boys, 45 percent had engaged in fire play. Yet, only 9 percent of those fires were reported to the fire department. The firesetting and fire play began at a very early age: 18 percent of the fires were set by children under the age of three. Firesetting and fire play, however, tapered off after age seven. Many of the boys understood the consequences of their fire action.

Firefighters and psychologists in Rochester, New York, discovered similar trends.[15] In an in-depth look at 474 fires set by 617 children aged 1 to 16 years, the Rochester group compiled the following statistics:

- Thirty-eight percent of the children in grades one through eight admitted to playing with matches or lighters at some point in their lives.
- Fourteen percent of the children in grades one through eight admitted to playing with matches or lighters during the current school year.
- Only 3.5 percent of the children started a fire to which the fire department responded. In other words, fire incident data only includes the "tip of the iceberg" of fires started by children.
- Fire play increased with age (in contrast to Kafrey's findings). Only 10 percent of six-year-olds had ever played with matches or lighters. By age 12, more than half of children had played with matches or lighters, and more than 20 percent of 12-year-olds were currently playing.
- The fires were serious: 47 percent caused structural damage, and 10 percent caused injury or death.
- Eighty-five percent of the children seen by the fire department were boys.
- Black children played with fire at a younger age and tended to observe other

children's fire play more often that white or Hispanic children.

- Children who live in single-parent homes are slightly more likely to play with fire. On the other hand, children whose parents were unemployed or earned a low income were much more likely to play with fire than children with more affluent parents.
- There was a strong sense of control over fire. In fact, almost eight out of ten children thought they could extinguish a small fire.
- Recidivism (repeated incidents by the same child) was quite low, only 3.4 percent.

> "The majority of children who are seen by the fire department have no serious problems, are motivated primarily by a mischievous curiosity, and lack understanding of the dangers of fire play."
>
> *Children and Fire*, Second Report of the Rochester, New York, Fire Department Fire-Related Youth Program Development Project, State of New York Office of Fire Prevention and Control, 1986.

PROBLEM CORRECTION

Firesetting and fire play are very different. Children's natural curiosity, the mischievousness of some children, and children's desire to experiment and explore lead to occasional episodes of fire play. Other children set fires repeatedly, collect firesetting tools (matches or lighters), and are often troubled about some situation at home or school.

Firesetting and fire play are both dangerous and must be stopped. The techniques for stopping the two actions, of course, are quite different.

Deciding whether a child is involved in firesetting or fire play is the first step in stopping the dangerous behavior. This decision process is called *assessment*. Because concerned parents call the fire department, the fire service often begins the assessment process.

In its simplest form, assessment involves determining why the fire activity happened (was the child curious and mischievous? angry? upset by troubles at home or at school?), how often the activity happened (once or perhaps twice versus several times), and the child's age (older children are expected to be less curious and more aware of the consequences of fire). The answers to these questions may pinpoint issues in the child's home, school, or relationships that a trained therapist will address.

As a rule of thumb, children who have played with fire once or twice will benefit from educational programs conducted by fire and life safety educators. Child firesetters, on the other hand, need the skills of a mental health professional. Educational intervention and referral to a mental health professional are both designed to stop the child's dangerous acts. Depending on the circumstances, it may be necessary to involve the juvenile justice system to stop the child's actions.

ASSESSMENT TECHNIQUES

The fire and life safety educator does not need to "start from scratch" in deciding whether a child's action is fire play or firesetting. Several time-tested assessment techniques are available.

For example, a U.S. Fire Administration Task Force prepared three firesetter handbooks[16,17,18] that were later revised by the International Association of Fire Chiefs (Figure 18.10). (NOTE : Despite the title of "firesetter handbooks," the three publications cover both firesetting and fire play.) The handbooks cover the psychology of a particular age group and give detailed guide-

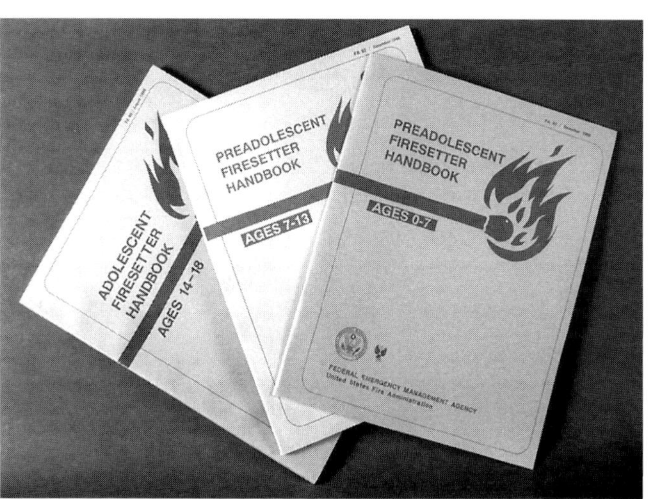

Figure 18.10 U.S. Fire Administration Firesetter Handbooks.

lines on interviewing children and their families. They also outline intervention strategies for fire play and provide direction on referring a child to a mental health professional. Finally, the handbooks give guidance on building a community coalition (of law enforcement personnel, medical and mental health professionals, and educators) to develop intervention strategies.

The fire and life safety educator can also adopt the assessment questions used by mental health professionals in their initial interview with a child or family.[19] This assessment includes questions such as the following:

- Was the fire deliberately set? Did an accidental fire result from extremely poor judgment or recklessness?
- What does the child say about intention and motive? Do the circumstances of the fire fit what the child says?
- Are the incidents repeated? Are the incidents repeated after educational intervention?
- How did the child react to the fire? attempt at extinguishment? remorseful?
- Were other children involved? Was there extreme peer pressure? gang activity?
- How did the family react?
- What is the overall family situation? Is the family having other difficulties? Is there any evidence of physical or sexual abuse? Is there any evidence of substance abuse?
- Has the child had other problems at home or at school?

Of course, fire and life safety educators are *not* mental health professionals. Fire and life safety educators should always involve mental health professionals in setting up their intervention and referral programs and practices. These questions at a screening interview are only designed to give a first impression about whether the child is involved in fire play or firesetting. The interview is just the first step in determining how serious the problem is and what the next steps should be. The next two sections address the topics of children involved in fire play and firesetting.

DEALING WITH CHILDREN INVOLVED WITH FIRE PLAY

Sometime during their career, fire and life safety educators will use education to stop children from playing with fire. The educational objective for this activity could be worded as follows:

> "The child and family will describe three new fire safety behaviors and explain in their own words why fire play cannot happen again."

Note that the fire and life safety educator's objective is educational. The objective is not to alarm the child or family, to punish the child, or to judge parenting skills.

(**NOTE**: See Chapter 10, "Developing the Program Curriculum," to learn about educational objectives.)

The child's age determines the behaviors that fire and life safety educators teach to a child who has been involved in fire play. The behaviors, though, are the same as for children who have not (yet) played with fire. There are two main differences between education for children who have played with fire and education for other children:

- Children who have played with fire often will receive their education one-on-one, rather than in a larger group of children.
- Parents and other family members of such children are more likely to take part in the education session.

For preschool children who have played with fire, critical behaviors from *Learn Not to Burn®: The Pre-School Program* include "Stay away from hot things that can hurt," "Tell a grown-up when you find matches or lighters," "Stop, drop, and roll if your clothes catch fire," and "Cool a burn". "Recognize the firefighter as a helper" may also be a key behavior (Figure 18.11).

In much the same way, elementary age children who have played with fire especially need to know behaviors such as "Uses matches and lighters safely," "Practices fire safety with flammable liquids," and "Encourages fire safe smoking habits."

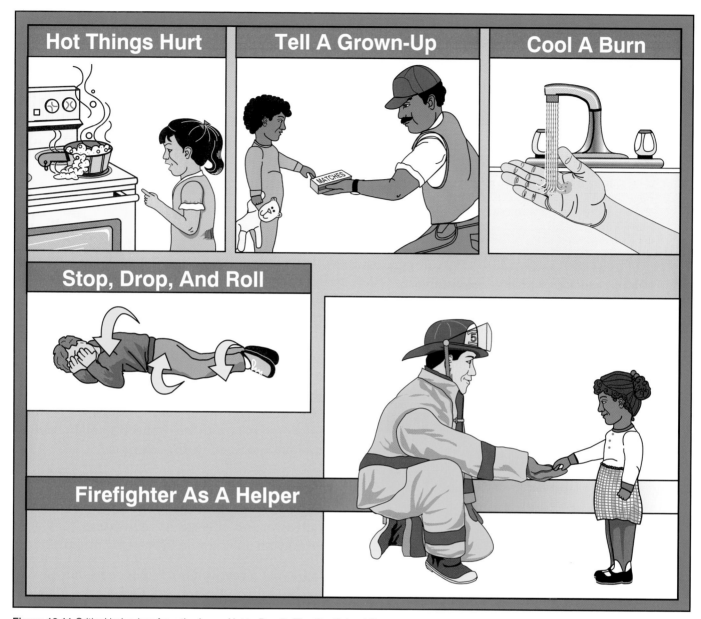

Figure 18.11 Critical behaviors from the *Learn Not to Burn®: The Pre-School Program*.

GETTING PROFESSIONAL HELP FOR FIRESETTERS

Children who are involved in firesetting need help beyond what even the most concerned and skillful fire and life safety educator can offer. Firesetters — those who intentionally and often repeatedly set fires for reasons other than curiosity or mischievousness — need care by a mental health professional.

This fact raises two issues for fire and life safety educators: 1) the need to develop a list of those to whom to refer the child and 2) how to tell the parents about the child's need for mental health care.

There are two types of referrals — public and private — depending on who will pay for mental health services. Public agencies may provide mental health services at no charge or for a small fee. Private practitioners charge a fee (which may be covered by health insurance). Public agencies that work with firesetters and their families include hospitals, clinics, child protective services and the juvenile justice system, and social service agencies. The staff at public agencies may include psychiatrists, psychiatric nurses, psychologists, and social workers. These same kinds of licensed professionals also may be in private practice. Fire and life safety educators

Suggestions for Educational Intervention

For ages 0-7*

- Ask the child how to help people not get hurt by fire. Discuss the child's ideas.
- Show appropriate teaching films, especially those showing danger to firefighters. Showing burn victims is NOT recommended for children in this age group.
- Invite the child to help prevent fires at home. Stress the child's responsibility in keeping people safe from fire. Have the child promise to tell a grown-up if matches and lighters are found or to use them only with adult supervision (depending upon the age of the child). Ask the child to explain, in his or her own words, why that is important. Assign a fire prevention task at home, such as emptying wastebaskets or checking to make sure the power light on the smoke detectors are lit.

For ages 7-13**

- Adopt educational strategies similar to those for younger children, but place more emphasis on the child's responsibility.
- Showing burn victims is not recommended for children under the age of 12. Use extreme caution in showing photos of burn victims to children aged 12-13 or in taking them to visit a burn center; get parents' permission, and consult with the child's therapist (if there is one).

* Adapted from *Preadolescent Firesetter Handbook, Ages 0-7*, United States Fire Administration, FA 83, December 1988.

** Adapted from *Preadolescent Firesetter Handbook, Ages 7-13*, United States Fire Administration, FA 82, December 1988.

About Scare Tactics and Saturation Tactics

Scare tactics are not effective education. Because they are concerned for the child's safety, some fire and life safety educators are tempted to show pictures of injured (or even dead) children or pets, to show burned toys, or to threaten the child with punishment, hospitalization, or painful medical treatment. Especially for young children, scare tactics may be overly frightening. Avoid scare tactics, and use good education.

Saturation tactics — such as forcing a child to light 200 matches or to light a lighter 100 times — were once used to satisfy a child's curiosity about fire. Saturation tactics were also seen as a way to make fire play boring and unpleasant. Saturation tactics are closer to punishment than education, and saturation tactics are "negative modeling" — they show exactly the act that the education program is trying to prevent! Saturation tactics are not recommended for use by the fire service or by other unlicensed people. These tactics are to be used only by trained mental health professionals as part of an entire treatment program.

need to have a current referral list of public agencies and private practitioners. The list can include information on whether private practitioners use a sliding scale, based on income and ability to pay.

Telling parents that their child needs psychological help can feel awkward and difficult. (See the sidebar, "Gaining Parents' Cooperation.")

CONCLUSION

Fire and life safety behaviors are the raw material that the educator uses to teach skills that the public can remember and use correctly, even during a life-threatening emergency. The behaviors can — and should — be taught in a variety of different ways, depending on the educational objective and on the audience. The age, developmental level, and cultural background of the audience are among the factors to consider when teaching fire and life safety behaviors. In many ways, the other chapters of this manual are devoted to how to teach the fire and life safety behaviors outlined in this chapter.

FOR MORE INFORMATION

The following publications are resources in which fire and life safety educators may find information on juvenile firesetting and fire play.

Robert G. Vreeland and Bernard M. Levin, "Psychological Aspects of Firesetting," Fires and *Human Behaviour* (2nd ed.), David Canter (ed.), David Fulton Publishers, London, 1990, pp. 31-46.

Wendy S. Grolnick, Robert E. Cole, Loretta Laurenitis, and Paul Schwartzman, "Playing with Fire: A Developmental Assessment of Children's Fire Understanding and Experience," *Journal of Clinical Child Psychology*, Vol. 19, No. 2, pp. 128-135, 1990.

Jessica Gaynor and C. Hatcher, *The Psychology of Child Firesetting*, Brunner/Mazel Publishers, New York, 1987.

Mary Jane Dittmar, "Juvenile Firesetting: An Old Problem Gets A New Look," *Fire Engineering*, December 1991, pp. 49+.

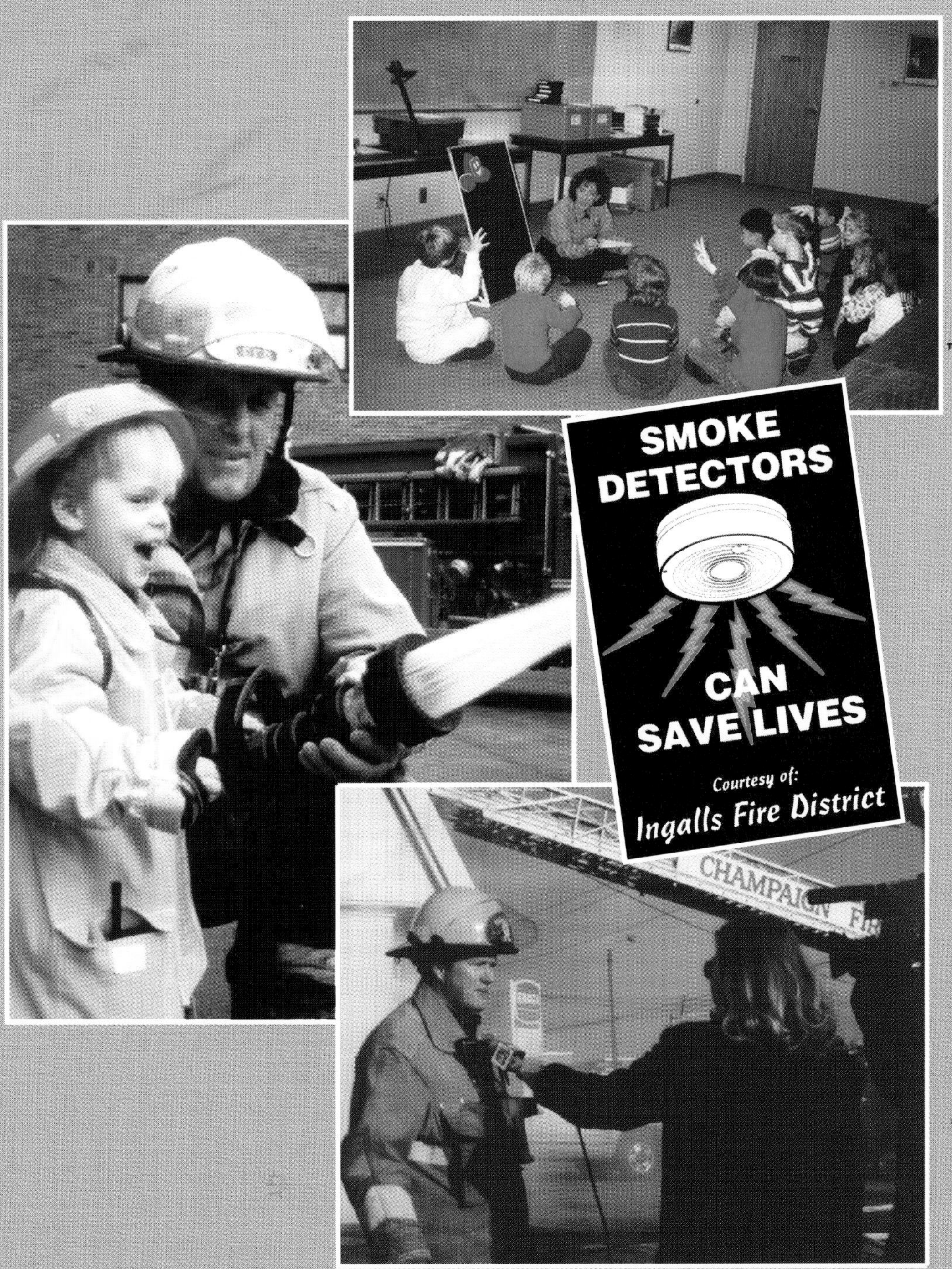
SMOKE
DETECTORS
CAN
SAVE LIVES
Courtesy of:
Ingalls Fire District
CHAMPAIGN

Appendices

Appendix A

Circumstances of Injury Classification in Children

Motor vehicle occupant deaths are those that occur in traffic and involve children who are passengers (or, occasionally, drivers) in cars or trucks.

Pedestrian traffic deaths refer to children who are struck and killed on public roads when not in or on a motor vehicle or bicycle.

Pedestrian nontraffic deaths occur off of public roads, for example in driveways and parking lots.

Motorcyclist deaths include all children categorized as occupants (riders) of motorcycles, regardless of whether the fatality occurred on public or private property.

Bicyclist deaths include any child on a vehicle that is operated solely by pedals and therefore exclude children riding motorized bicycles.

Other motor-vehicle-related deaths include those involving all-terrain vehicles (ATVs), snowmobiles, mopeds, and minibikes.

Total motor-vehicle-related deaths include all deaths in the previous six categories.

Air transport deaths include both commercial and private aviation.

Poisoning by solid or liquid, when fatal, typically involves medication or drugs (such as antidepressants, methadone, and cardiovascular drugs) or petroleum products (such as kerosene).

Poisoning by gas or vapor usually involves carbon monoxide from motor vehicle exhaust or less commonly from home heaters. Most deaths in house fires are actually due to carbon monoxide poisoning from smoke inhalation, but such deaths are classified with fire deaths.

Falls, although the most common cause of injury, are rarely fatal unless a child falls from a height or the head strikes a hard surface, such as concrete.

House fires cause 92 percent of all unintentional burn and fire-related deaths in children and therefore are analyzed as a specific category. House fires are the major cause of death in black children aged 1-9.

Drowning includes deaths related to boats (about 5 percent of childhood drownings) and drownings in bathtubs (about 9 percent).

Aspiration of food into the respiratory tract is most likely to be fatal if the food is round (hot dogs, grapes, peanuts, round candies, etc.).

Aspiration of other materials, as in the case of food, is most likely to cause fatal obstruction of the airway if the material is round (for example, balls, nipples from nursing bottles, etc.).

Suffocation occurs when the mouth and nose are covered (for example, by a plastic bag or fallen earth) or when oxygen is not available for other reasons.

Unintentional firearm deaths constitute about 40 percent of all gun deaths in the 0-14 year age group.

Electric current fatalities among children occur at home in about half of all cases; in about one-tenth of all cases, they involve contact with transmission lines.

Farm machinery causes about 85 percent of all machinery-related deaths in children and therefore is separately categorized. It is a major cause of childhood death in many farm states.

Medical or surgical deaths include those resulting from mistakes during medical or surgical care (which cause about 12 percent of deaths in this category), adverse reactions to drugs (10 percent), or, most commonly, surgical or medical procedures that result in abnormal reactions in a patient.

Other unintentional deaths include deaths from falling objects (about 80 annually), burns other than those from house fires, pedestrians killed by trains, children killed by a moving object or other person (for example, a baseball bat, air rifle pellet, or football player), animals being ridden, and falls from bicycles.

Suicide includes all deaths from intentionally self-inflicted injury. Death rates increase rapidly in the early teens.

Homicide includes deaths from child abuse, arson, and other intentional injuries such as those from shooting, strangulation, drowning, or knifing. Firearms are the most frequently used weapon. Homicide is the leading cause of injury death in the first year of life.

Unknown intent refers to deaths in which it is not determined whether the injury was unintentional or deliberately inflicted by the deceased or another person. Most of these deaths involve burns, drowning, or firearms.

Excerpted from Baker and Waller, "Circumstances of Injury Classification," *Childhood Injury — State-by-State Mortality Facts*, Johns Hopkins Injury Prevention Center, January 1989.

Appendix B

Public Service Announcements

Introduction

There are many ways to provide public service announcements. In order to coordinate and professionalize the process, it may be useful to make a schedule of ideas to be shared with the public. Decide whether the PSAs will be provided monthly, weekly, or quarterly. Create a schedule that includes the dates when the messages will be written, when they will be delivered to the media, and when they should be run. Include the topic of the message. Check with local media outlets to find out what format will be most useful. Is there a particular format to follow? Is providing facts all that is needed? Will someone within the fire department write or produce the actual print or broadcast PSA? Will media personnel help find a local celebrity to appear in the safety messages?

A few PSAs are included in this manual simply to move the fire and life safety educator along the right track. A creative fire and life safety educator will quickly learn which topics need to be covered in his or her community and will follow through with those ideas.

Sample PSA Schedule

Month	Date Written	Date Released	Date Used	Topic — Prevention
January				CO detection
February				Enhanced 9-1-1 system
March				Hot liquid burns
April				Leaf burning Storms/tornado
May				Home cleanup Flammable liquids
June				Bicycle safety Fireworks safety
July				Outdoor fire safety
August				"Matches are tools, not toys"
September				Fire Prevention Week activities
October				Fire Prevention Month using NFPA annual theme
November				Cooking safety
December				Holiday hints

A Dozen Ideas to Create PSAs For Radio Spots or Newspaper Filler

1. Replace smoke detectors every ten years, and replace batteries at least once a year.
2. Make your place fire safe:
   - Keep items a safe distance (three feet) from radiators, heaters, fireplaces.
   - Electric space heaters must meet the standards of a reputable testing facility.
   - Keep hot liquid foods out of the way of curious hands.
   - Store gasoline in approved metal containers away from heat or sparks.
3. Keep matches and lighters away from children. Fires don't just start—they are started.
4. Store cleaning supplies and poisons in a locked cupboard out of reach of children.
5. Seat Belts: On a hot day check the metal clips of the seat belt before buckling a child into the seat. Cover the clips with a towel or material to help keep them cool.
6. Get low and go—under the smoke, outside, to a designated meeting place.
7. Plan two ways out of each room in the home.
8. Once outside, stay at the meeting place. Never go back inside the building that is on fire.
9. Use oven mitts when removing foods from the microwave. Hot dishes and steam from foods heated in a microwave cause serious burns.
10. Don't lose your head. Use it! Wear a helmet when bicycling or motorcycling.
11. Keep fires in the fireplace. Have the chimney inspected and cleaned before winter.
12. Q & A—After an earthquake hits:
    A. Sit down, relax, and smoke a cigarette
    B. Sit down, relax, and listen to the radio
    C. Telephone Aunt Edith
    D. Drive over to see Aunt Edith

    Correct answer: B

Sample Public Service Announcements

The PSAs that follow are grouped according to type: either prevention, protection, or information. The text presented here is that of the main copy of the PSAs. Remember to provide the important additional information such as your name and phone number, run date, etc., when submitting PSAs.

Prevention PSAs

Bicycle Safety

Bicycle safely. Don't forget: Your small human-powered vehicle shares the road with much larger motor-powered vehicles. Use your head and wear a bicycle helmet. Ride in the designated bicycle lane. Ride with the traffic (on the right side of the road), and use hand signals to notify motor vehicles and others of your intentions.

-20-

****

Christmas

Planning a holiday party in your home, office, church, or school? Holiday parties often center around a live Christmas tree—and the [*your department or facility name*] reminds you that evergreen trees catch fire easily and burn furiously.

So, make safety as much a part of your holiday plans as the decorations or refreshments. Take these precautions:

- Purchase a small tree and keep it outdoors until just before Christmas.
- After bringing the tree indoors, remember to keep it moist and cool.
- Don't erect the tree near a stairway or elevator shaft that would produce a draft.
- Erect the tree away from any possible source of heat or sparks such as computers, copying machines, heaters or heater vents, light switches, electric trains, wood stoves, or fireplaces.
- Don't let the tree block a door or any exit.

- Be sure that all light sets and electric cords are in good condition and bear the UL label of fire and shock safety.
- Provide plenty of large, deep ashtrays for smokers—and don't allow smoking near the tree.
- Have someone in authority water and check the tree every day to determine whether or not it should be left up.
- When needles start to drop, take the tree down and discard it outdoors.
- Don't let fire come to your party! Plan to purchase and use a flame-retardant artificial tree in the coming years' celebrations.

-60-

****

Halloween

Boooooooooo! Is Halloween sneaking up on you? Make Halloween safe this year. The [*your department or facility name*] urges you to heed the following safety rules:

- Keep all matches, lighters, and candles out of the reach of children.
- Do not use lighted candles in jack-o-lanterns. Paint on faces instead, or use glue or toothpicks to attach fruit and vegetable features.
- Never place lighted candles in your windows or on your porch or steps where trick-or-treaters' costumes may contact them and ignite.
- Be sure that costumes are flame-retardant before your children put them on: Dip costumes into a solution of 4 ounces of boric acid and 9 ounces of borax to 1 gallon of water.
- Ensure that costumes do not hamper children's vision. Children must be able to see oncoming vehicles, curbs, steps, lighted candles, and hazardous costume props such as swords and wands.
- Escort young children on their trick-or-treat rounds.
- Provide older children with some candy from your own supply, and caution them against eating *any* other treats until all goodies have been inspected by you.

-60-

****

CO Poisoning

If you live in one of today's energy efficient homes, you may be at risk from carbon-monoxide poisoning. Protect yourself and your family with a carbon monoxide detector. Contact us at [*your department or facility name and phone number*].

-10-

****

Pedestrian Safety

Each year many children are hurt or killed while walking, running, or playing near the street. Parents: Here are a few tips for your children so they can be street smart.

- Stop at the curb and never run into the street.
- Before stepping from the curb, look for traffic left, right, and left again.
- Wait until traffic is clear and then carefully begin to cross; keep on looking both ways until you have safely crossed.

These rules are easy to understand and will help your children be street smart. A pedestrian safety message from this station and your local fire department.

-30-

****

Burn Prevention

Burns are life-long injuries. Sadly, almost all childhood burn injuries can be prevented. Here's some good advice for preventing burns: Keep hot foods and drinks away from the edge of tables, stoves, and counters. When cooking, keep your children away from the stove, and turn pot handles toward the back of the stove. Test bath water before giving your child a bath. A burn safety message from this station and your local fire department.

-30-

****

Bike Safety

Every child should know the rules of the road—the bike road, that is. Here are some riding do's to teach your children:

- Stop and look in every direction before riding onto a street.
- Ride as far to the right side of the road as possible.
- Obey all traffic lights and signs.
- Always walk the bike across intersections.

Remember Mom and Dad, your children are counting on you to keep them safe. Take time to teach them the rules of the road. A bike safety message from this station and your local fire department.

-30-

****

Fire Safety

Have you ever wondered what your children do when they're alone? Child fire play is the leading cause of fire in [*your city*]. Keep matches and lighters out of reach and sight. Talk to your children about the dangers of playing with fire. Most important, always be a fire-safe role model for your children. A fire safety message from this station and your local fire department.

-30-

****

Fireplace Safety

[Your department name] firefighters remind you to keep a fire safe fireplace.

- Have the fireplace cleaned professionally at least once a year, clearing out soot and creosote that can ignite and burn.
- Burn only seasoned dry hardwoods like oak, maple, birch, and hickory.
- Remove ashes in a metal container, and store them outside.
- Use a fireplace screen. It can prevent sparks and logs from slipping out and starting a fire.

Keep a fire safe fireplace.

-30-

****

Cooking Safety

If you leave the stove unattended when you're cooking, you could burn a **lot** more than your dinner.

When creating that special meal, stay in the kitchen. If you must leave, carry a pot holder with you as a reminder of the food on the stove.

Remember—the best time to stop a fire is before it starts.

The *[your department or facility name]* provides free education programs in an effort to keep you safe from burns and the ravages of fire. For more information, call *[telephone number of contact in your department or facility]*.

-30-

****

Electrical Outlet Safety

You might be shocked at just how easily an overloaded electrical outlet can start a fire.

Plug only one appliance into each outlet. Get rid of appliances with frayed or worn insulation. Avoid extension cords.

And, don't ever try to fool with the fuse box by jumping wires. That fuse box is your first line of defense against electrical fire.

Remember—the best time to stop a fire is before it starts.

This message is brought to you by the *[your department or facility name]*.

-30-

****

Wood-Burning Stoves

Wood-burning stoves are getting more popular all the time . . . but if you're not careful, they can be deadly. By following a few simple safety rules, you can keep the fire where it belongs . . . in the stove.

Be sure to have all connector pipes and chimneys inspected by professionals each year.

Never use gasoline, kerosene, charcoal starter, or other flammable liquids to light or kindle a fire.

Empty all ashes into a metal container with a tight-fitting lid.

Keep your family warm **and** safe this winter.

This message is brought to you by the *[your department or facility name]* and *[radio/television station]*.

-30-

****

Flammable Liquids

One gallon of gasoline equals the explosive power of six sticks of dynamite.

Gasoline vapors are heavier than air and settle to the floor or lowest point. The vapors then flow invisibly along the entire floor and can be ignited by a flame or spark anywhere in the garage.

For this reason, store gasoline in an approved safety can with a spring-valve closure, vapor vent, and pour spout—**away from heat or flame**.

The *[your department or facility name]* reminds you to check for hazards and make your home fire safe.

-30-

****

Chimney Cleaning

Birds and raccoons love to turn chimneys into their homes. Nests and animals block proper airflow through the fireplace and chimney—contributing to chimney fires. Chimney caps and screens can help keep the critters out and you safe.

The *[your department or facility name]* reminds you to keep your chimney clean and fire safe.

-30-

****

Protection PSAs

Family Fire Safety

Fire safety is a family affair. Sit down with your family, and plan fire escape routes. Teach your children safe escape behaviors such as feeling the door for heat before opening it and crawling low under smoke. Make sure that all family members know two ways out of each room. Practice Operation EDITH (Exit Drills in the Home).

-20-

****

Bike Safety

Did you know that the child who wears a helmet while riding a bike is ninety percent less likely to sustain a brain injury than the child without a helmet? Every child who rides a bike should wear an approved, properly fitted helmet. The helmet's safety strap should always be fastened. A properly fitted helmet is comfortable and does not slide around when the safety strap is fastened. A bike safety message from this station and your local fire department.

-30-

****

Residential Sprinklers

Building your dream home? **Insist** on a residential sprinkler system. It will lower your insurance rates and raise your life expectancy. Today's systems are effective, fail-safe, and tastefully inconspicuous. And, residential sprinklers are cheap—particularly when you look at the cost of **not** installing them. Call your local fire department for more information.

-30-

****

Smoke Detectors

(*15 seconds*) BEEEEEEEEEP....(*Sound effect: Sound of smoke detector alarm*)

Hear that sound? That's the sound of a working smoke detector, telling you it's ready to alert you if there's a fire. It's a sound that **could** save your life. Keep *your* smoke detectors working by testing them regularly. This message is brought to you by *[radio/television station]* and the *[your department or facility name]*.

-30-

****

Information PSAs

Statistical Information

[*Fifty Oklahomans*] have died in the first seven months of this year—not from cancer—not from automobile accidents—from fire. Fire is [*Oklahoma's second*] leading cause of accidental death. [*Sponsor's name*] and your local fire department urge you to "Learn Not to Burn®."

-15-

****

Fire Safety

Do you have a child between the ages of 1 and 14? Do you know that every year accidents take the lives of over 11,000 children in that age group? That's over three times the child death rate for any illness! In the home, the top child killer accident is fire . . . and since December and January are the worst months for fire deaths, the [*your department or facility name*] urges you to begin today taking the following safety precautions.

First, make your home as fire safe as possible, and keep hazards such as matches, hot liquids, and electric appliances out of children's reach. Second, make safety a part of every child's daily training. Remember, fire hazards may be an old story to you, but they're a new story to every child. Give that story a happy ending.

-60-

****

Appendix C
Example SOP for the Public Information Officer

UPPER HILLS	SECTION:	3111	PAGE: 1
FIRE DEPARTMENT	SUBJECT:	Public Information Officer	
Administrative			
Policy	DATE:	December 6, 1996	

PURPOSE

The purpose of this policy is to detail operational procedures for the Upper Hills Fire Department Public Information Officer (PIO).

SCOPE

This policy applies to release of all official Department information by the Public Information Officer to media and other organizations. This policy shall be adhered to by all members of the department unless otherwise approved by the Fire Chief.

PROCEDURE

Notification

1. The Public Information Officer shall be notified by the District Chief/Incident Commander of any injury or death to any fire department personnel or civilians at a fire, hazardous material, or special rescue incident; any evacuation of civilians due to unusual hazards; or any other situation which the Shift Commander or Incident Commander deems appropriate.
2. The Communication Center shall notify the Public Information Officer by pager or telephone of any fire requiring a multiple company response; any incident requiring two or more alarms; any high angle or special rescue incident; or any incident involving mutual aid with other fire departments.
3. The Investigations Section shall notify the Public Information Officer any time a civilian(s) is displaced from their residence or business due to fire damage; any situation in which a fire protection system contributed to the protection of life or property; or any other situation deemed appropriate or of interest to the media.

Release of Information

1. All release of information regarding policy issues of the department shall be coordinated through the Public Information Officer.
2. The Fire Chief shall be notified by the Public Information Officer of any significant incident before the release of information to the media.
3. The Fire Chief shall approve the release of any information which may be of special interest or involve other City departments.
4. The Public Communication Department shall be consulted prior to the release of any information which may impact public perception of the City or any of its departments. The Public Information Officer shall maintain an open channel of communication with the representative of the Public Communication Department and foster a positive relationship with that representative.
5. The Incident Commander or his/her representative may conduct on-scene interviews with local media regarding specific operations at any incident which does not require the Public Information Officer. However, any requests for other information by the media will be referred to the Public Information Officer.

Incident Command System

1. An Incident Commander may request the Public Information Officer at his/her discretion to assist with on-scene operations.
2. The Public Information Officer shall assume the role of "Information" within the Incident Command System. If the Public Information Officer is not present, the Incident Commander may assign a person to that function until the arrival of the Department Public Information Officer.
3. At incidents that do not require the response of the Public Information Officer, the Incident Commander, or his/her representative, will fulfill the function of "Information." *See Release of Information, Number 5 above.*
4. The Public Information Officer will coordinate all release of information with the Incident Commander prior to its release.
5. Any release of information at an emergency scene shall be done within the guidelines set forth in other sections of this policy.

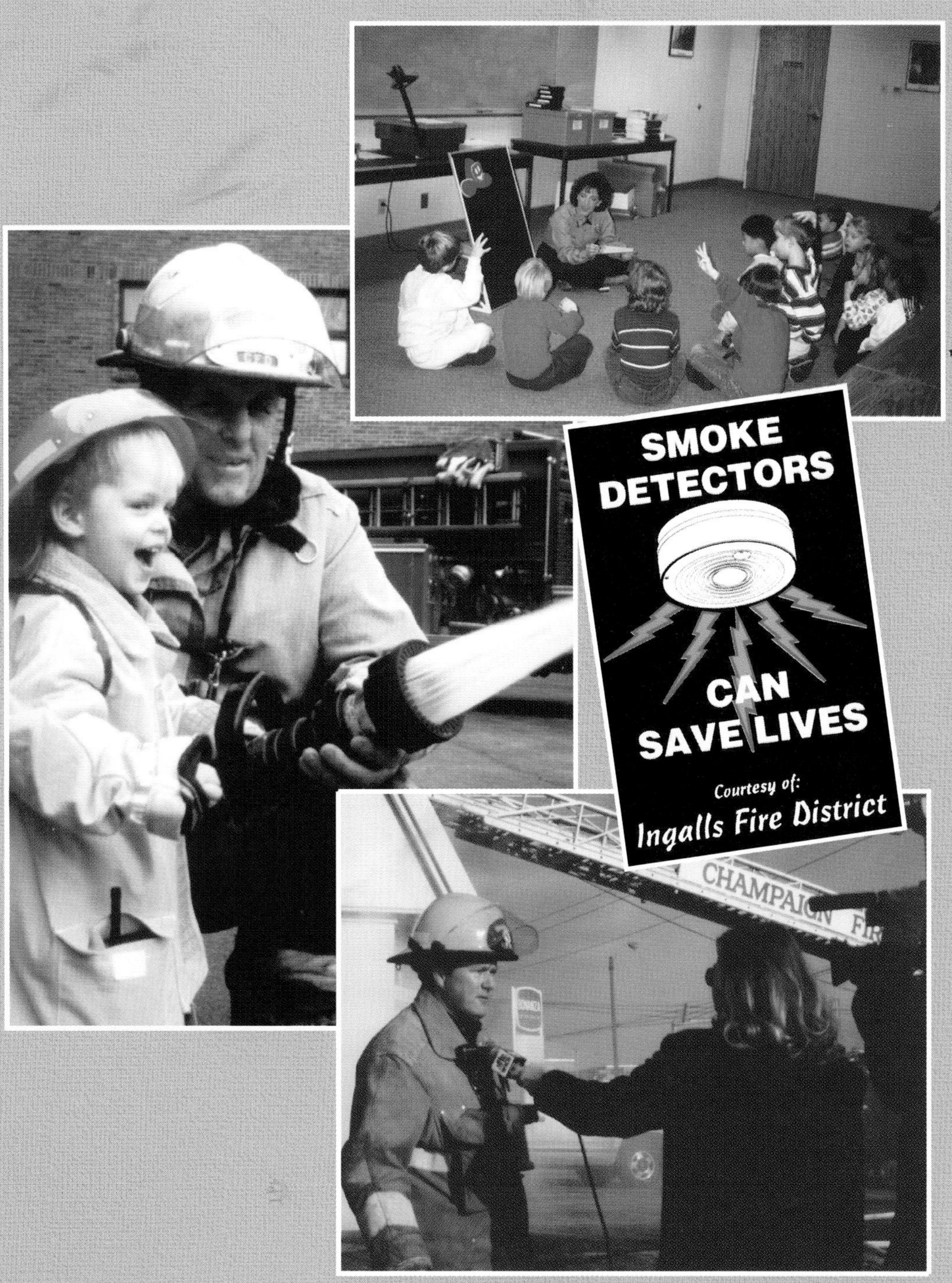
SMOKE
DETECTORS
CAN
SAVE LIVES
Courtesy of:
Ingalls Fire District
CHAMPAIGN

Glossary

Glossary

A

Accelerant
Flammable or combustible liquid used to initiate or increase the speed of fire.

Accident
Unplanned, uncontrolled event that results from unsafe acts of people or unsafe occupational conditions, either of which can result in an injury.

Acquired Immunodeficiency Syndrome (AIDS)
Fatal viral disease that is spread through direct contact with bodily fluids from a previously infected individual.

Active Listening
Method of listening characterized by maintaining eye contact with the message sender, imagining the sender's upcoming points, taking notes or mentally summarizing key points, paraphrasing especially important points, nodding the head, and thinking or saying something such as, "I understand."

Acute
Characterized by sharpness or severity; having rapid onset and relatively short duration.

Affective
Descriptive of a person's attitudes, values, and habits.

Affective Learning Domain
That aspect of learning that deals with attitudes, values, and habits.

Affiliation
Sociopsychological concept that shows that people tend to act as a group—even with people they do not know very well—and that generally no one leaves in an emergency until everyone leaves together.

AIDS
Acronym for acquired immunodeficiency syndrome.

Air Cylinder
Metal or composite container that holds compressed air for the breathing apparatus; also called the air tank.

Alarm
(1) Any signal indicating the need for emergency fire service response; (2) predetermined number of fire units assigned to respond to an emergency; (3) radio designation for dispatch center; for example, "Engine 65 to Alarm, we are returning and available."

Amphitheater Room Setup
Room arrangement in which the chairs are positioned in a slight semicircle to provide for better eye contact between the educator and the audience and to improve the audience's line of sight to a screen or video monitor; also called auditorium-style setup.

ANSI
Acronym for American National Standards Institute.

Apartment
NFPA subdivision of residential property classification: "buildings containing three or more living units with independent cooking and bathroom facilities, whether designated apartment houses, tenements, garden apartments, or by any other name."

Application
The third of the four teaching steps in which students use or apply what the educator has taught; the step in which students practice using new ideas, information, techniques, and skills.

Arson
Willful and malicious burning of one's property or the property of another; a criminal act of firesetting.

Arsonist
Person who commits an act of arson.

Asphyxiant
Any substance that prevents oxygen from combining in sufficient quantities with the blood or being used by body tissues.

Asphyxiation
Condition that causes death because of a deficient amount of oxygen and an excessive amount of carbon dioxide or other gas in the blood.

Audience
Person or persons receiving a message; also called the receiver.

Audiovisual Materials
Educational materials that can be heard as well as seen. (**NOTE:** This text includes flipcharts, mark-and-wipe boards, and chalkboards under the category of audiovisual materials even though there is no audio element involved.)

Auditorium-Style Room Setup
See Amphitheater Room Setup.

Autocratic Leadership
Leadership style in which the leader makes decisions independently of others, informing others only after the decision has been made.

Autoignition
Ignition that occurs when a solid, liquid, or gas is heated sufficiently to initiate or cause self-sustained combustion independently of the heat source.

Automatic Alarm
(1) Alarm actuated by heat, gas, smoke, flame-sensing devices, or waterflow in a sprinkler system conveyed to local alarm bells or the fire station; (2) alarm boxes that automatically transmit a coded signal to the fire station to give the location of the alarm box.

Automatic Fire Detection Systems
Heat, gas, and flame detectors used in nonresidential buildings.

Automatic Sprinkler System
System of water pipes, discharge nozzles, and control valves designed to activate during fires by automatically discharging enough water to control or extinguish a fire; also called sprinkler system.

Automatic Suppression Systems
Sprinkler, standpipe, carbon dioxide, and halogenated systems, as well as fire pumps, dry chemical agents and their systems, foam extinguishers, and combustible metal agents which sense heat, smoke, or gas and activate automatically.

Avoidance
Sociopsychological concept that shows that people feel that they can protect themselves — psychologically — by denying unpleasant situations; thus, during the first moments of a fire, people tend to search for other, safer explanations for the cues they see, smell, and hear.

Awareness Materials
Fire and life safety teaching materials that attempt to make the audience more aware of a problem or situation; sometimes called promotional materials.

B

Backdraft
Instantaneous explosion or rapid burning of superheated gases that occurs when oxygen is introduced into an oxygen-depleted confined space.

Baseline Data
Data and statistics before an education program starts; educators compare baseline data with data collected after the program has concluded to determine educational gain.

Beat
Regularly covered news area; similar to the regularly traversed area of a police officer's beat.

Behavior Change
Change in a person's actions because of an increase in knowledge.

Behavioral Objective
Measurable statement of behavior required to demonstrate that learning has occurred; also called educational objective, outcome objective, and enabling objective.

Bias
Highly personal or unreasoned distortion of judgment; prejudice.

Bill
Draft of a law presented to a legislature for enactment.

Bleed
Process in which ink seeps into adjoining areas on the same side of the paper.

Bleed Through
Process in which the ink seeps through to the other side of the paper.

Boarding House
NFPA subdivision of residential property classification: "building that provides sleeping accommodations for a total of 16 or fewer persons on either a transient or permanent basis, with or without meals, but without separate cooking facilities for individual occupants."

Body
Middle or main section of a fire and life safety educator's presentation.

Boilerplate
Standardized or formulaic language.

Brainstorm
Process of identifying as many ideas as possible without any initial evaluation, debate, agreement, or consensus.

British Thermal Unit (Btu)
Amount of heat energy required to raise the temperature of one pound of water one degree Fahrenheit.

Brochure
Small, folded booklet containing descriptive or advertising material; also called a folder or flyer.

Budget
Plan for action, with associated costs, for the coming year.

Building Code
List of rules, usually adopted by city ordinance, to regulate the safe construction of buildings.

Bunker Clothes
See personal protective equipment.

Bureaucratic Leadership
Style of leadership in which the leader has a low degree of concern for workers and production.

Burn Center
Medical facility designed, equipped, and staffed to treat severely burned patients.

Byline
Line at the beginning of a news story, magazine article, or book giving the author's name.

C

Canon
Group of rules, principles, or standards.

Capital Grant
Money gained through a large-scale fund-raising activity in which the funds raised will support a building or (occasionally) another so-called "capital expense" such as a large computer system.

Caption
Text under a photograph or illustration.

Carbon Monoxide (CO)
Colorless, odorless dangerous gas formed by the incomplete combustion of carbon; it attaches itself to hemoglobin much more easily than does oxygen, and thus decreases the blood's ability to carry oxygen.

Carbon Monoxide Poisoning
Sometimes lethal condition in which carbon monoxide molecules attach to hemoglobin, decreasing the blood's ability to carry oxygen.

Carboxyhemoglobin (COHb)
Hemoglobin saturated with carbon monoxide and therefore unable to absorb oxygen.

Case Study
Discussion in which a group reviews real or hypothetical events.

CD-ROM
Abbreviation for compact disc — read-only memory.

Cellulosic Materials
Organic materials, such as cotton or wood, composed of cells.

Celsius Scale
Temperature scale on which the freezing point is 0 degrees and the boiling point at sea level is 100 degrees; also known as centigrade scale.

Centigrade Scale
See Celsius scale.

Character
Written or printed alphabet letter or numeral.

Cheat Sheets
Slang for the pages or index cards of notes that fire and life safety educators carry with them to a presentation.

Chemical Burns
Those burns caused by contact with acids, lye, and vesicants such as tear gas, mustard gas, and phosphorus.

Chevron Room Setup
Room arrangement in which the chairs are positioned in a fan or V-formation, thus placing more members of the audience closer to the educator and allowing participants to see each other; sometimes called herringbone or fan-style setup.

Chronic
Of long duration or occurring over a period of time.

Class A Fire
Fire involving ordinary combustibles such as wood, paper, and cloth.

Class B Fire
Fire involving flammable and combustible liquids such as gasoline, kerosene, and propane.

Class C Fire
Fire involving energized electrical equipment.

Class D Fire
Fire involving combustible metals such as magnesium, sodium, and titanium.

Close
Conclusion or end of a fire and life safety presentation.

CO
Abbreviation for carbon monoxide.

Coalition
Formal, mutual relationship between or among organizations who agree to help each other in specific ways to reach a specific goal; relationship is often formalized with a written agreement that spells out what kind of help each organization will provide the other.

Coated Paper (Stock)
Paper that is coated with a substance that makes it less permeable, gives it a shiny look, and prohibits bleeding.

Code for Safety to Life from Fire in Buildings and Structures
NFPA 101; a building standard designed to protect lives in the event of a fire; also called *Life Safety Code*®.

Codes
Rules or laws used to enforce requirements for fire protection, life safety, or building construction.

Cognitive
Descriptive of knowledge or intellectual skills.

Cognitive Learning Domain
That aspect of learning that deals with knowledge and intellectual skills (facts and information).

COHb
Abbreviation for carboxyhemoglobin.

Combination Detection and Alarm Systems
Systems that have both fire and burglar alarms, with the fire alarm signal overriding the burglar alarm.

Combination Smoke Detector
Smoke-sensing device consisting of both photoelectric and ionization smoke detectors.

Communication
The ongoing process that educators and their audiences use to complete the exchange of information and attitudes about fire and life safety.

Communication Barriers
Poor listening habits or environments that get in the way of communication.

Communications Program
Computer software program that allows the user to create slides and other presentation visuals and materials.

Communication Vehicle
See medium.

Company
Basic fire fighting unit consisting of firefighters and apparatus; headed by a company officer.

Compartmentation Systems
Series of barriers designed to keep flames, smoke, and heat from spreading from one room or floor to another; barriers may be doors, extra walls or partitions, fire-stopping materials inside walls or other concealed spaces, or floors.

Complex Buildings
Structures such as manufacturing, health care, or multi-use buildings that are more structurally complex than single-family dwellings.

Computer Hardware
Computer equipment such as the computer itself, monitors, printers, modems, scanners, and CD-ROMs.

Computer Software
Computer programs such as word processors, spreadsheets, databases, graphics programs, and communications programs.

Condition
That part of an educational objective that tells under what conditions and with what resources the learner should be able to act.

Conduction
Transfer of heat energy from one body to another through a solid medium.

Conference Discussion
Discussion in which a group directs its thinking toward solving a common problem.

Conference-Table Room Setup
Room arrangement in which chairs are positioned around a long conference table.

Consensus
General agreement; the judgment or agreement arrived at by most of those in a group.

Consumable Materials
Those educational materials limited to one-time use because they are designed to be "consumed" or used up.

Consumer Product Safety Commission (CPSC)
U.S. federal agency that operates the National Electronic Injury Surveillance System (NEISS) database since 1972; data is based on a sample of hospital emergency rooms, focusing on the role of consumer products in fire and burn injuries.

Control Center
Communications or dispatch center used by the fire service for emergency communications; there are also mobile command posts that can be taken directly to the emergency scene to function as the incident operational control center.

Convection
Heat transfer by the movement of fluids or gases, usually in an upward direction.

Copyright Statutes
Laws designed to protect the competitive advantage developed by an individual or organization as a result of their creativity.

Cover Letter
Letter explaining or containing additional information about an accompanying communication.

CPSC
Abbreviation for the U.S. Consumer Product Safety Commission.

Criterion
(1) One of the three requirements of evaluation; (2) the standard against which learning is com-

pared after instruction; (3) the expected learning outcome.

Criterion-Referenced Testing
Measurement of individual performance against a set standard or criterion, not against other individuals; mastery learning is the key element of criterion-referenced testing.

CT
Abbreviation used for a measure of toxicity determined by multiplying exposure concentration (C) in ppm by the time of exposure (T) in minutes and expressed as the CT product or ppm per minute.

Curriculum
Sequence of presentations on fire and life safety education.

Curriculum Development
Using analysis, design, and evaluation to create a series of presentations that adhere to the four teaching steps and address the learning needs of a particular audience or program; sometimes called instructional design.

D

Data
Facts, numbers, and information used as a basis for reasoning, discussion, or calculation; singular datum.

Database
Computer software programs that serve as electronic filing cabinets and are used to create forms and record and sort information; databases can be used to develop mailing lists, organize libraries, customize telephone and fax lists, and track presentation and program outcomes.

dB
Abbreviation for decibel.

Decibel (dB)
Unit for expressing the relative intensity of sounds on a scale from 0 for the least perceptible sound to about 130 for the average pain level; degree of loudness.

Decoding
Translating a message to find its meaning.

Delegate
To assign responsibility or authority to another.

Delivery
See presentation.

Democratic Leadership
Leadership style in which the leader is team-oriented and gives authority to the group; the group makes suggestions and decisions; also called participative leadership.

Demography
The statistical study of human population, especially the size, density, distribution and other vital statistics of a group of people.

Demonstration
Teaching method in which the educator actually performs a task, usually explaining the procedure step-by-step.

Dermis
True skin; a dense elastic layer of fibrous tissue lying beneath the epidermis (the outer skin); and containing blood vessels, nerve fibers, hair follicles, muscular elements, oil and sweat glands, and receptor organs for the sensations of touch, pain, heat, and cold.

Desktop Publishing
Designing newsletters, brochures, and other print materials with a computer software program that enables the user to develop and lay out the text and graphics.

Directory
(1) Computer table of identifiers and references to the corresponding items or data; (2) a computer listing of files stored on a diskette.

Direct Question
Question aimed at one person in the audience.

Discussion
(1) Teaching method by which students contribute to the class session by using their knowledge and experience to provide input; the exchange of ideas between an educator and the audience;

(2) two-way communication between sender and receiver.

Dispatcher
Person who works in the communications center and processes information from the public and emergency responders.

Domains of Learning
Areas of learning and classification of learning objectives; often referred to as cognitive (knowledge), affective (attitude), and psychomotor (skill performance) learning.

Dormitory
NFPA subdivision of residential property classification: "buildings or spaces in buildings where group sleeping accommodations are provided for more than 16 persons who are not members of the same family in one room or a series of closely related rooms under joint occupancy and single management, with or without meals, but without individual cooking facilities."

DOT
Acronym for the U.S. Department of Transportation.

Dual-Issue Leadership
Leadership style in which the leader has a high degree of concern for both workers and production.

Duplex Occupancy
Type of two-family dwelling in which the families live side by side; one family occupies the left half of the structure and the other occupies the right half.

E

Education
Process of teaching, instructing, or training individuals in new skills or preparing individuals for some kind of action or activity; what teachers do to bring about learning in their students.

Educational Gain
Increase in knowledge, a positive change in behavior, or a positive change in the environment following a presentation or program.

Educational Materials
Any physical teaching aids, printed matter, audiovisual materials, and "props" that the educator uses to teach new fire and life safety skills to an audience; also called teaching aids.

Educational Objective
Teaching and learning goal that answers the question: "What will happen as a result of the education program?"; sometimes called instructional objective, behavioral objective, or learning objective.

Educator
Person charged with the responsibilities of conducting program presentations, directing the instructional process, teaching and demonstrating skills, imparting new information, leading discussions, and evaluating mastery to ensure that learning has taken place.

Egress
Place or means of exiting a structure.

Electrical Burns
Those burns caused by contact with electric current or power such as high-power wires or lightning.

Electrical Shock
Injury caused by electricity passing through the body; severity of injury depends upon the path the current takes, the amount of current, and the resistance of the skin.

Electronic Bulletin Board
Computer application that allows network users to communicate in specific subject areas (fire safety, education, public safety, health, travel, etc.); users can post messages and then other users of the bulletin board can respond.

Emergency Lighting
Lighting intended to back up exit lighting in the event it fails; *see* exit lighting.

Enabling Objective
Specific objective that allows the learner to achieve the presentation objective, and ultimately the program objective; also called outcome objective and behavioral objective.

Encoding
Putting a message into words.

End Impact
Ultimate goal of the fire and life safety educator: the decrease of fires and injuries; a long-term way of evaluating program effectiveness.

Energizers
Quick, attention-getting exercises that raise the energy level of participants (and perhaps the educator as well), promote readiness for learning, create excitement, overcome the effects of fatigue, and develop a sense of shared fun; sometimes called spice.

Engine
Fire department pumper.

Entertainment
Diverting or engaging public performance that may or may not be informational, educational, or result in learning.

Environment
(1) Circumstances, objects, and conditions by which one is surrounded; (2) the physical area in which an evaluation is done.

Environmental Change
Change in a learner's surroundings — particularly the home or workplace — following a fire and life safety outreach activity; *see* outreach activity.

Epidermis
Outer layers of the skin made up of an outer dead portion and a deeper living portion.

Established Burning
Fire stage in which fuel continues to burn without an external heat source.

Evacuation System
System intended to allow people to escape to safety during a fire; includes egress systems (exit access, exit, and exit discharge) as well as doors, panic hardware, horizontal exits, stairs, smokeproof towers, fire-escape stairs, escalators, moving sidewalks, elevators, windows, and exit lighting and signs.

Evaluation
Last of the four teaching steps in which the fire and life safety educator finds out whether the educational objectives have been met; process that examines the results of a presentation or program to determine whether the participants have learned the information or behaviors taught; consists of criteria, evidence, and judgment.

Evaluation Environment
Physical area in which an evaluation is done.

Evaluation Instrument
Physical means used to evaluate or test a learner's mastery of the educational objectives taught; may be written, oral, or performance-based.

Evaluation Strategy
Plan for conducting an evaluation, including the type of evaluation instrument to be used, the information or behaviors to be evaluated, and the methods used to interpret information provided through evaluation.

Exit
That portion of a means of egress that is separated from all other spaces of the building structure by construction or equipment and provides a protected way of travel to the exit discharge.

Exit Access
Portion of a means of egress that leads to the exit, i.e., hallways, corridors, and aisles.

Exit Discharge
That portion of a means of egress that is between the exit and a public way.

Exit Lighting
Lighting intended to help people see on their way out of a structure.

Exit Sign
Lighted sign indicating the direction/location of an exit from a structure.

Exothermic
Chemical reaction between two or more materials that changes the materials and produces heat, flames, and toxic smoke.

Exposure Concentration
Measure of toxicity expressed in parts per million (ppm) and abbreviated C.

Exposure Time
Exposure length expressed in minutes and abbreviated T.

F

Facepiece
That part of an SCBA that fits over the face and includes the head harness, facepiece lens, exhalation valve, and connection for either a regulator or a low-pressure hose; also called mask.

Faceshield
Protective shield attached to the front of a fire helmet; also called helmet faceshield.

Facilitator
Person in a group whose basic job is to stimulate others to participate in the group discussion.

Fact Sheet
List of facts and material that allow a reporter to write an in-depth article; a fact sheet may be several pages long and include historical perspective, anecdotal material, statistics, and local data.

Fahrenheit Scale
Temperature scale on which the freezing point is 32 degrees and the boiling point at sea level is 212 degrees.

Family Education Rights and Privacy Act of 1974
Legislation that provides that an individual's records are confidential and that information contained in these records may not be released without the individual's prior written consent.

Fan-Style Room Setup
See Chevron Room Setup.

Fatality
Someone who has died as the result of the incident.

Fax
To send a hard copy facsimile (copy) of print or illustrative material via the telephone lines.

Federal Emergency Management Agency (FEMA)
Federal agency responsible for emergency preparedness, mitigation, and response activities including natural, technological, and attack-related emergencies.

Federal Freedom of Information Act
Legislation used as a model for many state laws designed to make government information available to the public.

Feedback
In communications, responses that indicate that the receiver of a message has not only gotten the message but has understood it.

FEMA
Acronym for the Federal Emergency Management Agency.

FIDO
Acronym for the Fire Incident Data Organization.

File Server
Computer that contains the program files available to all workstations in a computer network.

Fire
Rapid oxidation of combustible materials accompanied by a release of energy in the form of heat and light.

Fire Behavior
See Fire Dynamics.

Fire Cause Determination
Process of establishing the origin and cause of a fire through careful investigation and analysis of the available evidence.

Fire Commissioner
See Fire Marshal.

Fire Department Emergency Communications Systems
Detection and alarm systems that transfer information from whomever reports a fire to fire service personnel.

Fire Detection Devices
Devices and connections installed in a building to detect smoke, heat, or flames.

Fire Detection System
System of detection devices, wiring, and supervisory equipment used to detect fire or the products of combustion and then signal that these elements are present.

Fire Door
Rated assembly designed to automatically close and cover a doorway in a fire wall during a fire.

Fire Drill
Training exercise practiced to ensure that the occupants of a building can exit the building in a quick and orderly manner in case of fire.

Fire Dynamics
Applying the tools of chemistry and physics to gain a technical understanding of how fires ignite, grow, and spread; also called fire behavior.

Fireground
Area around a fire and occupied by fire fighting forces.

Fire Hazard
Any material, condition, or act that may contribute to the start of a fire or increase the extent or severity of a fire.

Fire Incident Data Organization (FIDO)
One of the main sources of information (data, statistics) about fires in the United States; operated by NFPA; provides an in-depth look at certain fires, capturing almost all reported fires involving three or more civilian deaths, one or more firefighter deaths, or large dollar loss and including some other especially interesting fires such as high-rise fires.

Fire in the United States
USFA publication based largely on fire data submitted to NFIRS by roughly 13,000 fire departments; presented in an easy-to-understand format that relies heavily on the extensive use of charts and graphs.

Fire Load
Maximum amount of heat that can be produced if all the combustible materials in a given area burn; basic measurement of a fire's stored energy measured in Btu per pound per square foot.

Fire Loss in Canada
One of the main sources of information (data, statistics) about fires in Canada; compiled from data provided by the Association of Canadian Fire Marshals and Fire Commissioners and the government agency Statistics Canada.

Fire Marshal
Highest fire prevention officer of a state, province, county, or municipality; in Canada, this officer is sometimes called the fire commissioner.

Fireplay
Child's involvement with fire materials — usually lighting matches or lighters — without the approval or supervision of parents.

Fire Prevention
Division of a fire department responsible for conducting fire prevention programs of inspection, code enforcement, education, and investigation.

Fireproof
An outdated term for resistance to fire; a misnomer because all materials with the exception of water will burn at some point; other terms such as fire resistive or fire resistant should be used to indicate a material's degree of resistance to fire.

Fire Resistive
Ability of a structure or a material to provide a predetermined degree of fire resistance; usually according to building and fire prevention codes and given in hour ratings.

Fire Retardant
Chemical that is applied to a material and is designed to retard ignition or fire spread in that material.

Fire Risk
Number of incidents, injuries, or deaths per capita. (**NOTE:** Depending upon the source of information, the per capita unit may be one thousand people or one million people.)

Firesetting
Intentional act of lighting a fire that creates a disturbance or that harms people, animals, or objects.

Fire Tetrahedron
Model of the four elements required to create fire: fuel, heat, oxygen, and chemical chain reaction.

Fire Triangle
Model of the three elements necessary to sustain combustion: oxygen, heat, and fuel.

First-Degree Burn
Burn that affects only the skin's outer layer; characterized by redness and pain but does not blister or scar.

Fiscal
Having to do with finances and money.

Five-Step Planning Process
Systematic planning and action process composed of five steps: 1) identification of major fire problems, 2) selection of the most cost-effective objectives for the education program, 3) design of the program itself, 4) implementation of the program plan, and 5) evaluation of the fire safety program to determine impact.

Fixed-Temperature Heat Detector
Temperature-sensitive device that senses temperature changes and sounds an alarm at a specific point, usually 135°F [57°C] or higher.

Flame
Burning gas or vapor of a fire that is visible as light of various colors.

Flame Detector
Detection and alarm device that uses either infrared (IR) or ultraviolet (UV) light to detect flames; generally used in high-hazard areas; also called light detector.

Flame Resistant
Materials that are not susceptible to combustion to the point of propagating a flame AFTER the ignition source is removed.

Flammable
Capable of burning and producing flames.

Flammable Materials
Materials that will ignite easily and burn rapidly.

Flashover
Stage of a fire at which all surfaces and objects within a space have been heated to their ignition temperature, and flame breaks out almost at once over the surface of all objects in the space.

Flash Point
Minimum temperature at which a liquid gives off enough vapors to form an ignitable mixture with air near the liquid's surface.

Flat
Type of two-family dwelling in which the families live one above the other; one family occupies the entire ground floor (and basement if there is one) while the second family occupies the entire second floor (and attic if there is one) of a building.

Flesch Grade Level Index
See Flesch Reading Ease.

Flesch Reading Ease
Readability index; also called Flesch Grade Level Index.

Flipchart
Teaching aid consisting of a large easel and tablet.

Flyer
Another term for a brochure.

Folder
(1) Another term for a brochure; (2) a tabbed envelope in which to place a hard copy file; (3) a computer volume or directory which is just like a file folder, but instead of being stored in a file cabinet, it is stored on the computer hard drive or file server; inside the computer folders are the users' individual files.

Font
Typeface.

Formal Proposal
Written request for funding that describes the educator's organization, the problem to be solved, the solution to the problem (project plan), and the benefits of the project to the prospective donor, the target audience, and the community.

Formative Evaluation
Ongoing, repeated assessment during or after the presentation or program to determine the most effective instructional content, methods, aids, and testing techniques; evaluation of an individual presentation or evaluation of part of an overall program.

Four-Step Method of Instruction
Preparation, presentation and delivery, application, and evaluation; may be preceded by a fifth step, the pretest.

Free-Burning Stage
Second stage of burning in a confined area in which the fire burns rapidly, using up oxygen and building up heat that accumulates in upper areas at temperatures that may exceed 1,300°F (700°C).

Freewheeling Brainstorming
Type of brainstorming in which group members speak their ideas spontaneously, and ideas are recorded on flipcharts right away; most spontaneous form of brainstorming.

Fringe Benefit
Employment benefit (pension, health insurance, a paid holiday) granted by an employer to an employee without affecting the employee's basic wage rate; any additional benefit.

Fuel
Flammable and combustible substances available for a fire to consume.

Fuel Orientation
Position of the fuel (rug as a vertical wall hanging as opposed to rug on the floor, for example).

Full Color
Materials printed in at least four colors.

Funding
Fire department (or other organization) budget plus grants and in-kind contributions.

G

Gas- and Vapor-Testing System
Detection and alarm system used mainly in industry and manufacturing where there is a potential for large collections of combustible or flammable gases.

Gas-Sensing Detector
Detection and alarm device that uses either a semiconductor principle or a catalytic-element principle to detect fire gases.

General Support Grant
Money given with "no strings attached"; general support grant money may be applied to any legitimate operating expense, including salaries.

Grant
Gift of money to a nonprofit, tax-exempt organization or to a government organization.

Grantsmanship
Art of raising funds by developing grant proposals and receiving grants.

Graphics Program
Computer software program that allows the user to choose or create drawings and to combine text and art into materials that look professionally produced.

Grass Roots
Society at the local level as distinguished from the centers of political leadership.

Grid
Column layout method used by designers to structure the parts of a page; typical grids are one-, two-, or three-column formats, with uniform margins and uniform spacing between columns.

Guided Discussion
Type of discussion in which a group exchanges ideas directed toward reaching a common goal or conclusion.

Gunning FOG Index
Type of readability index.

H

Hard Copy
Paper copy as opposed to the copy stored in a computer or on a computer disc.

Hard News
News that has a time value so must be delivered immediately or it will become stale and no longer newsworthy.

Hazard
Condition, substance, or device that can directly cause injury or loss; the source of a risk.

Headline
(1) Head of a newspaper story or article, usually printed in larger type, that introduces and gives the gist of the story or article that follows; (2) to publicize highly.

Heat
Form of energy that is proportional to molecular movement; its intensity is measured in degrees of temperature.

Heat Energy Applied
Sum of the temperature of the heat source and the time of exposure.

Heat Flux
Scientific measurement of how much heat is available for transfer to human skin (or any other surface).

Heat Release Rate
Rate at which heat energy is generated by burning.

Heat Transfer
Flow of heat from a hot substance to a cold substance by convection, conduction, or radiation.

Helmet
Protective headgear worn by firefighters to provide protection from falling objects, side blows, the fire environment elements, and eye injuries.

Hemoglobin
Oxygen-carrying component of red blood cells.

Herringbone Room Setup
See Chevron Room Setup.

Hollow Square Setup
Room arrangement in which the chairs are positioned to form a square, with the chairs facing inward; similar to the U-shaped arrangement, but with this setup, the fire and life safety educator cannot walk into the center of the group.

Home Inspection
Process of educating residents about fire hazards by examining a residence for existing fire hazards and poor safety practices; process used as an evaluation instrument to determine the extent to which fire and life safety behaviors are being implemented in the community.

Hotel
NFPA subdivision of residential property classification: "buildings or groups of buildings under the same management in which there are more than 16 sleeping accommodations primarily used by transients for lodging with or without meals, whether designated hotel, inn, club, motel, apartment hotel, or by any other name."

Hot-Smoldering Phase
Fire stage in which the level of oxygen in a confined space is below that needed for flaming combustion; characterized by glowing embers, high heat at all levels of the room, and heavy smoke and fire gas production.

Household Fire Warning Systems
Detection and alarm systems that include single- and multiple-station smoke detectors as well as more complicated combination systems.

Hunter Model of Instruction
A method of instruction that emphasizes practice or application to achieve mastery of skills; developed by Madeline Hunter.

Hyperthermia
Abnormally high body temperature.

Hypothermia
Abnormally low body temperature.

Hypoxia
Condition caused by a deficiency in the amount of oxygen reaching body tissues.

I

IAFF
Abbreviation for the International Association of Fire Fighters.

ICS
Abbreviation for incident command system.

Ignition Temperature
Minimum temperature to which a fuel must be heated in order to start self-sustained combustion independent of the heating source.

Illustration
Educational method in which the fire and life safety educator shows the audience something; for instance, the parts of a smoke detector or how an overloaded electrical outlet looks.

Incendiary
Relating to or involving a deliberate burning of property.

Incident Command System (ICS)
Management system for controlling personnel, facilities, equipment, and communications so that different agencies can work together toward a common goal in an effective and efficient manner.

Incipient Phase
First stage of the burning process in a confined space in which the substance being oxidized is producing some heat, but the heat has not spread to other substances nearby and the oxygen content of the air has not been significantly reduced.

Informal Proposal
In-person request for funding.

Information
Facts, knowledge, data, or publicity; the raw material upon which a learner bases new educational skills and the change of learning.

Information Presentation
Presentation or delivery that covers theory and technical knowledge, such as the facts of fire growth and spread, and provides the background information (cognitive domain) that is often essential to performance skills development (psychomotor domain); sometimes called a technical lesson.

Informational Materials
Fire and life safety teaching materials that suggest an action or provide facts and figures; sometimes called promotional materials.

Injury in America
Resource book for fire and life safety educators that pinpoints the effects of injury and shows how fire and burns fit into the larger picture of injuries.

Injury/Loss Statistics
Facts and figures that reflect the effects of change; used for long-term evaluation of overall programs; the most reliable indicator of the success of a program.

In-Kind Contribution
Gifts of services, time, or products that do not involve money.

Inn
NFPA subdivision of residential property classification: "buildings or groups of buildings under the same management in which there are more than 16 sleeping accommodations primarily used by transients for lodging with or without meals, whether designated hotel, inn, club, motel, apartment hotel, or by any other name."

Instructional Design
See Curriculum Development.

Instructional Objective
See Educational Objective and Behavioral Objective.

International Association of Fire Fighters (IAFF)
Association that gathers data on on-duty firefighter deaths and injuries.

Inventory
Detailed, written, listing of equipment and materials on hand at a given time.

Ionization
Process by which an object or substance gains or loses electrons, thus changing its electrical charge.

Ionization Detector
Device that detects smoke by using a tiny amount of radioactive material to make the air within the detector conduct electricity.

J

Journal
See Log.

K

Keystoning
Distortion of the projected transparency image that happens when the projector and screen are not perpendicular to each other.

Kilowatt (kW)
Measurement of rate of heat release measured in the number of Btu per second (equivalent to ten 100-watt light bulbs).

Knowledge Change
Increase in a learner's understanding of fire and life safety practices.

kW
Abbreviation for kilowatt.

L

Laissez-Faire Leadership
Style of leadership in which the leader shares responsibility with the group, often relying on other people for suggestions and delegating a limited amount of decision making.

Lead
Introductory section (first few sentences) of a news story.

Leader's Guide
Publication of the National SAFE KIDS Campaign® that identifies and discusses seven fundamental steps in coalition-building.

Leadership
Knack of getting other people to follow you and to do willingly the things that you want them to do.

Learning
Knowledge gained through observation and study, resulting in a change of attitude or behavior.

Learning Environment
Physical facilities where the learning takes place.

Learning Objective
See Educational Objective and Behavioral Objective.

Learn Not to Burn® Curriculum
Curriculum developed by and available from the National Fire Protection Association in which 22 key fire safety behaviors for school children, as well as three "local option" behaviors, are established.

Learn Not to Burn®: The Pre-School Program
NFPA curriculum that addresses preschool children fire and life safety issues.

Lecture
One-way communication from the sender to the receiver; the educator talks to an audience but allows no exchange of ideas or verbal feedback.

Left Justified
See Ragged Right.

Legislation
Action of making official government rules and laws.

Legislative Strategy
Compromise between what some parties want and what all parties can live with.

Legislator
An elected official who makes laws.

Lesson
See Presentation.

Lesson Plan
Step-by-step guide for presenting a lesson or presentation; an outline of the material to be taught and the teaching procedures to be followed.

Lethal
Deadly; resulting in death.

Libel
Written or oral defamatory statement; the act, tort, or crime of making or publishing a libel against someone.

Life Safety Code®
See Code for Safety to Life from Fire in Buildings and Structures.

Light Detector
See Flame Detector.

Lobbying
Educating a person or an organization about your position on an issue or even urging the person or organization to adopt your position; more specifically, conducting activities aimed at influencing public officials, especially members of a legislative body on legislation.

Local Access Television
See Public Access Television.

Lodging House
NFPA subdivision of residential property classification: "building that provides sleeping accommodations for a total of 16 or fewer persons on either a transient or permanent basis, with or without meals, but without separate cooking facilities for individual occupants."

Log
Record book; to record information in a log or record book.

M

Maltese Cross
Symbol of the firefighter worn on the uniform or helmet.

Manage
To provide direction and leadership in order to achieve organizational objectives through effective and efficient application of resources.

Management
Process of accomplishing organizational objectives through effective and efficient handling of resources; official, sanctioned leadership.

Manager
Individual who accomplishes organizational objectives through effective and efficient handling of resources, both material and human.

Manipulative Lesson
See Practical Demonstration.

Maslow's Hierarchy of Needs
Theory put forth by Abraham Maslow that states that all human behavior is motivated by a drive to attain specific human needs in a progressive manner beginning with (1) physiological, (2) security, (3) social, (4) self-esteem, and (5) self-actualization.

Mask
See Facepiece.

Mass Media
Publications, broadcasts, and visuals that reach large numbers of individuals and usually carry advertising; the four primary mass media are newspapers, television, radio, and magazines — with computer fast closing for a fifth primary mass medium.

Masthead
Printed (usually boxed) section in a newspaper or periodical that gives the title and pertinent details of ownership, editorship, advertising rates, and subscription rates.

Matching Grant
Grant in which the funder agrees to give an amount that is equal to (or a specific ratio of) the amount that another funder gives.

Mean
Average score of a set of scores; calculated by adding all test scores and dividing by the total number of scores.

Means of Egress
Safe, continuous path of travel from any point in a structure to a public way; composed of three parts: the exit access, the exit, and the exit discharge.

Mechanical Heat Energy
Friction heat and heat of compression from the moving parts of machines such as belts and bearings.

Media
See Medium.

Media Advisory
Advisory of specific event or program to be held in the future; conversely, a news release discusses something that has already happened.

Media Kit
Packet containing information about the public fire and life safety educator's own organization.

Medium
Vehicle for sending a message; plural media; also called communications vehicle.

Megawatt (MW)
Measurement of rate of heat release equal to 1,000 kilowatts (equivalent to ten thousand 100-watt bulbs).

Message
Information, attitude, or opinion transmitted to another person or persons.

Middle-of-the-Road Leader
Leader who is moderately concerned with both production and workers.

Mitigate
To cause to become less harsh or hostile; to make less severe or painful; to alleviate.

Mixed Occupancy
According to NFPA, "an occupancy in which two or more classes of occupancy occur in the same building or structure and are intermingled so that separate safeguards are impracticable."

Modem
Device that converts digital data from a computer to an analog signal that can be transmitted on a telephone line.

Motel
NFPA subdivision of residential property classification: "buildings or groups of buildings under the same management in which there are more than 16 sleeping accommodations primarily used by transients for lodging with or without meals, whether designated hotel, inn, club, motel, apartment hotel, or by any other name."

Motivation
See Preparation.

MW
Abbreviation for megawatt.

N

National Burn Information Exchange (NBIE)
Voluntary registry of specialized burn-care facilities; established at the University of Michigan Burn Center, NBIE's database had grown by early 1986 to include the medical records of almost 95,000 burn patients from 130 hospitals.

National Fire Codes® (NFC)
Series of volumes published by the National Fire Protection Association containing the current consensus standards prepared by various committees and adopted by the Association.

National Fire Incident Reporting System (NFIRS)
One of the main sources of information (data, statistics) about fires in the United States; under NFIRS, local fire departments collect fire incident data and send these to a state coordinator; the state coordinator develops statewide fire incident data and also forwards information to the USFA; begun by FEMA.

National Fire Protection Association (NFPA)
Nonprofit educational and technical association devoted to protecting life and property from fire by developing fire protection standards and electrical codes and by educating the public.

National Highway Traffic Safety Administration (NHTSA)
Agency within the U.S. Department of Transportation (DOT) that publishes annual summary reports of fatal highway accidents.

National Institutes for Occupational Safety and Health (NIOSH)
Government agency under the Centers for Disease Control and Prevention, U.S. Department of Health and Human Services, that helps ensure that the workplace and associated equipment are safe; investigates workplaces and recommends safety measures and reports of on-the-job fire injuries.

National SAFE KIDS Campaign®
Nationwide coalition with the goal of reducing preventable injuries to children.

National Transportation Safety Board (NTSB)
Agency within the U.S. Department of Transportation (DOT) that maintains a fire-related data base on aircraft and railway accidents, as well as highway accidents involving hazardous materials injuries.

NBIE
Abbreviation for the National Burn Information Exchange.

Needs Analysis
Assessment of training needs identifying the gap between what exists and what should exist.

Network
Informal group of persons with a mutual interest who communicate with each other to share ideas, information, and resources.

Networking
Communicating and creating linkages between people and clusters of people.

News Pegs
Another name for the news values that editors use to decide whether the information given them is newsworthy; some of the news pegs that editors use to evaluate a story are timeliness, proximity, conflict, progress, consequence, uniqueness, and human interest.

News Release
Short, factual description of an event or an issue written or outlined by a fire and life safety educator and given to one of the mass media for publication or airing.

News Value
See News Pegs.

NFC
Abbreviation for National Fire Codes®.

NFIRS
Acronym for the National Fire Incident Reporting System.

NFPA
Abbreviation for National Fire Protection Association.

NFPA Fire Department Survey
Annual survey in which the NFPA gathers data and statistics about fires in the United States.

NFPA Life Safety Code©
See Code for Safety to Life from Fire in Buildings and Structures.

NHTSA
Abbreviation for the U.S. National Highway Traffic Safety Administration.

NIOSH
Acronym for National Institutes for Occupational Safety and Health.

Nonflammable
Incapable of combustion under normal circumstances; usually used when referring to liquids or gases.

Nonprofit
Legal status that the U.S. Internal Revenue Service may give to an organization after the IRS has reviewed a written application; nonprofit, tax-exempt organizations are sometimes called 501 (c) 3 organizations, after the section of the Internal Revenue Code that describes them.

NTSB
Abbreviation for the U.S. National Transportation Safety Board.

Nuclear Heat Energy
Energy generated when atoms are either split apart (fission) or combined (fusion).

O

Objective
(1) Purpose or educational goal of a presentation or program; 2) unbiased; dealing with facts or interpreting results without distorting with personal feelings, prejudices, or interpretations.

Objective Test
(1) Test in which the results are scientifically accurate or correct and cannot be influenced by outside factors; (2) term used loosely to describe tests that contain short-answer items such as multiple-choice, true/false, and matching that require little or no subjectivity in answering or evaluating.

Observation
Actually seeing or watching a learner's behaviors in a natural setting; as a means of evaluation, direct observation provides very reliable information on the effects of programs.

Occupancy
General fire service term for a building, structure, or residency.

Occupational Safety and Health Administration (OSHA)
Federal agency within the U.S. Department of Labor that develops and enforces standards and regulations for safety in the workplace.

One- and Two-Family Dwellings
NFPA subdivision of residential property classification: "buildings containing not more than two dwelling units in which each living unit is occupied by members of a single-family unit with no more than three outsiders, if any, accommodated in rented rooms."

Open-Ended Question
Question that requires more than a yes or no answer.

Opening
Beginning or motivational part of a fire and life safety educator's presentation.

Operation School Burning
Series of fire tests in Los Angeles that analyzed physiological effects of fire in schools and determined tenability.

OSHA
Acronym for Occupational Safety and Health Administration.

Outcome Objective
Desired student performance resulting from a lesson or presentation.

Outreach Activity
Method the public fire and life safety educator uses to reach an audience, generally a direct presentation.

Overhead Expenses
Those expenses necessary for routine administration of a project, program, or department.

Oxygen Deficiency
Insufficient oxygen to support life or flame; at least 16 percent oxygen is needed for flame production and human life.

Oxygen-Deficient Atmosphere
Any atmosphere containing less than the normal 21 percent oxygen found in atmospheric air.

Overhead
See Transparency.

Overhead Projector
Simple machine used to project a transparency onto a screen.

Overhead Question
Question aimed at the whole group, rather than one person in the group.

Oxidation
Chemical reaction in which oxygen combines with other substances; fire, explosions, and rusting are examples of oxidation.

P

Panic
As defined by the University of Maryland: "a sudden and excessive feeling of alarm or fear, usually affecting a body of persons, originating in some real or supposed danger, vaguely apprehended, and leading to extravagant and injudicious efforts to secure safety."

Participative Leadership
See Democratic Leadership.

Parts per Million (ppm)
Ratio of the volume of contaminants (parts) compared to the volume of air (million parts).

Passive-Sentence Index
Readability index that computes reading level by determining the percentage of passive sentences within a passage.

Patient
Someone who is receiving medical care.

PC
Abbreviation for personal computer.

Per Capita
Per unit of population.

Percentage
Way of interpreting evaluation results by expressing a part of a whole in hundredths.

Performance/Behavior
That part of an educational objective that tells what learners must do to show what they have learned.

Performance Test
See Skills Test.

Personal Protective Equipment (PPE)
General term for the equipment worn by firefighters and rescuers; includes helmet, coat, gloves, pants, boots, eye protection, protective hood, SCBA, and a personal alert safety system (PASS device); also called bunker clothes, protective clothing, turnout clothing, or turnout gear.

Personnel Management
Decision making concerning the effective use of human resources within an organization so that organizational and individual goals are met.

Photoelectric Smoke Detector
Device that uses a small light source — either an incandescent bulb or a light-emitting diode (LED) — to detect smoke by shining light through the detector's chamber: smoke particles reflect the light into a light-sensitive device called a photocell.

Physiological
(1) Of or relating to an organism's healthy and normal functioning; (2) first and most basic group of needs in Maslow's Hierarchy of Needs, that is, those needs related to personal survival — such as food, water, and shelter that are essential to sustain life; Maslow's physiological needs also include escaping from situations, such as a fire, that are immediately life-threatening.

Pica
Print measurement equal to 12 points or 1/6 of an inch.

Placard
(1) Diamond-shaped sign affixed to each side of a vehicle transporting hazardous materials; placard indicates the primary class of the material, and, in some cases, the exact material being transported; (2) diamond-shaped 704 placard affixed to a structure to inform of fire hazards, life hazards, special hazards, and reactivity potential.

Point
Print measurement unit of about 1/72 inch.

Position Description
Written description of a specific employee position that spells out the expectations of the job, the activities that are needed to meet those expectations, and the qualifications needed to fill the job.

PPE
Abbreviation for personal protective equipment.

ppm
Abbreviation for parts per million.

Practical Demonstration
Method of teaching psychomotor skills, such as installing a smoke detector or using a portable fire extinguisher safely; sometimes called a manipulative lesson.

Preparation
First of the four teaching steps and the one in which the educator prepares the student to learn; getting the students' attention and letting them know why the material is important to them; arousing curiosity, developing interest, and developing a sense of personal involvement on the part of the student; closely linked to the term motivation.

Prerequisite
Something that is necessary to an end or to carrying out a function; knowledge or skill required before the learner can acquire additional or more complex knowledge or skill.

Prescriptive Test
(1) Test given at the beginning of instruction (pretest) to determine what the individual or audience already knows; (2) test given remedially.

Presentation
Single delivery of fire and life safety information; the second of the four teaching steps in which the educator teaches a class or individual and transfers facts and ideas; a commitment by the presenter to help the audience do something; also called lesson or delivery.

Presentation Program
Computer software program that enables the user to create audiovisuals, primarily paper masters that can become slides or overhead transparencies; some programs project slides directly onto the computer screen.

Press Release
Written news release.

Pretest/Posttest
Prescriptive evaluation instrument used to compare knowledge or skills either before (pretest) or after (posttest) a presentation or program.

Print Materials
Printed materials such as brochures (also called flyers or folders), posters, fact sheets, coloring books, activity sheets, educational card or board games, and pretests/posttests; sometimes called consumable materials.

Products of Combustion
Materials produced and released during burning.

Program
Comprehensive strategy that addresses fire and life safety issues via educational means.

Project Grant
Money given for a very specific activity or for very specific expenses, such as the purchase of fire safety educational videotapes for use in community schools.

Promotional Materials
See Awareness Materials and Informational Materials.

Prop
Object used during a fire and life safety presentation that the audience can see, touch, smell, or hear, i.e., a burned remnant from a home fire, a piece of melted glass, a manual fire alarm pull station, or a smoke detector.

Proposal
Document or request that describes what accomplishments the applicant promises to achieve in return for the investment of the sponsor's funds.

Prospect
Local business and other resource that may be a possible source of funding.

Protective Clothing
See Personal Protective Equipment.

Protective Signaling Systems
Detection and alarm systems that transfer information from a specific place in a fire-involved building to some remote monitoring station.

Psychomotor
Descriptive of physical, hands-on activities; actions that a student must be able to do or perform.

Psychomotor Learning Domain
That aspect of learning that deals with hands-on performance skills.

Pull Box
Manual fire alarm activator.

Q

Qualitative Evaluation
Assessment method that does not use numbers and that relies on the fire and life safety educator's experience, judgment, and interpretation.

Quantitative Evaluation
Assessment method that uses numbers to compare different materials and methods, is likely to be more sophisticated than qualitative methods, and involves formal testing.

R

Radiated Heat
See Radiation.

Radiation
Transfer of heat energy through air by electromagnetic waves; also called radiated heat.

Ragged Left
Type alignment in which the right margins of all lines of type end at the same vertical place but the left edges of the lines end at different places, creating a "ragged" left margin but a straight right margin; also called right justified.

Ragged Right
Type alignment in which the left margins of all lines of type begin on the same vertical place but the right edges of the lines end at different places, creating a "ragged" right margin but a straight left margin; also called left justified.

Rate Compensated Heat Detector
Temperature-sensitive device that sounds an alarm at a preset temperature, regardless of how fast temperatures change.

Rate-Of-Rise Heat Detector
Temperature-sensitive device that sounds alarm when the temperature changes at a preset value, such as 12°F to -15°F per minute.

Reactivity
Ability of two or more chemicals to react and release energy and the ease with which this reaction takes place.

Readability Index
System for measuring how easy (or difficult) a passage is to read.

Receiver
Person or persons to whom a message is directed in the communications process; also called audience.

Relay Question
Question from the audience that the educator sends back to the audience.

Residential Board and Care Facility
NFPA subdivision of residential property classification; "a building or part thereof that is used for lodging or boarding of four or more residents, not related by blood or marriage to the owners or operators, for the purpose of providing personal care services."

Residential Occupancy
According to NFPA, "those occupancies in which sleeping accommodations are provided for normal residential purposes and include all buildings designed to provide sleeping accommodations."

Restricted Grant
See Project Grant.

Rhetorical Question
Question to which an answer is not expected.

Right Justified
See Ragged Left.

Right of Privacy
See Family Education Rights and Privacy Act of 1974.

Risk
Likelihood of suffering harm from a hazard; exposure to a hazard; the potential for failure or loss.

Role
Sociopsychological concept that says that the role or status someone has in a building determines that person's response to a fire or other emergency.

Role-Playing
Discussion in which a group acts out various scenarios.

Rollover
Condition in which unburned combustible gases released during the incipient burning phase accumulate at ceiling level where they are pushed away from the fire and mix with oxygen; when they reach their ignition temperature, they ignite and expand very rapidly to roll across the ceiling.

Rooming House
NFPA subdivision of residential property classification: "building that provides sleeping accommodations for a total of 16 or fewer persons on either a transient or permanent basis, with or without meals, but without separate cooking facilities for individual occupants."

Round-Robin Brainstorming
Method of brainstorming in which each member of a group offers an idea in turn, with participants electing to pass on any round, until everyone has passed a turn; ideas are recorded as soon as they are stated.

S

Safety Officer
(1) Fire officer whose primary function is to administrate safety within the entire scope of the fire department operations; (2) member of the incident command system command staff.

Sampling Error
Measure of the error created because estimates are based on a sampling of fire losses rather than on a complete census of the fire problem; also called a standard error.

Sans Serif
Typeface in which the letters have no serif; literally "without" serif. (**NOTE:** This typeface is sans serif.)

Saturation Tactics
Practice of having a person (usually a child) who has played with fire repeat an act (such as lighting a match) until the person's curiosity is satisfied and the act becomes boring; no longer a recommended practice.

Save
Life that has been saved as a direct result of a public fire and life safety education program.

Scald
Those burns caused by contact with hot fluids or steam.

Scare Tactics
Practice of frightening a child who has played with fire by showing the child pictures of injured or dead children, pets, or burned toys; or to threaten the child with punishment, hospitalization, or painful treatment; not a recommended practice.

SCBA
Abbreviation for self-contained breathing apparatus.

SCUBA
Acronym for self-contained underwater breathing apparatus.

Sealed, Pneumatic, Line-Type Heat Detector
Heat-sensitive device that depends on the presence of normal pressure at normal temperatures.

Second-Degree Burn
Burn that extends to the dermis, causes skin blisters, and may scar.

Security
Second need in Maslow's Hierarchy of Needs; need concerned with personal safety and future physical comfort; similar to physiological needs, but encompassing long-term dangers or dangers that are not immediately threatening.

Self-Actualization
Highest need in Maslow's Hierarchy of Needs; the need to become all one is capable of becoming.

Self-Contained Breathing Apparatus (SCBA)
Protective breathing device worn in hazardous atmospheres; also called air mask or air pack.

Self-Contained Underwater Breathing Apparatus (SCUBA)
Protective breathing device worn by divers to allow them to explore underwater environments; generally called SCUBA gear or underwater breathing gear.

Self-Esteem
Second highest need in Maslow's Hierarchy of Needs; the need to have self-respect and respect for others, to have social status within the group, and to be recognized for one's worth or value.

Sender
Person who sends or transmits a message in the communications process; also called the source.

Serif Font
Typeface (like the one in this manual) in which the letters are adorned with short angled lines called serif.

Service Learning
Educational trend that tries to connect young people to the community in which they live through community service projects.

Single-Issue Leader
Leader who is very concerned about either production needs or worker needs.

Skills Test
Evaluation instrument used to assess the individual's ability to perform a specific physical behavior; also called a performance test.

Slander
False and defamatory oral statement about a person.

Slip Brainstorming
Type of brainstorming in which each person in the group independently and anonymously writes ideas on a slip of paper and the slips are then collected and organized.

Smoke-Control System
Engineered system that uses mechanical fans to produce airflows and pressure differences across smoke barriers to limit and direct smoke movement.

Smoke Obscuration
Act of being hidden by smoke.

Smoldering Phase
See Hot-Smoldering Phase.

Social Need
Middle need in Maslow's Hierarchy of Needs; the need to belong to a group or to have some means of identification.

Soft News
News that can be printed or broadcast today, tomorrow, or next week because it does not have a time value.

Solar Heat Energy
Energy transmitted from the sun in the form of electromagnetic radiation.

Solicit
To approach with a request.

SOP
Abbreviation for standard operating procedure.

Source
See Sender.

Spice
Attention-getter or energizer that gets the audience's attention during a fire and life safety presentation.

Spontaneous Combustion
See Spontaneous Ignition.

Spontaneous Heating
Heating resulting from chemical or bacterial action in combustible materials that may lead to spontaneous ignition.

Spontaneous Ignition
Combustion of a material initiated by an internal chemical or biological reaction producing enough heat to cause the material to ignite; also called spontaneous combustion.

Spreadsheet
Computer software program that allows the user to deal with numbers and create graphs such as in developing budgets, monitoring presentations delivered, and keeping an inventory current.

Sprinkler System
See Automatic Sprinkler System.

Sprinkler System Supervision Systems
See Waterflow Alarms.

Standard
That part of an educational objective that tells the minimum level the learner should meet in accomplishing the performance/behavior.

Standard Error
See Sampling Error.

Standard Operating Procedure (SOP)
Standard method in which an organization or department carries out routine functions; usually these procedures are written in a policies and procedures handbook.

Statistics
Numerical data.

Stop, Drop, and Roll
Fire and life safety behavior to be performed when one's clothing or hair catches fire.

Strategic Planning
Process for identifying long-term goals and objectives for a program or department (usually for a period of five years).

Subhead
Headline that is subordinate to or of lesser importance than the main headline; generally printed in smaller type than the main headline.

Summative Evaluation
Comprehensive approach to evaluation using test results, educator's observations, and the program statistics to determine total program effectiveness; evaluation of the overall program following its completion.

Sunshine Laws
Local, state, or provincial laws which require public notification and open attendance of government meetings.

Supervise
To oversee the work of others or another.

Survey
Evaluation instrument used to identify the behavior and/or attitude of an individual or audience both before and after a presentation.

Suspicious Fires
Fires that may be incendiary or caused by arsonists.

T

Target Audience
Group of people who will receive the fire and life safety education presentation; this may not always be the group of people identified as a high-risk group; rather it may be those who influence or control the high-risk group.

Task Force
Group of individuals convened to analyze, investigate, or solve a particular problem.

Tax-Exempt
See Nonprofit.

Teaching Aids
See Educational Materials.

Team Teaching
Classroom method in which two or more instructors work together—combining their individual content, techniques, and materials—to meet a single educational objective.

Technical Lesson
See Information Presentation.

Tenability
Determination of whether or not people can remain unhurt or escape a fire area without serious injury.

Tenement
NFPA subdivision of residential property classification: "buildings containing three or more living units with independent cooking and bathroom facilities, whether designated apartment houses, tenements, garden apartments, or by any other name."

Tetrahedron
See Fire Tetrahedron.

Thermal Burns
Those burns caused by contact with flames, hot objects, and hot fluids (scalds and steam burns).

Thermoelectric-Effect Heat Detector
Heat-sensitive device that measures electrical resistance changes that correspond with temperature changes.

Third-Degree Burn
Full-thickness burn that penetrates the epidermis, dermis, and underlying tissue, leaving skin charred or white and leathery, and accompanied by an initial loss of pain or sensation to the area because of destroyed nerve cells.

Toxicity
Ability of a substance to do harm within the body.

Transfer of Learning
Process of applying what has been learned in one situation to a new situation.

Transparency
Educational visual printed on acetate or mylar and projected onto a screen for common viewing; sometimes called an overhead.

Turnout Clothing
See Personal Protective Equipment.

Turnout Gear
See Personal Protective Equipment.

U

Unrestricted Grant
See General Support Grant.

USFA
Abbreviation for the United States Fire Administration, which operates within the Federal Emergency Management Agency (FEMA); formerly the National Fire Prevention and Control Administration (NFPCA).

U-Shaped Room Setup
Room arrangement in which the chairs are placed in a U-shape, allowing learners to see one another and allowing the educator to walk into the center of the group or to face the audience from the open end of the configuration.

V

Victim
Either a fatality or a casualty.

Vesicant
Agent that causes blistering.

Vital Signs
Indicators of a patient's condition that reflect body temperature, pulse, respirations, and blood pressure.

Volunteer
Anyone, inside or outside the fire department, who helps with fire and life safety education programs.

Visual Aid
See Educational Materials.

W

Waterflow Alarms
Detection and alarm systems that detect when sprinklers activate; also called waterflow detectors and sprinkler system supervision systems.

Word Processor
Computer software program used with a personal computer and designed specifically for creating text documents; usually allows the user to justify or align type, to use boldface or italics, to choose a typeface from a large selection, and to add, delete, and rearrange blocks of type.

Index